PULMONARY AND RESPIRATORY DISEASES AND DISORDERS

NON-INVASIVE MECHANICAL VENTILATION COMPLICATIONS

ESSENTIALS FOR TREATMENT AND PREVENTION

PULMONARY AND RESPIRATORY DISEASES AND DISORDERS

Additional books and e-books in this series can be found on Nova's website under the Series tab.

PULMONARY AND RESPIRATORY DISEASES AND DISORDERS

NON-INVASIVE MECHANICAL VENTILATION COMPLICATIONS

ESSENTIALS FOR TREATMENT AND PREVENTION

ANTONIO M. ESQUINAS, MD, PHD
EDITOR

nova
Medicine & Health
New York

Library of Congress Cataloging-in-Publication Data

ISBN: 978-1-53619-515-6

Published by Nova Science Publishers, Inc. † New York

CONTENTS

PREFACE

Noninvasive mechanical ventilation has managed to establish itself as the treatment option for a wide variety of causes of acute and chronic respiratory failure in different settings in hospital and home noninvasive mechanical ventilation. In the last decades, we have discovered its positive effects on gas exchange and symptoms such as dyspnea control, widely contrasted against endotracheal intubation. However, although this wide range of beneficial effects have been described, pathophysiology, diagnosis, prevention and treatment of noninvasive mechanical complications could not be forgotten for a correct application as they clearly affect patient outcome and mortality.

Nowadays, there is a scarce number of publications analyzing noninvasive mechanical ventilation complications and this book is the first dedicated to its analysis. This book brings together a broad multidisciplinary vision of common and unusual complications, thus it serves as the original and essential scientific published reference on noninvasive mechanical ventilation complications.

The present book has been structured to offer through its sections and chapters an exhaustive and in-depth analysis of noninvasive mechanical ventilation complications, mechanisms, direct or indirect factors determinants, key recommendations for the early diagnosis and treatment for most frequent applications from multidisciplinary perspective. Finally, we analyze noninvasive mechanical ventilation complications and how they impact in short- and long-term complications and mortality. The book concludes analyzing evidence in diagnosis, prevention and treatment.

We believe that the readers of this book will find in it an essential reference for a correct application of noninvasive mechanical ventilation, and thus be able to improve results and prognosis. Only the precise knowledge of complications of noninvasive mechanical ventilation will allow us to achieve a proper application to success.

Chapter 1 - Non-invasive ventilation (NIV) has been widely used for acute and chronic respiratory failure. Compared to traditional invasive mechanical ventilation, NIV has the benefit of improving patients' outcomes with fewer complications than with invasive procedures, which include sedation, infections and patient discomfort. However,

NIV is regularly associated with negative consequences that are often unpleasant or life-threatening, and patients should be extensively monitored to reduce possible complications.

Chapter 2 - Patient compliance and tolerance is the key factor for the success of the noninvasive ventilation (NIV). There are many factors that influence this. Staff training and careful application of the interface makes a difference in improving the compliance, preventing complications and improving adherence to the therapy. Respiratory Therapist plays a major role in the treatment of patients who require NIV. Non-Compliance to the therapy makes it difficult to continue with NIV and patient may end up having worsened respiratory failure requiring invasive ventilation. Compliance and adherence to home mechanical ventilation using NIV is also a concern for the respiratory care providers.

Chapter 3 - When we talk about non-invasive mechanical ventilation (NIMV), we are referring to a type of ventilatory support treatment that falls between conventional oxygen therapy and invasive mechanical ventilation. With this type of treatment, positive pressure is administered through a non-invasive interface, such as a face mask, to try to achieve good ventilation for the patient instead of an invasive interface (endotracheal tube, tracheostomy). Non-invasive mechanical ventilation is indicated in both patients with acute and chronic respiratory failure. Despite being a simple technique with a high number of indications, it is not exempt from possible complications. In this chapter we will focus on the oronasal symptoms, which, even though they are minor complications, we must know.

Chapter 4 - NIV presents complications that are not common but that we should be aware of. One of them is parotitis, which is due to multiple causes, the most defended being the increase in intraoral pressure due to the application of positive airway pressure, and this leads to obstruction of the Stensen's duct. Other complications are ocular, mostly due to persistent leakage from a poorly fitting mask.

Chapter 5 - This chapter highlights the side effects of NIMV and in particular the pressure ulcers created by the devices used to ventilate the patient. The need to contain air leaks, which are more commonly encountered during mechanical ventilation at high pressure levels, induces health professionals to increase the tightening of the masks on the patient's face. This tightening, while on the one hand reduces the air leaks, on the other hand increases the contact pressure on the face with the possibility of skin damage. Various severity levels of pressure ulcers are cited and the pathophysiological mechanisms that induce skin damage are explained. The main factors are: pressure and cutting forces, friction on the skin, humidity, time, the characteristics of the mask, the anatomy of the face, the fragility and subtlety of the skin and bacterial pollution. The diagnosis, based on careful visual observation, can also make use of the help of specific instruments to classify the lesions. Prevention is implemented with the identification and removal of possible critical contact points, with the right choice of the best mask, with the possible rotation of the same and with the use of devices to reduce the contact pressure. Lesion treatment involves dressing and applying ointments, creams, alginate or hydrocolloid or protease-based gels. However, a recent and extensive meta-analysis has failed to be an adequate and certain guide for therapeutic choices.

Chapter 6 - The strengths and the weaknesses of non-invasive ventilation (NIV) are all located at the same point: the patient-ventilator interface. On the one hand, the interface avoids the need for intubation and all the mechanical or infective complications of invasive ventilation. On the other hand, NIV interfaces cause many problems and risks of complications. Interface-related complications can be the main reason for NIV failure, by making patients unable to endure the process. The main NIV interface complications reported in scientific literature are discomfort, pressure ulcers on the face, skin rashes, claustrophobia, noise, CO_2 re-breathing, and dyssynchrony with ventilators. The aim of this chapter is to describe and discuss the complications caused by the most common NIV interfaces in adult patients during their stay in hospital (helmet, full-face masks, oro-nasal masks, nasal masks), and suggest the most reasonable solutions to prevent and overcome their adverse effects. Given that the perfect interface has yet to be developed, healthcare professionals should acquire in-depth knowledge of the characteristics of every available NIV interface, with its potential advantages and disadvantages. This is the only way to optimize the management of patients on NIV support and achieve the desired outcomes.

Chapter 7 - One of the most recognized complications of mechanical ventilation is barotrauma, referring to the manifestations of extra-alveolar air, such as subcutaneous emphysema, pneumopericardium, pneumomediastinum, pneumoperitoneum and even pneumocephalus. Barotrauma results from positive pressure mechanical ventilation and is caused by alveolar rupture due to overdistension. This allows the passage of air into the perivascular sheath and tissue dissection into the mediastinum and subcutaneous tissue. Increased pressures can also lead to pleural rupture and subsequently a pneumothorax. Clinical manifestations range from absent symptoms and subtle radiographic signs, as in interstitial emphysema, to respiratory distress and cardiac arrest caused by a tension pneumothorax. The occurrence of barotrauma in non-invasive mechanical ventilation (NIV) is much lower when compared to invasive mechanical ventilation. Nonetheless any patient can develop barotrauma, especially in the presence of predisposing lung disease such as acute respiratory distress syndrome (ARDS), obstructive pulmonary disorders and interstitial lung disease.

Chapter 8 - Secretion accumulation may cause atelectasis, increased work of breathing, ventilation/perfusion mismatch and can lead to infection. Various factors may contribute for retained secretions on the mechanically ventilated patient such as immobility, altered state of consciousness, secretion viscosity and increased production of sputum. To avoid the failure of NIV, airway clearance techniques and secretion management measures should be carried out. Manual techniques, via chest percussion and the application of vibration, and postural drainage are of greatest importance on the patient that is unable to cooperate. The active cycle of breathing and autogenic drainage technique can be modified for use during NIV treatment. High-frequency chest wall oscillation involves compression of the thorax at a high frequency and, in intrapulmonary percussive ventilation, a pneumatic device delivers small volumes of air at high frequencies, both promoting the vibration and mobilization of secretions. Heated humidification may also aid the clearance of thick and viscous sputum. The state of hydration of the patient should always be kept in mind, as it can influence the viscosity of the secretions. The use of mucolytic agents, bronchodilators, and antibiotics, when necessary, should be considered. Finally, flexible bronchoscopy may play a role in the setting of large amounts of secretions.

Chapter 9 - Secretion accumulation may cause atelectasis, increased work of breathing, ventilation/perfusion mismatch and can lead to infection. Various factors may contribute for retained secretions on the mechanically ventilated patient such as immobility, altered state of consciousness, secretion viscosity and increased production of sputum. To avoid the failure of NIV, airway clearance techniques and secretion management measures should be carried out. Manual techniques, via chest percussion and the application of vibration, and postural drainage are of greatest importance on the patient that is unable to cooperate. The active cycle of breathing and autogenic drainage technique can be modified for use during NIV treatment. High-frequency chest wall oscillation involves compression of the thorax at a high frequency and, in intrapulmonary percussive ventilation, a pneumatic device delivers small volumes of air at high frequencies, both promoting the vibration and mobilization of secretions. Heated humidification may also aid the clearance of thick and viscous sputum. The state of hydration of the patient should always be kept in mind, as it can influence the viscosity of the secretions. The use of mucolytic agents, bronchodilators, and antibiotics, when necessary, should be considered. Finally, flexible bronchoscopy may play a role in the setting of large amounts of secretions.

Chapter 10 - Aspiration pneumonia is a major, serious and life-threatening complication of NIV. The incidence of aspiration pneumonia in patients with NIV has been reported in about 5% of cases, and the mortality rate has been very high. Developed aspiration pneumonia is very difficult to treat, so it is necessary, before applying NIV, to consider all risk factors that could lead to its development.

Chapter 11 - Non-invasive ventilation (NIV) as supportive therapy in acute respiratory failure has become popular. But concerns exist for potential complications due to ventilator support and patient effort interaction. Ventilator-induced lung injury (VILI) and effort-induced lung injury (EILI) are two of those complications. They have some common pathophysiologic pathways only with different origin of applied forces to the lung. In fact this two entities co-exist and may aggravate lung injury. Usually the ratio between PaO_2/FiO_2 is diminished in lung pathology of various aetiologies this possibly correlating with lung heterogeneity with local variability in lung compliance. This heterogeneity exacerbates the negative effects of both positive (ventilator) and negative (patient) intrapleural pressure. Correlation between higher tidal volume and NIV failure has been established. But although pathophysiologic mechanisms suggest lung injury occurrence with higher tidal volumes, that has not been undoubtedly demonstrated. Reviewing VILI and EILI mechanisms, its differences, and the importance of both tidal volume and PaO_2/FiO_2, may help us optimize monitoring and therapeutic actions to both prevent or minimize lung injury in NIV setting.

Chapter 12 - Non Invasive Ventilation (NIV) has vastly developed and grown in the last decades becoming one of the main treatments used both in acute respiratory failure (ARF) and in chronic respiratory failure (CRF). There are a lot of factors which determine the success or failure of NIV, from a good patient selection to medical expertise and choosing the right interface. Finding a suitable interface for each patient and each situation is essential to the success of the treatment.

Chapter 13 - Non-invasive ventilation (NIV) is a therapy treatment that has been successfully applied for global respiratory failure. A cause of failure of non-invasive mechanical ventilation as therapy is rebreathing. It consists of rebreathing the expired air, which causes a poor removal of the carbon dioxide. It has a direct impact on the clinical worsening of the patient. The rebreathing of carbon dioxide is influenced by a large number of different factors such as the type of mask, the number of branches used in the ventilatory circuit, the level of espiratory positive airway pressure (EPAP), the tidal volume, the use of an expiratory port or an antirebreathing valve, the expiratory time, the respiratory rate of the patient and the degree of adaptation of the patient to non-invasive mechanical ventilation. The use of anti-rebreathing valves is recommended when using low EPAPs. If it is not possible to use an anti-rebreathing valve, EPAP greater than 8 cm H2O should be used to avoid rebreathing.

Chapter 14 - Assisted mechanical ventilation (MV) is applied early, following the critical stage of the critical disease, to eliminate the injurious consequences of controlled MV, most reputably the rise of ventilator-induced diaphragmatic dysfunction. The development of patient-ventilator asynchrony often counteracts the advantages of assisted MV. Patient-ventilator asynchrony happens when both the beginning and/or finish of mechanical breath is not in time accord with the beginning and finish of neural inspiration, respectively, or if the measurement of mechanical assist does not respond to the patient's respiratory need. As patient-ventilator asynchrony has been correlated with several adverse results and can unfavourably impact patient result, every effort should be performed to identify and change this occurrence at the bedside. Patient-ventilator asynchrony is usual during mechanical ventilation. Asynchrony reduces the comfort, increases mechanical ventilation and intensive care unit stays, and it could lead to worse results. To identify patient-ventilator dyssynchronies, the physician should estimate patient comfort and carefully investigate the pressure and flowtime waveforms, accessible on the ventilator screen of every modern ventilators. Contemporary ventilators give several modifiable settings to promote patient-ventilator synergy. New comparative modes of ventilation are likewise very helpful in enhancing patient-ventilator interaction.

Chapter 15 - Non-invasive Mechanical Ventilation has had an exponential advance in the last four decades, offering us great advantages for the treatment of ventilatory support in patients with both acute and chronic respiratory failure. It avoids in many cases to arrive to invasive ventilation; and we can control and monitor with the different ventilatory parameters that it has. In the recent years, many technological advances have been added with different NIV equipment that allows us to perform an optimal and narrow monitoring of the ventilatory parameters, up to the point where it is possible to carry out telemonitoring and to connect telematically with these equipment and to be able to assess the various ventilatory parameters, make the corresponding adjustments in a safe manner, as well as to assess compliance, adhesion, evolution, detect early and treat acute exacerbation, disease progression, minimize and treat adverse effects and avoid complications.

Chapter 16 - In general, NIMV is well tolerated hemodynamically, presumably due to the lower levels of insufflation pressures used, compared with invasive ventilation. The use of NIMV for a short period of time, not in the long term, has effects on heart rate, systolic blood pressure and systemic vascular resistance, depending on the type of patient and the clinical situation. When initiating non-invasive mechanical ventilation (NIMV), many changes occur which end up affecting the patient haemodynamically. These hemodynamic effects are the result of positive airway pressure being transmitted to the surrounding structures of the thorax. The extent to which this occurs varies according to chest wall and lung compliance. Systolic volume can be compromised during NIMV because of the alteration that preload suffers due to thoracic pressure augmentation. It decreases venous return due to a pressure increased nearby RA. Additionally, LV's distensibility. This decreased preload compromises cardiac output as it affects RV. However, the use of NIMV can trigger significant hypotension and decreased cardiac output in patients with a previously altered haemodynamic state, especially with hypovolemia or with underlying heart disease without adequate drug therapy.

Chapter 17 - Compared with invasive mechanical ventilation, noninvasive ventilation (NIV) achieves the same physiological benefits of reduced work of breathing and improved gas exchange. Furthermore, it avoids complications of intubation and increased risks of ventilator-associated pneumonia especially in patients with comorbidities. Use of NIV has spread in recent years, due in part to the change in patient profile: over time, the number of patients with baseline pathologies increases, due to the increasing age of the population and the possibility of applying NIV in patients to patients who previously required invasive measures.

Chapter 18 - Hypercapnia is a term that refers to the elevation of the partial pressure of carbon dioxide (PaCO2) above the value of 45 mmHg. This will occur if the gas exchange process that takes place in the lungs is compromised. Hypercapnia will result in acid-base balance disturbances due to the relationship between CO2 and hydrogen carbonate (HCO3) known as the pH buffering system. Hypercapnic respiratory failure is more commonly determined by the reduction of alveolar ventilation than by the increase of the rate of CO2 production. There are many causes of hypercapnic that include among others pre-existing lung conditions, thoracic wall deformities and neuromuscular disorders. Clinical examination is important part of the diagnostic process together with a detailed personal history. Diagnostic imaging tests, as well as laboratory tests, may be useful in discovering the etiology of hypercapnia. Treatment will depend on the cause of hypercapnic failure and instructions must be followed as given for the best possible outcome. Various prevention strategies exist in order to avoid more serious complications.

Chapter 19 - Chronic obstructive pulmonary disease (COPD) is one of the main causes of morbidity and mortality worldwide. Non-invasive ventilation (NIV) has been applied in the last decades for the treatment of exacerbations and end-stage COPD with remarkable results in the improvement of quality of life, lung function and survival. However, the use of NIV, and particularly high intensity-NIV, may result in some complications. The most frequent complications associated to NIV treatment in COPD patients include hemodynamic effects, the *deventilation syndrome*, pulmonary barotrauma, auto-positive end-expiratory pressure (auto-PEEP) and ventilator-associated pneumonia, which are addressed in this chapter. Although complementary studies are needed to clarify the reported complications, and in some cases the data is still sparce, clinicians should be aware of the risks associated with NIV in this particular subset of patients. Yet, current guidelines strongly recommend the use of NIV in patients with acute exacerbations of COPD.

Chapter 20 - The impact of these neuromuscular disorders on the respiratory muscles and the upper airway results in swallowing and breathing problems, as well as the appearance of ineffective cough, all of which leads to a higher risk of recurrent respiratory infections. Most patients need to exceed hours of continuous use of NIV, with pressure ulcers, irreversible malformations, dryness in the nasopharyngeal mucosa, sleep disorders, and many other complications. Special equipment is also needed in order to adapt ventilation for day, night or social activities, besides a backup one in case of failure. Finally, an early diagnosis of the pathology and its complications are essential in order to avoid failure of NIV.

Chapter 21 - Positive airway pressure is a well-known treatment for multiple sleep breathing disorders. In order to choose the best therapy for each patient it is important to recognize the different pathophysiology beside each clinical entity (sleep apnoea, obesity hypoventilation syndrome,), but also the more common adverse events of therapy to avoid and solve them. CPAP and APAP are the first line therapies in moderate to severe OSAS, servoventilation is an adequate therapy for CSA with Cheyne Stokes respiration and bilevel pressure or CPAP could be used in OHS. Although the differences between equipments and modalities for each pathology, the side effects are usual very similar. The majority of side effects are in relation with the interface or the pressure administered, and a careful follow-up is essential to identify and resolute the common problems with ventilation. Finally, is also important to know that some serious but rare adverse events have been reported as pneumothorax, pneumocephalon and massive epistaxis.

Chapter 22 - Acute respiratory failure (ARF) is the most frequent and challenging complication in onco-hematologic patients. Early referral to ICU, multidisciplinary cooperation, new therapeutic, large application of NIV has contributed to improve the prognosis of malignancies complicated by ARF. Among all, non-invasive ventilation (NIV) has been considered crucial for the "turning point" in the mortality of critically ill patients with malignancies as it averts IMV-associated life-threatening complications The actual evidence suggests benefits from a trial of "prophylactic" CPAP or NIV in the early phase of ARF in onco-hematologic patients without multiple organ dysfunctions. However, delayed intubation after prolonged NIV failure is associated with poor hospital survival. Concerning the setting, starting early CPAP/NIV in the ward to reduce ICU admission is still controversial. Finally, NIV is feasible as "palliation" in selected terminally onco-hematologic patients.

Chapter 23 – Non-invasive mechanical ventilation (NIMV) is a therapeutic procedure that aims to supplement or improve ventilatory function. In recent decades its benefit and multiple indications have been demonstrated in the treatment of patients with chronic heart failure (CHF) and acute complications. However, the use of this therapy in patients with chronic heart failure, is not exempt from risks and complications, so it must be carefully individualized and requires close monitoring when ischemic heart disease and/or arterial hypotension also coexist. Special mention requires the revision of the indication of servo ventilation in patients with severe chronic heart failure, due to its possible adverse effects.

Chapter 24 - Non-invasive ventilation (NIV) has to be used meticulously in patients with terminal illnesses. Evidence supporting the palliative role of NIV in end-stage lung diseases is still lacking. In patients with respiratory failure and limited life-expectancy, NIV helps to reduce dyspnea and opiate requirements and has more acceptability than conventional oxygen therapy. Facial skin breakdown, claustrophobia, aerophagia, aspiration, discomfort, dead space, dryness, and persistent leak are known complications of NIV, which pose more challenges to the intended purpose of palliative care. However, it helps the patient feel more comfortable and perhaps improve communication abilities. In the past decade, the use of palliative NIV has increased substantially.

Chapter 25 - Non-invasive ventilation (NIV) during endoscopic procedures has been considered an extremely useful and safe approach for either diagnostic or therapeutic purpose. Bronchofiberoscopy, carried out for difficult intubation and to perform bronchoalveolar lavage and biopsies, is one of the upper endoscopic exams in which NIV is used the most. In clinical practice peri-procedural NIV improves oxygenation operating with masks that allow the insertion of endoscopic probes. The full face Janus mask is a device with an opening covered by a membrane and two separable halves with a midline port that allows the insertion of endoscopic probes into patients mouth or nose, without interrupting continuous positive airway pressure. To reduce patients unpleasant sensations during the procedure, a mild degree of sedation is usually administered, which furthermore compared with general anesthesia, results in no need for hospitalization, reducing costs and complications. Despite these advantages, NIV support is not free of complications, especially because the unprotected airway may lead to a higher risk of aspiration and the occurrence of cough, when under sedation, might cause intraprocedural anatomic lesions. Hypoventilation and desaturation may also be associated with the procedure, resulting in its no completion or leading to acute respiratory failure and intubation. Bronchoalveolar lavage (BAL) is known to induce significant hypoxemia and therefore previous severe hypoxemia may represent a contraindication for this procedure. Additionally, the indications to perform endoscopic maneuvers in the cardiac and gastrointestinal settings are clearly expanding because they represent a considerable less invasive approach compared with surgical interventions.

Chapter 26 - Non-invasive respiratory support methods have been increasingly used in recent years for patients receiving treatment for acute respiratory failure. Avoiding invasive methods provides better results here, as in every field of medicine. However, patients with respiratory distress are not intubated at the right time and delayed intubation causes an increase in mortality. Various preoxygenation methods are applied to avoid hypoxemia during the apnea period after anesthesia induction until intubation occurs in patients undergoing surgery. The apnea period, which is limited to only a few minutes in healthy lungs, is very short in lung diseases. Therefore, preoxygenation is of particular importance before the intubation of patients with respiratory failure. Preoxygenation is the process of filling lung reserves with oxygen. Determining which method to use in which patient for preoxygenation is an issue that should be considered, as it can directly affect patient outcomes.

Chapter 27 - Non-invasive respiratory support methods have been increasingly used in recent years for patients receiving treatment for acute respiratory failure. Avoiding invasive methods provides better results here, as in every field of medicine. However, patients with respiratory distress are not intubated at the right time and delayed intubation causes an increase in mortality. Various preoxygenation methods are applied to avoid hypoxemia during the apnea period after anesthesia induction until intubation occurs in patients undergoing surgery. The apnea period, which is limited to only a few minutes in healthy lungs, is very short in lung diseases. Therefore, preoxygenation is of particular importance before the intubation of patients with respiratory failure. Preoxygenation is the process of filling lung reserves with oxygen. Determining which method to use in which patient for preoxygenation is an issue that should be considered, as it can directly affect patient outcomes.

Chapter 28 - Weaning in the clinical history of an intubated and ventilated patient with mechanical ventilation is an extremely delicate moment. Several studies have been performed to understand the appropriate time to wean and how to perform weaning correctly and safely. In this regard, the spontaneous breathing trial has been developed, which makes it possible to understand whether the patient is able to breathe independently or not. This test, together with the overall clinical evaluation of the patient, allows to decide whether to proceed with the extubation. However, a proportion of extubated patients experience respiratory failure and require reintubation. These are usually complex patients with a variety of comorbidities and in 50% of cases, they die. In recent years it is becoming increasingly common to use NIV immediately after extubation, even before any respiratory failure can occur. The use of non-invasive mechanical ventilation seems to significantly reduce the mortality of extubated patients and the risk that they will experience reintubation.

Chapter 29 - Non-invasive ventilation (NIV) allows to mechanically ventilate a patient by means of a full-face or nasal mask instead of an endotracheal tube. The main benefits are decreases in the intubation rate, mortality rate, and number of infectious complications, particularly pneumonia. In most studies of NIPPV in the ICU setting, the main outcome measure has been the need for tracheal intubation. For those patients who avoid intubation, the main advantage is the avoidance of artificial airway complications. Several studies document a lower infection rate (nosocomial pneumonia and sinusitis) with NIPPV, which may be related to the maintenance of the protective glottic barrier. Other advantages include reduced need for sedative medications. Some NIPPV trials have demonstrated reductions in ICU length of stay, ICU mortality, or in-hospital mortality. This chapter is intended to explore the applications and benefits of NIV in postoperative patients, especially in those undergoing neurosurgery, thoracic and abdominal surgery.

Chapter 30 - Non-invasive ventilation is currently one of the most commonly used support methods in hypoxaemic and hypercapnic acute respiratory failure. Data suggests that the prevalence of delirium it is higher in the subset of patients requiring NIV for acute respiratory failure than in a population of general medical inpatients. The development of agitation and the deterioration of mental status, such as in delirious patients, decreases the ability to cooperate and tolerate NIV, potentially increasing the risks for NIV failure and subsequent intubation. Agitation, intolerance, and patient–ventilator asynchrony are factors implicated in NIV failure for which judicious sedation is recommended. Sedation during NIV should be performed with no/minimal respiratory depression and no/minimal impairment of the upper airway.

Chapter 31 - The utility of non-invasive ventilation (NIV) in the emergency departments (ED) may reduce mortality and morbidity, provided the right approach for the right patient at the right time. More important is the balance between clinical outcome and prevention of untoward complications, which decides the success of NIV in the ED.

Complications in the initial hours of stabilization are mostly related to patient-NIV asynchrony, interfaces, and high airflows. Fatal complications, like barotraumas and pulmonary aspiration are few and may occur rarely. ED clinicians are expected to balance the cart of physiological homeostasis by understanding the patients' clinical demand against the potential complications of NIV, which are preventable.

Chapter 32 - High flow nasal oxygen therapy (HFNO) through specially designed nasal cannula is a novel non-invasive breathing device that has caught the imagination of intensivists worldwide. This device is being used in many acute and chronic situations with further emerging fields of application including pediatric population. However, with wider usage various problems are coming into our purview - the most worrisome of which is generation of unpredictable pharyngeal pressure with alveolar over distension. The safe practitioner should be thorough about every nitty-gritty while applying these devices - from looking at the evidence regarding its use in a particular scenario, diligently monitoring the patient parameters and device function throughout duration of therapy, and act judiciously when problems arise including escalation of therapy or on the other hand abandoning this therapy altogether for an alternate therapy as the situation demands. Some problems are relatively minor while others are really life-threatening, and can develop during short term as well as at long term use of these devices. This article highlights the vital practice points and important complications of HFNO from published articles till date.

Chapter 33 - Complications of Non-Invasive Ventilation are similar both in paediatric and adult patients. The real incidence is still unknown, it varies between 10 - 20% according to previous papers, being skin lesions the most common. Major complications are serious yet very uncommon: barotrauma, aspiration pneumonia or hemodynamic effects. Minor complications are more frequent: skin and mucosal lesions, gastric distention, and irritative conjunctivitis.

Chapter 34 - Non-invasive mechanical ventilation (NIV) at home has been widely used since 1981 to date in both children and adults. There are several complications reported in the literature, the most frequent being conjunctivitis and skin lesions, the rarest being malar hypoplasia. There are several theories to explain this complication in pediatrics. When using NIV for chronic pediatric patients, it should be kept in mind that children's faces are in process of development. The treatment involves a multidisciplinary team of pediatricians, dentists, surgeons, and speech therapists.

Chapter 35 - Noninvasive ventilation has been used as a short term adjunct to the main therapy in acute critical settings like pneumonia, postoperative hypoxemia or acute exacerbation of chronic obstructive pulmonary disease. In these cases, typically, a short trial of NIV is commonly applied. Subsequently, careful evolution of the patient is required to assess the positive (or negative) effects of the treatment to continue the NIV or not. However, NIV can also be employed for longer durations as in sleep apnea, chronic obstructive pulmonary disease and neuromuscular disorders. NIV improves daytime sleepiness, lung functions and gas exchange in Obstructive Sleep Apnea Syndrome and. End stage Chronic Obstructive Pulmonary Disease (COPD) patients commonly develop hypercapnic respiratory failure. Eventually, fatigue, daytime headache, dyspnea and impaired Quality of Life (QoL) is encountered. Long term NIV application may partially alleviate these symptoms and improves QoL and reduce mortality improves oxygenation, decreases dyspnea and increases walking distance. Neuromuscular Disorders (NMDs) are heterogeneous group of diseases and their response to NIV differs. Commonly, Work of Breathing (WoB) is significantly increased at the expense of already weakened respiratory muscles. The imbalance between the WOB and the muscle capacity elicits a typical pattern of rapid shallow breathing. Some disorders such as Spinal Muscular Atrophy or mitochondrial diseases requires very early respiratory support. On the other hand, respiratory failure may develop slowly and gradually or they may never require respiratory support during the course. Air leaks and pressure wounds due to interfaces can be encountered in long term NIV. In conclusion, long term NIV therapy is a significant burden both to the patient and to the caregivers. Its success relies on a collaboration between the patient, the caregiver and the clinician.

Chapter 36 - Non-invasive ventilation is more utilised in acute respiratory failure to prevent endotracheal intubation and invasive ventilation, however, failure rates of NIV include selection of patients, intervention, careful monitoring and a skilled team. The pathophysiology of NIV failure is difficult to prevent and some cases early diagnosis are important for example Patient–ventilator asynchrony, Upper airway disorerders, secretions and bronchial aspiration are key determinants

Chapter 37 - Failure of Non Invasive Ventilation (NIV) can potentially be associated with prolonged invasive mechanical ventilation (MV) and increased mortality. Correct selection of patients for NIV treatment is essential, since the application of NIV should not delay endotracheal intubation but avoid it. The aim of this review is to analyze the determinants of outcomes in pathologies in which NIV has proven to be the treatment of choice.

Chapter 38 - Non-invasive ventilation (NIV) appeared in 1927 as a result of the invention of the iron lung by Drinker and Shaw. Patients needing this type of treatment have shown to benefit from fewer hospital admissions, shorter stays, and fewer sleep breathing disorders; nevertheless, for some diseases like amyotrophic lateral sclerosis (ALS) or Duchenne muscular dystrophy, there are discrepancies concerning the utility of NIV with regards to the patient's quality of life. Noteworthy, since 1995, the WHO highlights the importance of quality of life as a significant factor for one's existence. Accordingly, it is necessary to create specific tools to measure the quality of life of patients requiring chronic NIV.

Chapter 39 - The use of non-invasive mechanical ventilation has become widespread for acute and chronic respiratory failure. With its use, it is often possible to reduce the number of patients who require invasive mechanical ventilation, with the advantages that this entails, especially associated with avoiding some of the complications of the procedure. This represents significant economic savings, because although non-invasive ventilation is not without risks, these are in any case less in number and in severity than those associated with invasive mechanical ventilation. In this chapter we will review different studies carried out throughout history in which an attempt has been made to evaluate the benefits of non-invasive mechanical ventilation, as well as an economic analysis of its cost-effectiveness.

Chapter 40 - The education and training of medical personnel on NIMV is crucial to ensure success, reduce complications and improve outcomes for patients with respiratory failure. Patients with respiratory failure who require NIMV are by definition critically ill patients; they need to be managed by experienced personnel with skills in respiratory therapy capable to deal with ventilator settings, patient response, respiratory equipment, and monitoring preventable NIMV failure. Understanding respiratory physiology, knowledge of how a ventilator works and interacts with abnormal patient physiology is vital. Effective and safe use of NIMV depends on careful selections of the patient, but also trained personnel. Education programs ensure basic training in NIMV management, and these skill translate into improve patients care and better outcomes. Although many educational centers give training on NIMV, mainly in the ICU and respiratory field, specialized courses are not as common as they should be. To acquire in-depth knowledge that would let physicians to understand and manage NIMV, specialized courses and training are needed. Even though training programs should be adapted to previous knowledge, it is vital to put up skills in progressive manner to ensure understanding of NIMV related topics. All personnel involved in day-to-day care of patients requiring NIMV may get a minimum skill in the management of these patients; these include not only physicians but also nurses, respiratory therapist, and physiotherapists.

Chapter 41 - For patients in need of ventilatory assistance, non-invasive mechanical ventilation has proven an increase in survival rate in patients with acute respiratory insufficiency or chronic obstructive pulmonary disease, as well as lees need for invasive ventilation. Nevertheless, as with any other technique, there are several contraindications and complications which we will explain in this chapter, as being aware of them and with the correct formation of the staff in charge we can make these complications to be recognized and we can take actions to palliate them.

Chapter 42 - Noninvasive ventilation is an important resource for preventing orotracheal. Noninvasive ventilation has the advantages of reducing patient discomfort, and procedural complications. However, noninvasive ventilation is associated with frequent uncomfortable or even life-threatening adverse effects (aerophagia, nasal skin injury, ventilator-induced lung injury; patient-ventilator asynchrony; nasal and eye irritation, bronchoaspiration risks, hypotension, and pneumothorax), and patients should be thoroughly screened beforehand to reduce potential severe complications. Even complications common to both noninvasive ventilation and invasive mechanical ventilation occur less frequently in patients undergoing noninvasive ventilation. Thus, noninvasive ventilation is associate with a reduced need for invasive mechanical ventilation and significant outcome and minor complications. Noninvasive ventilation should be applied by a trained and experienced team, taking constantly into account the potential complications.

In: Non-Invasive Mechanical Ventilation Complications
Editor: Antonio M. Esquinas
ISBN: 978-1-53619-515-6

Chapter 1

COMPLICATIONS DURING NON-INVASIVE MECHANICAL VENTILATION: EPIDEMIOLOGY, DEFINITIONS, CLASSIFICATIONS

***Jaber S. Alqahtani*[1,*] *and Abdulelah M. Aldhahir*[2]**
[1]Department of Respiratory Care,
Prince Sultan Military College of Health Sciences,
Dammam, Kingdom of Saudi Arabia
[2]Respiratory Care Department,
Faculty of Applied Medical Sciences,
Jazan University, Jazan, Saudi Arabia

ABSTRACT

Non-invasive ventilation (NIV) has been widely used for acute and chronic respiratory failure. Compared to traditional invasive mechanical ventilation, NIV has the benefit of improving patients' outcomes with fewer complications than with invasive procedures, which include sedation, infections and patient discomfort. However, NIV is regularly associated with negative consequences that are often unpleasant or life-threatening, and patients should be extensively monitored to reduce possible complications.

Keywords: non-invasive ventilation, mechanical ventilation, complications, pressure ulcers

* Corresponding Author's E-mail: Alqahtani-Jaber@hotmail.com/Jaber@psmchs.edu.sa.

1.1. Introduction

Non-invasive ventilation (NIV) in acute respiratory failure (ARF) has been the preferred therapy for the last two decades. Throughout intensive care facilities, as well as in larger hospitals and home environments, the use of NIV has increased for patients with severe and recurrent respiratory problems [1-3]. NIV involves supplying the patient with a supportive pressure boost via a non-invasive interface, without invasive endotracheal intubation [4]. There have been several reports that NIV improves dyspnea and gas exchange, and decreases the incidence of tracheal intubation. NIV also decreases the duration of stay in the intensive care unit (ICU) or hospital, and decreases morbidity and mortality of patients with severe and persistent respiratory disease associated with invasive mechanical ventilation (IMV) [5]. While the overall treatment success of NIV is high, the failure rate ranges between 18% and 40%. Two reasons are attributed to this: the first is that the optimum NIV procedure needed to manage respiratory failure is not fully understood, both in terms of NIV modality and the skills necessary to apply it. The second factor is related to the seriousness of patient's illness, despite the optimal NIV procedure having been applied [6].

Various forms of ventilation systems and interfaces can be used to provide NIV support. Health care providers who use such intervention play a crucial role in selecting appropriate interfaces and setting the parameters to prevent potential respiratory problems [7]. Successful NIV relies on a variety of factors, including patient selection, comorbidities, NIV experience and patient response to NIV. While the majority of patients respond well to NIV, it is not entirely free of serious adverse effects and complications. Increasing awareness of common complications, prediction of factors, and therefore timely identification and care of unexpected incidents will improve NIV compliance [1, 8]. The literature mentions several complications of NIV, both major and minor. Major complications may contribute to mortality or increased morbidity, such as pneumonia and hemodynamic effects, while minor complications are mild or temporary side effects related to features specific to NIV, for instance masks, gas flow and ventilators. Knowledge of these complications helps clinicians to select appropriate patients, equipment and monitoring techniques. The purpose of this chapter is to provide a thorough overview of all possible NIV-related complications, both minor and major. It will also discuss the management of such complications.

1.2. Definitions of NIV Associated Complications

The incidence of severe complications associated with invasive ventilation can be minimized by using NIV. However, NIV can produce several complications that range from minor (e.g., interface-related problems) to serious (e.g., aspiration and hemodynamic effects). According to the literature, serious or major complications are defined as those that can lead to death or increased disease, such as hemodynamic instability, barotrauma, and pneumonia. However, these complications are rare if skillful clinicians, who have carefully assessed patients, apply NIV. On the other hand, minor complications are defined as those common problems relating to features unique to NIV, such as masks, helmets, gas flow and ventilators. Usually, they are mild or temporary side effects. In the next section of this chapter, all these complications will be discussed in detail. (Figure 1)

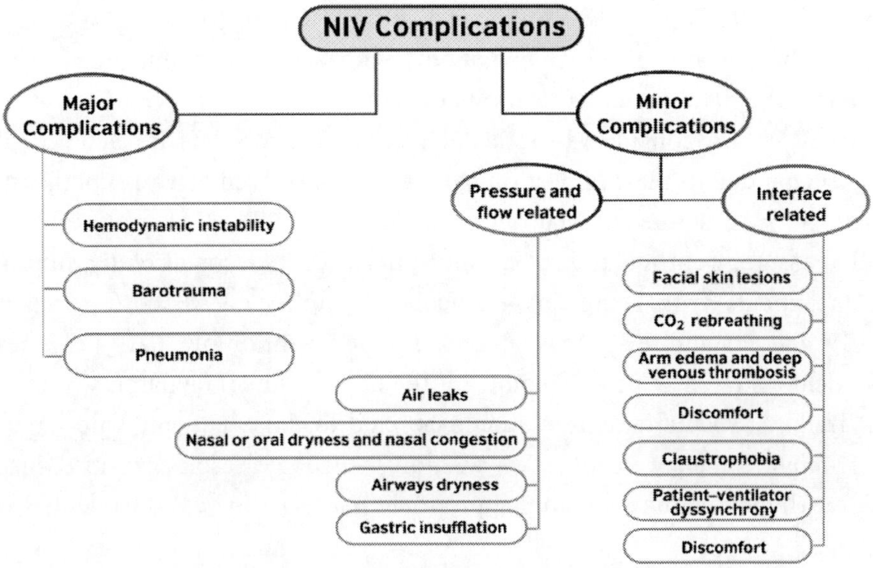

Figure 1. Major and minor complications related to NIV.

1.3. Major Complications Associated with NIV

1.3.1. Hemodynamic Effects

NIV may have a serious, unfavorable impact on hemodynamic, especially in patients with unstable cardiac output, but this rarely occurs. The use of positive pressure ventilation to the upper airway during NIV causes an increase in the intrathoracic pressure. Consequently, venous return and left ventricular filling are reduced, which eventually leads to a reduction in right ventricular preload and after load. In such cases hypotension can occur in susceptible patients [9-11]. In healthy subjects, NIV and continuous positive airway pressure (CPAP) reduce stroke volume (SV) and cardiac output (CO) without heart rate alteration, while systemic vascular resistance simultaneously increases. These anomalous changes also occur in COPD patients with acute ventilatory failure or individuals with a high risk of respiratory distress development [9-14]. In stable COPD patients without cardiovascular abnormalities, bi-level positive airway pressure support ventilation (Bi-PAP; IPAP 15 cm H_2O and EPAP 5 cm H_2O) resulted in CO reduction, without heart rate and arterial pressure (AP) changes [15]. Similar findings resulted from COPD patients who had severe hypercapnic respiratory failure, but with different BiPAP settings (IPAP 12 cm H_2O and EPAP 2 cm H_2O) [16].

It is evident that NIV has a negative impact on cardiac patients. In COPD patients who had severe respiratory failure and fluid depletion, a reduction in the cardiac index by more than 15% was observed during pressure support ventilation (PSV) [17]. In contrast, PSV (PS of 15 cm H_2O and PEEP of 5 cm H_2O) and CPAP (5 cm H_2O) did not affect heart rate, CO, or mean AP either in patients with acute lung injury or patients who required NIV immediately after extubation [18, 19].

NIV or CPAP are considered the standard treatment options for acute cardiogenic pulmonary edema due to their impact on cardiac function even after discontinuation [20, 21]. In patients with acute left ventricular impairment, CPAP reduces left ventricular transmural pressure, ventricular preload and afterload, and concurrently improves CO [22, 23]. In patients with acute congestive heart failure, CPAP of 5 to 15 cm H_2O improves SV and CO and this effect remains despite cessation of CPAP [22]. In general, NIV has demonstrated a considerable influence on hemodynamics during acute respiratory failure. Special attention should be paid to those patients who have chronic ventricular impairment, severe illnesses with an inadequate respiratory rate, insufficient blood volume (hypovolemia), and to inappropriate pharmacological treatment [18].

1.3.2. Barotrauma

Barotrauma is a serious well-recognized complication during positive pressure ventilation but is less likely to occur (less than 5%) during NIV [4, 24]. Barotrauma has been identified and reported in patients with COPD, acute lung injury, cystic fibrosis, interstitial lung disease, or neuromuscular disorders and may appear in different forms, such as pneumothorax [25-27]. To minimize the risk of developing barotrauma, pressure-controlled (PC) ventilation with peak inspiratory pressure (PIP) $\leq$ 30 cm H_2O should be considered, especially in the presence of reduced lung compliance. Attention should also be paid to the inspiratory and expiratory ratio, allowing adequate expiratory time to avert air-trapping, premature termination of expiration or breath stacking. Additionally, excessive PEEP should be avoided to prevent auto-PEEP and patient- ventilator dyssynchrony [26, 27].

1.3.3. Pneumonia

NIV-associated pneumonia is a serious complication that may be encountered during NIV. Around 6% of patients who use NIV develop nosocomial-acquired pneumonia [5].

During intubation, it is fully understood that IMV increases the risk of nosocomial infection by suppressing mucus clearance techniques [24]. Tracheal intubation is an independent factor predisposing to pneumonia in adult patients with low levels of neutrophils [28]. It has been reported that NIV lowers the risk of ventilator-associated pneumonia (VAP) by five times, mainly for patients with comorbidities or immunodeficiency diseases [8, 24, 29-33]. Additionally, when compared to IMV, NIV was associated with significantly lower VAP incidence: 0% vs. 8% [34]. NIV also reduces the risk of VAP occurrence for patients with respiratory failure who require some form of ventilatory support for up to two days [34, 35]. NIV is associated with a lower mortality rate among patients with hypoxemic or hypercapnic respiratory failure, pulmonary edema, or COPD, compared with IMV [36, 37].

Aspiration pneumonia may occur during NIV as a result of gastric contents, excessive secretions, or foreign materials in 5% of patients [24, 32, 33]. Therefore, Fowler's position is recommended for those with a greater risk of aspiration pneumonia [24]. Patients with upper airway dysfunction, those unable to clear secretions or those who require sedation should not be considered for NIV [32, 33]. Special precautions should be taken for patients who are susceptible to vomiting, nausea, or gastric aspiration [24].

1.4. Minor Complications Associated with NIV

1.4.1. Complications Related to the Interface

1.4.1.1. Facial Skin Lesions

At the site of interface interaction, nasal skin lesions (pressure injuries) may develop after using NIV for longer periods [4]. Nasal lesions induce the most mask problems, which happens in 5% to 50% of patients [5]. Pressure injuries occur in bone prominence regions due to physical friction between the interfaces and the skin of the patient. Pressure injuries have been identified by the European Pressure Ulcer Advisory Panel (2014) as skin damage or underlying tissue damage confined to a specific region, usually induced by bone prominence [38]. Factors that may intensify pressure damage include incremental tightening of the strap tension, increased positive pressure and increased air volume in the mask cushions [6, 39]. The key trigger for pressure ulcers, according to research, is lack of knowledge and comprehension of skin function, of how many times the NIV system should be attached and how to maintain a proper mask seal without progressively increasing strap strain. Effective detection of patients with a high risk of developing pressure ulcers at the start of NIV is critical for initiating preventive treatment to reduce the occurrence of such injuries [6]. Use of humidification in NIV may increase the likelihood of facial skin pressure ulcers, as shown by the detrimental impact of the underlying skin barrier mechanism and related inflammatory response patterns [39]. Therefore, those who use NIV with humidification should be closely monitored to safeguard skin integrity because wet skin is at greater risk of maceration and friction injuries. It is important to preserve the skin by keeping it dry and clean to avoid maceration and reduce friction. Routine interface repositioning, a 10-minute break if the patient can tolerate it, and rotating various types of mask are important, particularly for patients at high risk of pressure injuries [6, 40]. Proper interface selection, understanding of and correct evaluation of patient-related risk factors are important for avoiding skin pressure lesions.

1.4.1.2. Carbon Dioxide Rebreathing

Rebreathing carbon dioxide during NIV is very common and may increase CO_2 accumulation and raise the burden on ventilatory muscles by increasing the work of breathing [41-47]. Rebreathing CO_2 may be caused by the interface, circuit, concentration of the end tidal CO_2, mode, level of PEEP, and respiratory rate (RR) or cycle of NIV [42, 43]. Ventilator circuit and interface appear to add extra dead space, which predisposes to CO_2 accumulation or rebreathing during NIV [41, 47]. The amount of dead space when using a facial or nasal interface is small in comparison to the tidal volume, unlike helmet masks, which add a significant amount of dead space volume due to the larger internal volume in comparison to the tidal volume [43, 44, 48]. To minimize CO_2 rebreathing, a high flow gas system is advocated rather than decreasing the size of the helmet mask, which does not prevent CO_2 rebreathing during CPAP [43, 46]. Some types of home care ventilators induce CO_2 rebreathing because of the single-lumen circuit for both inspiration and expiration, and lack of an exhalation valve in the mask. It is recommended to use a double-lumen circuit and an interface with an exhalation port as an alternative to single-lumen circuit with an exhalation valve [42]. Several remedies can be implemented to prevent CO_2 rebreathing, such as choosing the appropriate interface, reducing RR and providing sufficient tidal volume, adequate expiratory time and PEEP [43].

1.4.1.3. Arm Edema and Deep Venous Thrombosis

Edema is rarely reported during helmet NIV and is caused by an increase in fluid filtration that usually occurs in the upper extremities and worsens due to failure in the lymphatic drainage [48, 49]. The NIV helmet is designed with two armpit braces and two hooks, which may result in venous stasis and eventually edema [48]. Malnourished and cachexic patients are predisposed to such incidence, which may lead to deep venous thrombosis, especially in the axillary vein [48]. In the case of deep venous thrombosis, anticoagulant therapy is recommended to avoid its occurrence. Special attention should be paid to the armpit braces to avoid excessive compression.

1.4.1.4. Discomfort

Although NIV is considered more convenient than invasive ventilation, intolerance or discomfort remains an issue that affects up to 50% of patients and is responsible for almost 33% of NIV failures [4, 24, 50-58]. Discomfort during NIV usually occurs in patients due to different factors, such as modes of ventilation and NIV interface [1, 4, 8, 24]. When different models of masks were utilized during NIV, the mouthpiece was the most intolerable interface compared to oronasal and nasal masks [59]. Intolerance may be induced by tightening the mask's straps, which compresses all attachment systems against the skin, to promote patient-ventilator dyssynchrony and minimize air leaks [59, 60]. Different strap systems or masks should be implemented in such a case to reduce the level of discomfort.

Generally, PSV is more comfortable that volume-controlled (VC) ventilation and is considered the preferred mode of ventilation in acute settings [61]. Optimizing PS is crucial for patients' comfort as excessive or insufficient PS is linked to high levels of discomfort [62, 63].

Judicious sedation during NIV may be used to diminish the level of discomfort without altering respiratory function, but this remains controversial and insufficient evidence is provided [64, 65].

1.4.1.5. Claustrophobia

Claustrophobia may occur at first as slight discomfort, but may progress to a suffocated or restricted feeling. Claustrophobia occurs in almost 20% of patients, and it is impossible to start or continue NIV when claustrophobia is present [1, 3, 4, 24, 48, 66, 67]. Face masks are more likely than nasal masks to cause claustrophobia, which might be a chronic condition due to negative past experiences [2, 8, 60, 68]. In such situations, using an appropriate interface is crucial for minimizing claustrophobia.

1.4.1.6. Patient-Ventilator Dyssynchrony

Ideally, NIV should be synchronized, cycling off and triggering with patients' needs to avoid wasted inspiratory efforts [69]. In reality, a delay in inspiration is noticed between the start of the inspiratory effort and the beginning of the inspiratory pressure increase [44, 70]. Additionally, a delay in expiration is noticed between inspiratory flow attaining 25% of its peak value and the expected end of PIP boost [44, 70]. In patients with ARF who receive mask NIV, double and auto-triggering, late and premature cycling, and ineffective breaths were detected and observed, which resulted in patient-ventilator dyssynchrony (PVD) [71]. PVD is considered one of the most common complications during NIV and was noticed in 43% of patients with ARF [71]. Several factors play a major role in patient-ventilator dyssynchrony, such as mode of ventilation, patient and interface [44, 70, 72]. PVD is less common with a nasal/oronasal mask than a mouthpiece [70]. Auto-triggering may be a result of water in the circuit and random noise, whereas premature cycling is caused by inappropriate inspiratory times, and ineffective breaths may be caused by dynamic hyperinflation, inspiratory muscle weakness and low respiratory drive [70, 71]. Other factors that may play a crucial role in PVD are air leakage, tidal volume and PS level [71, 72]. Higher PS delays the expiratory cycle, whereas lower PS prematurely activates the expiratory cycle while the inspiratory muscle is still contracting, leading to a non-triggered breath [69, 71]. Appropriate ventilatory support and identifying the cause of PVD are pivotal for optimizing patients' ventilatory support and comfort.

1.4.1.7. Noise

Noise may overreach the acceptable level in ICU settings during NIV and may result in discomfort, sleep interruption and tinnitus, temporary auditory threshold shift or hearing loss [73-75]. The NIV interface influences the level of noise; helmet NIV has a significantly higher noise level than mask NIV [73, 74]. The noise level inside the helmet can reach 100 decibels (dB). In contrast, the noise level inside NIV facial and nasal masks is below 60 dB, which is similar to the usual ICU noise level. The cause of noise during helmet NIV is the turbulent gas flow while the noise in NIV masks is induced by the NIV machine [73]. Noise can be minimized in several ways, such as using a heat and moisture exchanger (HME), attaching sound traps to the inspiratory circuit, and using earplugs [60, 73].

1.4.2. Complications Related to Pressure and Flow

1.4.2.1. Air Leaks

One of the most common complications during NIV is air leakage, which usually occurs because of the interface's sealing feature [4, 47, 59]. Appropriate interfaces are crucial in minimizing air leaks, which are usually large with small masks and small with helmets or larger masks [48, 59, 76]. During air leakage, arterial oxygen saturation (SaO_2) and FiO_2 decreased, and auto-triggering of ventilator, patient-ventilator dyssynchrony and rebreathing occurred, all of which reduce the chances of NIV success [76-78]. Air leaks can be minimized when appropriate NIV interfaces are selected and fitted properly [76-78]. Fitting an NIV interface tightly may lower the proportion of leaks and improve ventilation, but care should be taken as skin damage and discomfort may arise [4, 47, 48, 76]. In COPD patients with stable hypercapnia, minimum air leaks were noticed during PC ventilation, lower PIP and a similar volume was delivered compared with VC ventilation. During NIV, compensating for air leaks usually adds additional volume which may cause some side effects, such as eye conjunctivitis, throat dryness and sleep disruption [78]. Reducing tidal volume or inspiratory pressure may also minimize air leaks [79].

1.4.2.2. Nasal or Oral Dryness and Nasal Congestion

During nasal CPAP or using a nasal mask, congestion and dryness of the upper airway may occur. Around 20% of NIV patients developed oral/nasal dryness, while around 50% developed nasal congestion [1, 4, 8, 24, 80]. Air leaks through the mouth usually impair nasal mucosa's ability to humidify the inspired gas and consequently lead to oral/nasal dryness. Dryness of nasal mucosa is encountered, further inflammation mediators released, and resistance and congestion increase which further reduces patient comfort level and lowers tidal volume [80, 81]. Several strategies should be considered to minimize upper airway dryness and congestion while using NIV.

1.4.2.3. Airway Dryness

Atelectasis and mucus plugs may occur during NIV due to dry and unheated gases, which alter the mucosa of a patient's airway [81]. Thick secretions are a serious issue as they may prolong NIV and induce a life-threatening obstruction of the airway [82]. The humidity of dried gas is usually low compared with the desired humidification level during ventilator use: 5 mg H_2O versus 10 to 15 mg H_2O of absolute humidity [81]. However, regardless of the benefits of humidification with respect to tolerance and comfort in COPD patients who require long-term ventilatory support, the controversy remains about weather humidification should be routinely provided during acute care settings [81]. Heated humidifiers and heat and moisture exchangers (HME) are the main kinds of humidification systems used during NIV in the short term and the long term [81]. HMEs add additional dead space when attached into the ventilatory circuit, and subsequently increase the work of breathing and minute ventilation during PSV when compared with headed humidifiers [83, 84].

1.4.2.4. Gastric Insufflation

Gastric insufflation affected up to 40% of NIV patients [5, 24]. The volume distribution between stomach and lungs during NIV depends on airway resistance and varies with inspiratory flow rate and time, tidal volume and head position [85]. A tidal volume of 800 to 1,200 ml, low compliance, high airway resistance, and insufficient inspiratory time all increase the chance of gastric insufflation, whereas a tidal volume of 500 ml or below is considered effective and safe to reduce gastric insufflation incidence [85]. During gastric insufflation, gastric distension occurs and compresses the lungs, which reduces lung compliance and requires higher ventilation pressure [85]. Gastric insufflation may occasionally induce vomiting and aspiration of gastric contents, which can lead to several serious complications, such as, but not limited to, pulmonary aspiration and stomach rupture [4, 86]. Ideally, higher airway pressure of more than 25 cm H_2O should be avoided but if used, patients should be in a sitting position with no food for at least half an hour [4, 86].

Conclusion

NIV has many benefits, from providing ventilatory support to reducing the incidence of nosocomial pneumonia (although not all studies promote this perspective) and avoiding intubation, which makes it more attractive in acute care settings. NIV complications range from minor to somewhat severe, but if applied by a skillful team these can be minimized. NIV exaggeration should be averted and carefully monitored until the patients is stabilized. Careful sedation may be considered since conflicting data is presented in the literature. Patient selection, device choice and an appropriate management strategy should strictly follow the available guidelines to deliver the best care for patients.

Key Messages

- NIV is preferred to IMV where possible, but its usage may cause minorto serious complications.
- The issues related to features particular to NIV such as masks, helmets, gas flow and ventilators, are classified as minor complications.
- Serious or major NIV complications may result in death or increasing illness such as hemodynamic instability, barotrauma and pneumonia.
- In promoting preventive therapy, successful identification of patients at an elevated risk of experiencing minor or significant side effects at the start of NIV is crucial to mitigating the incidence of these harmful effects.
- Setting standards for the treatment of NIV patients with ARF based on available evidence and establishing minimum standards are essential to ensuring that patients receive optimal NIV care.

References

[1] Evans, TW. International Consensus Conferences in Intensive Care Medicine: non-invasive positive pressure ventilation in acute respiratory failure. Organised jointly by the American Thoracic Society, the European Respiratory Society, the European

Society of Intensive Care Medicine, and the Societe de Reanimation de Langue Francaise, and approved by the ATS Board of Directors, December 2000. *Intensive Care Med.*, 2001, 27(1), 166-78.

[2] Garpestad, E; Brennan, J; Hill, NS. Noninvasive ventilation for critical care. *Chest.*, 2007, 132(2), 711-20.

[3] Ferrer, M; Esquinas, A; Leon, M; Gonzalez, G; Alarcon, A; Torres, A. Noninvasive ventilation in severe hypoxemic respiratory failure: a randomized clinical trial. *American journal of respiratory and critical care medicine.*, 2003, 168(12), 1438-44.

[4] Mehta, S; Hill, NS. Noninvasive ventilation. *American journal of respiratory and critical care medicine.*, 2001, 163(2), 540-77.

[5] Carron, M; Freo, U; BaHammam, AS; Dellweg, D; Guarracino, F; Cosentini, R; et al. Complications of non-invasive ventilation techniques: a comprehensive qualitative review of randomized trials. *Br J Anaesth.*, 2013, 110(6), 896-914.

[6] Alqahtani, JS; AlAhmari, MD. Evidence based synthesis for prevention of noninvasive ventilation related facial pressure ulcers. *Saudi Med J.*, 2018, 39(5), 443-52.

[7] Caples, SM; Gay, PC. Noninvasive positive pressure ventilation in the intensive care unit: A concise review. *Read Online: Critical Care Medicine | Society of Critical Care Medicine.*, 2005, 33(11).

[8] Nava, S; Hill, N. Non-invasive ventilation in acute respiratory failure. *Lancet.*, 2009, 374(9685), 250-9.

[9] Valipour, A; Schneider, F; Kossler, W; Saliba, S; Burghuber, OC. Heart rate variability and spontaneous baroreflex sequences in supine healthy volunteers subjected to nasal positive airway pressure. *Journal of applied physiology* (Bethesda, Md: 1985)., 2005, 99(6), 2137-43.

[10] Jardin, F; Farcot, JC; Boisante, L; Curien, N; Margairaz, A; Bourdarias, JP. Influence of positive end-expiratory pressure on left ventricular performance. *The New England journal of medicine.*, 1981, 304(7), 387-92.

[11] Montner, PK; Greene, ER; Murata, GH; Stark, DM; Timms, M; Chick, TW. Hemodynamic effects of nasal and face mask continuous positive airway pressure. *American journal of respiratory and critical care medicine.*, 1994, 149(6), 1614-8.

[12] Maestroni, A; Aliberti, S; Amir, O; Milani, G; Brambilla, AM; Piffer, F; et al. Acute effects of positive end-expiratory pressure on left ventricle diastolic function in healthy subjects. *Internal and emergency medicine.*, 2009, 4(3), 249-54.

[13] Leithner, C; Podolsky, A; Globits, S; Frank, H; Neuhold, A; Pidlich, J; et al. Magnetic resonance imaging of the heart during positive end-expiratory pressure ventilation in normal subjects. *Critical care medicine.*, 1994, 22(3), 426-32.

[14] Leech, JA; Ascah, KJ. Hemodynamic effects of nasal CPAP examined by Doppler echocardiography. *Chest.*, 1991, 99(2), 323-6.

[15] Summers, RL; Patch, J; Kolb, JC. Effect of the initiation of noninvasive bi-level positive airway pressure on haemodynamic stability. *Eur J Emerg Med.*, 2002, 9(1), 37-41.

[16] Ambrosino, N; Nava, S; Torbicki, A; Riccardi, G; Fracchia, C; Opasich, C; et al. Haemodynamic effects of pressure support and PEEP ventilation by nasal route in patients with stable chronic obstructive pulmonary disease. *Thorax.*, 1993, 48(5), 523-8.

[17] Diaz, O; Iglesia, R; Ferrer, M; Zavala, E; Santos, C; Wagner, PD; et al. Effects of Noninvasive Ventilation on Pulmonary Gas Exchange and Hemodynamics during Acute Hypercapnic Exacerbations of Chronic Obstructive Pulmonary Disease. *American journal of respiratory and critical care medicine.*, 1997, 156(6), 1840-5.

[18] Confalonieri, M; Gazzaniga, P; Gandola, L; Aiolfi, S; Porta, RD; Frisinghelli, A; et al. Haemodynamic response during initiation of non-invasive positive pressure ventilation in COPD patients with acute ventilatory failure. *Respiratory Medicine.*, 1998, 92(2), 331-7.

[19] Kilger, E; Briegel, J; Haller, M; Frey, L; Schelling, G; Stoll, C; et al. Effects of noninvasive positive pressure ventilatory support in non-COPD patients with acute respiratory insufficiency after early extubation. *Intensive Care Medicine.*, 1999, 25(12), 1374-80.

[20] Nieminen, MS; Böhm, M; Cowie, MR; Drexler, H; Filippatos, GS; Jondeau, G; et al. Executive summary of the guidelines on the diagnosis and treatment of acute heart failure: The Task Force on Acute Heart Failure of the European Society of Cardiology. *European Heart Journal.*, 2005, 26(4), 384-416.

[21] Hill, NS; Brennan, J; Garpestad, E; Nava, S. Noninvasive ventilation in acute respiratory failure. *Critical care medicine.*, 2007, 35(10), 2402-7.

[22] Baratz, DM; Westbrook, PR; Shah, PK; Mohsenifar, Z. Effect of nasal continuous positive airway pressure on cardiac output and oxygen delivery in patients with congestive heart failure. *Chest.*, 1992, 102(5), 1397-401.

[23] Chadda, K; Annane, D; Hart, N; Gajdos, P; Raphaël, JC; Lofaso, F. Cardiac and respiratory effects of continuous positive airway pressure and noninvasive ventilation in acute cardiac pulmonary edema. *Critical care medicine.*, 2002, 30(11), 2457-61.

[24] Gay, PC. Complications of noninvasive ventilation in acute care. *Respir Care.*, 2009, 54(2), 246-57, discussion 57-8.

[25] Gupta, D; Nath, A; Agarwal, R; Behera, D. A prospective randomized controlled trial on the efficacy of noninvasive ventilation in severe acute asthma. *Respir Care.*, 2010, 55(5), 536-43.

[26] Carron, M; Gagliardi, G; Michielan, F; Freo, U; Ori, C. Occurrence of pneumothorax during noninvasive positive pressure ventilation through a helmet. *J Clin Anesth.*, 2007, 19(8), 632-5.

[27] Haworth, CS; Dodd, ME; Atkins, M; Woodcock, AA; Webb, AK. Pneumothorax in adults with cystic fibrosis dependent on nasal intermittent positive pressure ventilation (NIPPV): a management dilemma. *Thorax.*, 2000, 55(7), 620-2.

[28] Celis, R; Torres, A; Gatell, JM; Almela, M; Rodriguez-Roisin, R; Agusti-Vidal, A. Nosocomial pneumonia. A multivariate analysis of risk and prognosis. *Chest.*, 1988, 93(2), 318-24.

[29] Brochard, L; Mancebo, J; Wysocki, M; Lofaso, F; Conti, G; Rauss, A; et al. Noninvasive ventilation for acute exacerbations of chronic obstructive pulmonary disease. *The New England journal of medicine.*, 1995, 333(13), 817-22.

[30] Antonelli, M; Conti, G; Rocco, M; Bufi, M; De Blasi, RA; Vivino, G; et al. A Comparison of Noninvasive Positive-Pressure Ventilation and Conventional Mechanical Ventilation in Patients with Acute Respiratory Failure. *New England Journal of Medicine.*, 1998, 339(7), 429-35.

[31] Ferrer, M; Esquinas, A; Arancibia, F; Bauer, TT; Gonzalez, G; Carrillo, A; et al. Noninvasive ventilation during persistent weaning failure: a randomized controlled trial. *American journal of respiratory and critical care medicine.*, 2003, 168(1), 70-6.

[32] Hess, DR. Noninvasive positive-pressure ventilation and ventilator-associated pneumonia. *Respir Care.*, 2005, 50(7), 924-9, discussion 9-31.

[33] Kohlenberg, A; Schwab, F; Behnke, M; Geffers, C; Gastmeier, P. Pneumonia associated with invasive and noninvasive ventilation: an analysis of the German nosocomial infection surveillance system database. *Intensive Care Med.*, 2010, 36(6), 971-8.

[34] Guerin, C; Girard, R; Chemorin, C; De Varax, R; Fournier, G. Facial mask noninvasive mechanical ventilation reduces the incidence of nosocomial pneumonia. A prospective epidemiological survey from a single ICU. *Intensive Care Med.*, 1997, 23(10), 1024-32.

[35] Nourdine, K; Combes, P; Carton, MJ; Beuret, P; Cannamela, A; Ducreux, JC. Does noninvasive ventilation reduce the ICU nosocomial infection risk? A prospective clinical survey. *Intensive Care Med.*, 1999, 25(6), 567-73.

[36] Carlucci, A; Richard, JC; Wysocki, M; Lepage, E; Brochard, L. Noninvasive versus conventional mechanical ventilation. An epidemiologic survey. *American journal of respiratory and critical care medicine.*, 2001, 163(4), 874-80.

[37] Girou, E; Brun-Buisson, C; Taille, S; Lemaire, F; Brochard, L. Secular trends in nosocomial infections and mortality associated with noninvasive ventilation in patients with exacerbation of COPD and pulmonary edema. *Jama.*, 2003, 290(22), 2985-91.

[38] Haesler, E. National pressure ulcer advisory panel, european pressure ulcer advisory panel and pan pacific pressure injury alliance. *Prevention and treatment of pressure ulcers: quick reference guide.*, 2014.

[39] Alqahtani, JS; Worsley, P; Voegeli, D. Effect of Humidified Noninvasive Ventilation on the Development of Facial Skin Breakdown. *Respiratory Care.*, 2018, 63(9), 1102.

[40] Schallom, M; Cracchiolo, L; Falker, A; Foster, J; Hager, J; Morehouse, T; et al. Pressure ulcer incidence in patients wearing nasal-oral versus full-face noninvasive ventilation masks. *American Journal of Critical Care.*, 2015, 24(4), 349-56.

[41] Schettino, GPP; Chatmongkolchart, S; Hess, DR; Kacmarek, RM. Position of exhalation port and mask design affect CO2 rebreathing during noninvasive positive pressure ventilation. *Critical care medicine.*, 2003, 31(8), 2178-82.

[42] Szkulmowski, Z; Belkhouja, K; Le, QH; Robert, D; Argaud, L. Bilevel positive airway pressure ventilation: factors influencing carbon dioxide rebreathing. *Intensive Care Med.*, 2010, 36(4), 688-91.

[43] Taccone, P; Hess, D; Caironi, P; Bigatello, LM. Continuous positive airway pressure delivered with a "helmet": effects on carbon dioxide rebreathing. *Critical care medicine.*, 2004, 32(10), 2090-6.

[44] Racca, F; Appendini, L; Gregoretti, C; Stra, E; Patessio, A; Donner, CF; et al. Effectiveness of mask and helmet interfaces to deliver noninvasive ventilation in a human model of resistive breathing. *Journal of applied physiology* (Bethesda, Md: 1985)., 2005, 99(4), 1262-71.

[45] Fodil, R; Lellouche, F; Mancebo, J; Sbirlea-Apiou, G; Isabey, D; Brochard, L; et al. Comparison of patient-ventilator interfaces based on their computerized effective dead space. *Intensive Care Med.*, 2011, 37(2), 257-62.

[46] Patroniti, N; Foti, G; Manfio, A; Coppo, A; Bellani, G; Pesenti, A. Head helmet versus face mask for non-invasive continuous positive airway pressure: a physiological study. *Intensive Care Med.*, 2003, 29(10), 1680-7.

[47] Gonzalez, J; Sharshar, T; Hart, N; Chadda, K; Raphaël, JC; Lofaso, F. Air leaks during mechanical ventilation as a cause of persistent hypercapnia in neuromuscular disorders. *Intensive Care Medicine.*, 2003, 29(4), 596-602.

[48] Antonelli, M; Pennisi, MA; Pelosi, P; Gregoretti, C; Squadrone, V; Rocco, M; et al. Noninvasive positive pressure ventilation using a helmet in patients with acute exacerbation of chronic obstructive pulmonary disease: a feasibility study. *Anesthesiology.*, 2004, 100(1), 16-24.

[49] McDonagh, PF. The microvascular pathophysiology of chronic venous insufficiency. *Yale J Biol Med.*, 1993, 66(1), 27-36.

[50] Barbé, F; Togores, B; Rubí, M; Pons, S; Maimó, A; Agustí, AG. Noninvasive ventilatory support does not facilitate recovery from acute respiratory failure in chronic obstructive pulmonary disease. *Eur Respir J.*, 1996, 9(6), 1240-5.

[51] Conti, G; Antonelli, M; Navalesi, P; Rocco, M; Bufi, M; Spadetta, G; et al. Noninvasive vs. conventional mechanical ventilation in patients with chronic

obstructive pulmonary disease after failure of medical treatment in the ward: a randomized trial. *Intensive care medicine.*, 2002, 28(12), 1701-7.

[52] Mehta, S; Jay, GD; Woolard, RH; Hipona, RA; Connolly, EM; Cimini, DM; et al. Randomized, prospective trial of bilevel versus continuous positive airway pressure in acute pulmonary edema. *Critical care medicine.*, 1997, 25(4), 620-8.

[53] Gray, A; Goodacre, S; Newby, DE; Masson, M; Sampson, F; Nicholl, J. Noninvasive ventilation in acute cardiogenic pulmonary edema. *The New England journal of medicine.*, 2008, 359(2), 142-51.

[54] Wood, KA; Lewis, L; Von Harz, B; Kollef, MH. The use of noninvasive positive pressure ventilation in the emergency department: results of a randomized clinical trial. *Chest.*, 1998, 113(5), 1339-46.

[55] Honrubia, T; García López, FJ; Franco, N; Mas, M; Guevara, M; Daguerre, M; et al. Noninvasive vs conventional mechanical ventilation in acute respiratory failure: a multicenter, randomized controlled trial. *Chest.*, 2005, 128(6), 3916-24.

[56] Nava, S; Gregoretti, C; Fanfulla, F; Squadrone, E; Grassi, M; Carlucci, A; et al. Noninvasive ventilation to prevent respiratory failure after extubation in high-risk patients*. *Critical care medicine.*, 2005, 33(11), 2465-70.

[57] Confalonieri, M; Calderini, E; Terraciano, S; Chidini, G; Celeste, E; Puccio, G; et al. Noninvasive ventilation for treating acute respiratory failure in AIDS patients with Pneumocystis carinii pneumonia. *Intensive Care Med.*, 2002, 28(9), 1233-8.

[58] Hill, NS. Saving face: better interfaces for noninvasive ventilation. *Intensive Care Med.*, 2002, 28(3), 227-9.

[59] Tarabini Fraticelli, A; Lellouche, F; L'Her, E; Taillé, S; Mancebo, J; Brochard, L. Physiological effects of different interfaces during noninvasive ventilation for acute respiratory failure*. *Critical care medicine.*, 2009, 37(3), 939-45.

[60] Chiumello, D; Pelosi, P; Carlesso, E; Severgnini, P; Aspesi, M; Gamberoni, C; et al. Noninvasive positive pressure ventilation delivered by helmet vs. standard face mask. *Intensive Care Med.*, 2003, 29(10), 1671-9.

[61] Hess, DR. The Evidence for Noninvasive Positive-Pressure Ventilation in the Care of Patients in Acute Respiratory Failure: A Systematic Review of the Literature. *Respiratory Care.*, 2004, 49(7), 810.

[62] Chiumello, D; Pelosi, P; Croci, M; Bigatello, LM; Gattinoni, L. The effects of pressurization rate on breathing pattern, work of breathing, gas exchange and patient comfort in pressure support ventilation. *European Respiratory Journal.*, 2001, 18(1), 107.

[63] Vitacca, M; Bianchi, L; Zanotti, E; Vianello, A; Barbano, L; Porta, R; et al. Assessment of physiologic variables and subjective comfort under different levels of pressure support ventilation. *Chest.*, 2004, 126(3), 851-9.

[64] Rocco, M; Conti, G; Alessandri, E; Morelli, A; Spadetta, G; Laderchi, A, et al. Rescue treatment for noninvasive ventilation failure due to interface intolerance

with remifentanil analgosedation: a pilot study. *Intensive Care Med.*, 2010, 36(12), 2060-5.

[65] Clouzeau, B; Bui, HN; Vargas, F; Grenouillet-Delacre, M; Guilhon, E; Gruson, D; et al. Target-controlled infusion of propofol for sedation in patients with non-invasive ventilation failure due to low tolerance: a preliminary study. *Intensive Care Med.*, 2010, 36(10), 1675-80.

[66] Kirakli, C; Cerci, T; Ucar, ZZ; Erer, OF; Bodur, HA; Bilaceroglu, S; et al. Noninvasive assisted pressure-controlled ventilation: as effective as pressure support ventilation in chronic obstructive pulmonary disease? *Respiration.*, 2008, 75(4), 402-10.

[67] Conti, G; Cavaliere, F; Costa, R; Craba, A; Catarci, S; Festa, V; et al. Noninvasive positive-pressure ventilation with different interfaces in patients with respiratory failure after abdominal surgery: a matched-control study. *Respir Care.*, 2007, 52(11), 1463-71.

[68] Gregoretti, C; Confalonieri, M; Navalesi, P; Squadrone, V; Frigerio, P; Beltrame, F; et al. Evaluation of patient skin breakdown and comfort with a new face mask for non-invasive ventilation: a multi-center study. *Intensive Care Med.*, 2002, 28(3), 278-84.

[69] Spahija, J; de Marchie, M; Albert, M; Bellemare, P; Delisle, S; Beck, J; et al. Patient-ventilator interaction during pressure support ventilation and neurally adjusted ventilatory assist. *Critical care medicine.*, 2010, 38(2), 518-26.

[70] Costa, R; Navalesi, P; Spinazzola, G; Ferrone, G; Pellegrini, A; Cavaliere, F; et al. Influence of ventilator settings on patient-ventilator synchrony during pressure support ventilation with different interfaces. *Intensive Care Med.*, 2010, 36(8), 1363-70.

[71] Vignaux, L; Vargas, F; Roeseler, J; Tassaux, D; Thille, AW; Kossowsky, MP; et al. Patient-ventilator asynchrony during non-invasive ventilation for acute respiratory failure: a multicenter study. *Intensive Care Med.*, 2009, 35(5), 840-6.

[72] Kondili, E; Xirouchaki, N; Georgopoulos, D. Modulation and treatment of patient-ventilator dyssynchrony. *Curr Opin Crit Care.*, 2007, 13(1), 84-9.

[73] Cavaliere, F; Conti, G; Costa, R; Proietti, R; Sciuto, A; Masieri, S. Noise exposure during noninvasive ventilation with a helmet, a nasal mask, and a facial mask. *Intensive Care Med.*, 2004, 30(9), 1755-60.

[74] Cavaliere, F; Conti, G; Costa, R; Spinazzola, G; Proietti, R; Sciuto, A; et al. Exposure to noise during continuous positive airway pressure: influence of interfaces and delivery systems. *Acta Anaesthesiol Scand.*, 2008, 52(1), 52-6.

[75] Gabor, JY; Cooper, AB; Crombach, SA; Lee, B; Kadikar, N; Bettger, HE; et al. Contribution of the intensive care unit environment to sleep disruption in mechanically ventilated patients and healthy subjects. *American journal of respiratory and critical care medicine.*, 2003, 167(5), 708-15.

[76] Vargas, F; Thille, A; Lyazidi, A; Campo, FR; Brochard, L. Helmet with specific settings versus facemask for noninvasive ventilation. *Critical care medicine.*, 2009, 37(6), 1921-8.

[77] Miyoshi, E; Fujino, Y; Uchiyama, A; Mashimo, T; Nishimura, M. Effects of gas leak on triggering function, humidification, and inspiratory oxygen fraction during noninvasive positive airway pressure ventilation. *Chest.*, 2005, 128(5), 3691-8.

[78] Storre, JH; Bohm, P; Dreher, M; Windisch, W. Clinical impact of leak compensation during non-invasive ventilation. *Respiratory Medicine.*, 2009, 103(10), 1477-83.

[79] Cosentini, R; Brambilla, AM; Aliberti, S; Bignamini, A; Nava, S; Maffei, A; et al. Helmet Continuous Positive Airway Pressure vs Oxygen Therapy To Improve Oxygenation in Community-Acquired Pneumonia: A Randomized, Controlled Trial. *Chest.*, 2010, 138(1), 114-20.

[80] Richards, GN; Cistulli, PA; Ungar, RG; Berthon-Jones, M; Sullivan, CE. Mouth leak with nasal continuous positive airway pressure increases nasal airway resistance. *American journal of respiratory and critical care medicine.*, 1996, 154(1), 182-6.

[81] Branson, RD; Gentile, MA. Is Humidification Always Necessary During Noninvasive Ventilation in the Hospital? *Respiratory Care.*, 2010, 55(2), 209.

[82] Wood, KE; Flaten, AL; Backes, WJ. Inspissated secretions: a life-threatening complication of prolonged noninvasive ventilation. *Respir Care.*, 2000, 45(5), 491-3.

[83] Lellouche, F; Maggiore, SM; Lyazidi, A; Deye, N; Taillé, S; Brochard, L. Water content of delivered gases during non-invasive ventilation in healthy subjects. *Intensive Care Med.*, 2009, 35(6), 987-95.

[84] Jaber, S; Chanques, G; Matecki, S; Ramonatxo, M; Souche, B; Perrigault, PF; et al. Comparison of the effects of heat and moisture exchangers and heated humidifiers on ventilation and gas exchange during non-invasive ventilation. *Intensive Care Med.*, 2002, 28(11), 1590-4.

[85] De Keulenaer, BL; De Backer, A; Schepens, DR; Daelemans, R; Wilmer, A; Malbrain, MLNG. Abdominal compartment syndrome related to noninvasive ventilation. *Intensive Care Medicine.*, 2003, 29(7), 1177-81.

[86] Luria, O; Reshef, L; Barnea, O. Analysis of non-invasive ventilation effects on gastric inflation using a non-linear mathematical model. *Resuscitation.*, 2006, 71(3), 358-64.

In: Non-Invasive Mechanical Ventilation Complications
Editor: Antonio M. Esquinas
ISBN: 978-1-53619-515-6

Chapter 2

DISCOMFORT, COMPLIANCE, ADHERENCE, DETERMINANTS AND PREVENTION OF USING NIV

Saumy Johnson[1], Carol Mathews[1] and Savitha Joseph,[2]
[1]Respiratory Therapy, Inaya Medical College, Riyadh
[2]Kuwait Oil Company Hospital, Kuwait

ABSTRACT

Patient compliance and tolerance is the key factor for the success of the noninvasive ventilation (NIV). There are many factors that influence this. Staff training and careful application of the interface makes a difference in improving the compliance, preventing complications and improving adherence to the therapy. Respiratory Therapist plays a major role in the treatment of patients who require NIV. Non-Compliance to the therapy makes it difficult to continue with NIV and patient may end up having worsened respiratory failure requiring invasive ventilation. Compliance and adherence to home mechanical ventilation using NIV is also a concern for the respiratory care providers.

INTRODUCTION

Noninvasive ventilation (NIV) in the current clinical practice is inevitable and is often applied in Intensive Care Units, Emergency Departments, step-down units and respiratory wards. NIV is established as the standard of care in treating patients with respiratory failure. The term 'Non-Invasive" itself points out the definition of NIV as a ventilatory modality which provides positive pressure ventilation (PPV) without the use of an invasive artificial airway devices like endotracheal tube (ETT) or a tracheostomy tube (TT) [1-5]. The major interfaces used for the delivery of the NIV are oronasal or nasal mask, full face mask and helmets etc.

The use of the NIV and its advantages over the conventional invasive techniques are extensively researched since its inception. Several studies have shown the success of NIV in reducing the work of breathing and enhancing gas exchange which ultimately curtailed the incidence of tracheal intubation and its associated complications. The highlighted benefits of the NIV over invasive ventilation are reduction in the length of Intensive Care Unit (ICU) and hospital stay, morbidity and mortality [6-8].

Despite of these advantages, many patients fail to tolerate NIV and even develop life threatening adverse effects. NIV failure rates range from 18% to 40% in an acute care setting. One of the key factors leading to NIV failure is patient discomfort, which reflects the NIV intolerance and a decline in controlling respiratory distress. Hence the main outcome of NIV failure is the extended need for intubation and its associated complications [9-10]. Cheng SL et al. in their research evaluated the compliance to the home NIV in sixty-five patients. A questionnaire on symptomatology and adverse effects associated with home NIV was administered. It was found that the Mean daily use was 7.3 ± 2.9 h/day and median percentage of days on which home NIV was used for ≥ 4 h/day was 96.7% [11].

The efficacy of therapy varies depending on several factors like patient selection, underlying pathology, use of appropriate equipment and interface, clinician experience, environmental factors, psychological factors, personal beliefs and experiences etc. These factors predict the success or failure of NIV in patients [4-10].

RECOMMENDATIONS

1	Assessment of patient comfort and pain is to be completed at least second hourly and documented	Consensus	Holanda [11] MA et al., 2009
2	Assessment of patient tolerance for higher levels of the NIV is to be completed at least hourly until the highest level of compliance reached	Consensus	Holanda [11] MA et al., 2009
3	The choice of mask is influenced by: • patient comfort • clinical effectiveness • equipment availability.	Evidence C	Patroniti N et al., [12]

Devices vary in functionality due to differences in technology (Figure 1) and operating systems. Few existing equipment related problems causing NIV intolerance are incorrect mode selection, inadequate leak compensation, CO_2 rebreathing, patient ventilator asynchrony, absence of continuous monitoring of parameters, lack of oxygen blenders and proper alarms systems. Additionally, the ventilators provided with single limb or the double limb circuits, location of the exhalation port, etc., has an impact on patients and may determine the NIV tolerance level. Air pressure and flow related complications such as air leaks, nasal congestion and gastric distension are virtually universal during NIV which lead to patient discomfort to the therapy.

Patient Comfort and Compliance to Therapy

Patient comfort and enhanced compliance are key factors in determining successful application of non-invasive ventilation. Factors that contribute to patient comfort and compliance include [1, 13]:

- Choice of suitable interface
- Levels of pressure applied
- Position of the patient
- Synchrony of ventilation
- Pharmacotherapy for dyspnea, anxiety and pain
- Humidification
- Palliation of symptoms.

The Visual Analog scale could be used to assess patient's comfort. Visual analogue scale (0-10): 10 representing maximum comfort, as if you were breathing without a mask; 0 indicates maximum discomfort you could imagine.

Staff Training

It is important to give awareness about the care of NIV patients among the nurses and the Respiratory Therapists so that the complications could be minimized. There are many studies in the literature which states that the knowledge about the application of the NIV is poor among the healthcare professionals [14-23].

Simulation based staff training has been shown to be effective in terms of both resource utilization and reducing the time of initiation of the NIV [24, 25]. The British Thoracic society's guideline is a comprehensive document to guide the use of the NIV [26]. Workshops and hands on training will offer a chance for the participants to play the role as patient and feel the mask fitting, helmet fitting and the positive pressure breathing and they can feel how exactly the patient may feel when the mask is on. These experiences provide the trainees with a unique awareness that can help them to manage real NIV situations at the patients' bedside [27].

How You Do It Is More Important Than Where You Do It

There are variations in the practice of NIV in different parts of the world. A survey by Lari, F et al., in Italy [28] found that there are still variations in the practice of the NIV. Similar results are seen in India as well [29]. Though many physicians use it, a marked variation in the patterns relating to actual deployment of NIV, site of initiation, protocols for initiation, and monitoring of patients were noted. Respiratory Therapists have a key role to play in the initiation and management of patients who are on the NIV.

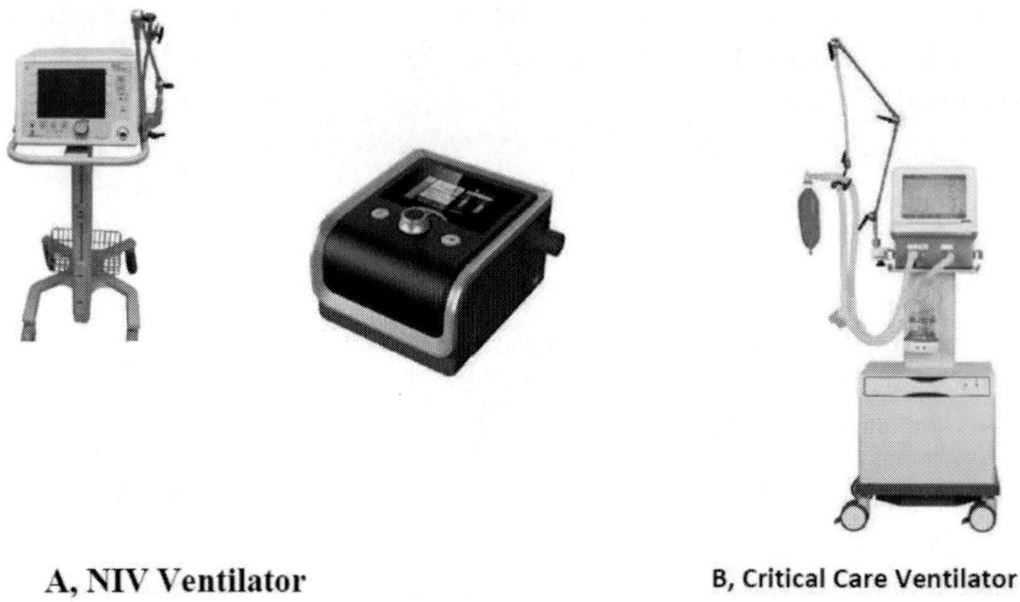

Figure 1. A NIV Ventilator, B: Critical Care Ventilator.

A major challenge faced by the clinician on the application of NIV is interface selection. It's essential to choose an appropriate interface as it connects the equipment via circuit to the patient. The main six categories of interfaces used commercially for NIV delivery (Figure 2) are:

1. Nasal mask; covers the whole nose
2. Oronasal mask; covers the mouth and nose
3. Total Face mask; seals the entire face
4. Nasal pillows; applied externally to the nares
5. Mouthpiece; placed in the mouth of the patient
6. Helmet; the whole head is placed in a hood and has a collar that seals.

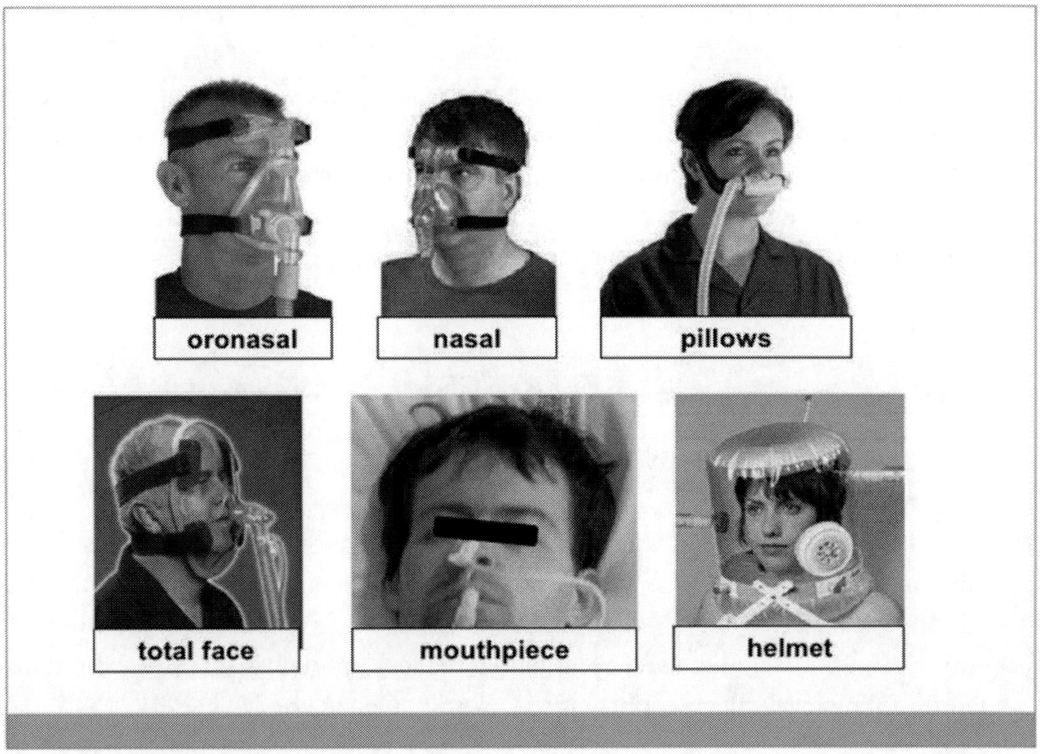

Figure 2. NIV Interfaces.

Each interface has its own advantages and disadvantages. The main interface related problems causing patient discomfort includes claustrophobia, eye irritation, CO_2 rebreathing, facial skin lesions, air leaks due to poorly fitted mask, aerophagia, noise, nasal or oral dryness etc. Approximately 10-15% of patients face NIV intolerance due to adjustments in strap tension, repositioning and inability to handle copious secretion and mask placement instability etc. Pressure ulcers related to the use of the NIV are an increasing clinical problem due to the increased acceptance of the intervention. Estimated Prevalence of grade I pressure ulcers have been at 5-50% after a few of hours and 100% after 48 hours [29].

Selection of the interface has always been dependent on the facial anatomy, breathing pattern and the patient's level of comfort. Another frequent problem associated with the interface is air leaks due to nasogastric feeding tubes, beards or absence of dentures. Patient comfort and enhanced compliance while using an interface could underline the success of non-invasive ventilation [30-31].

The patient related problems leading to intolerance to NIV can itself be the severity of the disease, development of aspiration pneumonia, barotrauma and hypotension associated with the initiation of NIV, anxiety, fear of death, personal perception, limitations to physical activities and mobility, socio economic factors 32-34 etc. The patient ventilator asynchrony can occur due to poor respiratory drive, weak respiratory muscles and poor cough reflex, existing chronic lung disease etc., shows an impact on NIV tolerance.

Hence, compatibility of a chosen interface or the ventilator with the patient should be evaluated while using the NIV to determine the success or failure of the therapy. NIV tolerance is multifaceted and mainly depends on the selection of patients, equipment and the interface. Routine assessment of the patients on NIV is mandatory and a contributing factor to ensure patient comfort and enhance compliance to the therapy.

REFERENCES

[1] Nava S, Hill N. Non-invasive ventilation in acute respiratory failure. *Lancet* 2009; 374(9685): 250-9.

[2] Roberts, C M, J L Brown. Non-invasive ventilation in chronic obstructive pulmonary disease: management of acute type 2 respiratory failure. *Clin. Med.* 2008;8(5):517-21.

[3] Auriant I, et al. Noninvasive ventilation reduces mortality in acute respiratory failure following lung resection. *Am. J. Respir. Crit. Care Med.* 2001; 164:1231–1235.

[4] Gul Gursel et al. Factors associated with noninvasive ventilation response in the first day of therapy in patients with hypercapnic respiratory failure. *Ann. Thorac. Med.* 2012 Apr-Jun; 7(2): 92–97. doi: 10.4103/1817-1737.94531.

[5] Brill A K. How to avoid interface problems in acute noninvasive ventilation. *Breathe* 2014 10: 230-242; DOI: 10.1183/20734735.003414.

[6] Brill A K. Choosing the interface. In: Anita K S, editor. Noninvasive ventilation. *ERS Practical*. 2015; pp 26–34.

[7] Khaled Hussein. Efficacy and troubleshooting of noninvasive ventilation. *The Egyptian Journal of Chest Diseases and Tuberculosis,* Vol. 67 No. 4, October-December 2018.

[8] Ngandu, H et.al. Experiences of noninvasive ventilation in adults with hypercapnia respiratory failure: a review of evidence. *Eur. Respir. Rev.* 2016; 25: 451–471 | DOI: 10.1183/16000617.0002-2016.

[9] An-Kwok Ian Wong et.al. Consequences and Solutions for the Impact of Communication Impairment on Noninvasive Ventilation Therapy for Acute Respiratory Failure: A Focused Review. *Crit. Care Expl.* 2020; 2e0121 DOI: 10.1097/CCE.0000000000000121.

[10] Cheng S L, Chan V L, Chu C M. *Compliance with home non-invasive ventilation. Respirology.* 2012 May;17(4):735-6. doi: 10.1111/j.1440-1843.2012.02169.x. PMID: 22420583.

[11] Holanda M A, Reis R C, Winkeler G F, Fortaleza S C, Lima J W, Pereira E D. Influence of total face, facial and nasal masks on short-term adverse effects during noninvasive ventilation. *J. Bras. Pneumol.* 2009;35(2):164-73.

[12] Patroniti N, Foti G, Manfio A, Coppo A, Bellani G, Pesenti A. Head helmet versus face mask for non-invasive continuous positive airway pressure: a physiological study. *Intensive Care Med.* 2003;29(10):1680-7.

[13] Plant P, Owen J, Elliott M. Early use of non-invasive ventilation for acute exacerbations of chronic obstructive pulmonary disease on general respiratory wards: a multicentre randomised controlled trial. *The Lancet.* 2000;355 (9219):1931-5.

[14] Lopez-Campos J L, Garcia Polo C, Leon Jimenez A, Arnedillo A, Gonzalez-Moya E, Fenandez Berni J J. Staff training influence on non-invasive ventilation outcome for acute hypercapnic respiratory failure. *Monaldi Arch. Chest Dis.* 2006; 65:145–151.

[15] Hess D R. How to initiate a noninvasive ventilation program: bringing the evidence to the bedside. *Respir. Care* 2009; 54:232–243.

[16] Karim H R, Burns K E, Ciobanu L D, El-Khatib M, Nicolini A et al. Noninvasive ventilation: education and training.A narrative analysis and an international consensus document. *Adv. Respir. Med.* 2019;

[17] Cox C E, Carson S S, Ely E W, Govert J A, Garrett J M, Brower R G et al. Effectiveness of medical resident education in mechanical ventilation. *Am. J. Respir. Crit. Care Med.* 2003; 167:32–38.

[18] Nicolini A, Santo M, Ferrera L, Ferrari-Bravo M, Barlascini O, Perazzo A. The use of non-invasive ventilation in very old patients with hypercapnic respiratory failure because of COPD exacerbation. *Int. J. Clin. Pract.* 2014; 68:1523–1529.

[19] Bierer G B, Soo Hoo G W. Noninvasive ventilation for acute respiratory failure: a national survey of Veterans Affairs Hospitals. *Respir. Care* 2009; 54:1313–1320.

[20] Davies J D, Gentile M A. What does it take to have a successful noninvasive ventilation program? *Respir. Care* 2009; 54:53–61.

[21] Tallo F S, Abib S C, Negri A J, Filho P C, Lopes R D, Lopes A C. Evaluation of self-perception of mechanical ventilation knowledge among brazilian final-year medical students, residents and emergency physicians. *Clinics (Sao Paulo)* 2017; 72:65–70.

[22] Simonelli C, Paneroni M, Vitacca M. An implementation protocol for non invasive ventilation prescription: the physiotherapist role in an Italian Hospital. *Respir. Care* 2012; 58:662–668.

[23] Scala R, Windisch W, Kohnlein T, Cuvelier A, Navalesi P, Pelosi P, European Respiratory Society Respiratory Intensive Care Assembly.Targeting European Respiratory Society Group Activities: A Survey of the Noninvasive Ventilatory Support Group. *European Respir. Rev.* 2014; 23:258–260.

[24] McQueen S, Dickinson M, Pimblett M. Human patient simulation can aid staff training in non-invasive ventilation. *Nurs Times* 2010; 106:20.

[25] Kramer N, Meyer T J, Meharg J, Cece R D, Hill NS. Randomized, prospective trial of noninvasive positive pressure ventilation in acute respiratory failure. *Am. J. Respir. Crit. Care Med.* 1995; 151:1799–1806.

[26] British Thoracic Society Standards of Care Committee. Non-invasive ventilation in acute respiratory failure. *Thorax* 2002; 57:192–211.

[27] Brill A K, Moghal M, Morrell M J, Simonds A K. Randomized crossover trial of a pressure sensing visual feedback system to improve mask fitting in noninvasive ventilation. *Respirology* 2017; 22:1343–1349.

[28] Lari, F., Gilioli, F., Ongari, M., & Ballardini, G. (2020). The use of non-invasive ventilation for acute respiratory failure in general medical wards: a regional Italian survey. *Italian Journal of Medicine*, 14(2), 62-68.

[29] Chawla R, Sidhu U S, Kumar V, Nagarkar S, Brochard L. Noninvasive ventilation: A survey of practice patterns of its use in India. *Indian J. Crit. Care Med.* 2008; 12:163–169.

[30] Carron M, Freo U, BaHammam A S, et al. Complications of non-invasive ventilation techniques: a comprehensive qualitative review of randomized trials. *Br. J. Anaesth.* 2013; 110(6): 896-914.

[31] Carron M., U. Freo et.al Complications of non-invasive ventilation techniques: a comprehensive qualitative review of randomized trials. *British Journal of Anaesthesia* 110 (6): 896–914 (2013) doi:10.1093/bja/aet070.

[32] Khilnani G C, Banga A, Sharma S K. Predictors of need of mechanical ventilation and reintubation in patients with acute respiratory failure secondary to chronic obstructive pulmonary disease. *Indian J. Crit. Care Med.* 2006;10:88-94.

[33] Vignaux L et.al. Patient–ventilator asynchrony during non-invasive ventilation for acute respiratory failure: a multicenter study. *Intensive Care Med.* (2009) 35:840–846 DOI 10.1007/s00134-009-1416-5.

[34] Hadil A Otair et.al. Ventilator- and interface-related factors influencing patient-ventilator asynchrony during noninvasive ventilation. *Ann. Thorac. Med.* 2020; 15:1-8.

In: Non-Invasive Mechanical Ventilation Complications ISBN: 978-1-53619-515-6
Editor: Antonio M. Esquinas

Chapter 3

Complications during Non-Invasive Mechanical Ventilation: Nasal Symptoms, Sinus Congestions, Oronasal Drying

***Marta Ruiz Pérez de la Blanca*[1,*],**
***Elena María Jiménez González*[1]**
***and Cristina Palma Rodríguez*[1]**
[1]UGC Urgencias, Hospital Comarcal de Baza, Granada, Spain

Abstract

When we talk about non-invasive mechanical ventilation (NIMV), we are referring to a type of ventilatory support treatment that falls between conventional oxygen therapy and invasive mechanical ventilation. With this type of treatment, positive pressure is administered through a non-invasive interface, such as a face mask, to try to achieve good ventilation for the patient instead of an invasive interface (endotracheal tube, tracheostomy).

Non-invasive mechanical ventilation is indicated in both patients with acute and chronic respiratory failure. Despite being a simple technique with a high number of indications, it is not exempt from possible complications. In this chapter we will focus on the oronasal symptoms, which, even though they are minor complications, we must know.

Keywords: non-invasive ventilation, complications, nasal symptoms, sinus congestions, oronasal drying

* Corresponding Author's E-mail: mariaperezdela@hotmail.com.

1. Introduction

The benefits of using non-invasive ventilation are widely demonstrated in situations of acute and chronic respiratory failure. The initiation of NIMV treatment in the case of acute insufficiency should be as early as possible, since delays in it lead to clinical deterioration of the patient and an increased probability of failure [2].

In most cases, it is in the hospital emergency services where the treatment with NIMV is started, subsequently being maintained in intensive care services, internal medicine or pulmonology if the patient continues to require it. Some studies suggest that the use of prehospital NIMV in patients with acute respiratory failure may reduce mortality and the need for intubation in these patients [2].

Be that as it may, the success of the VMNI depends to a great extent on the presence of expert personnel in its management; the placement of a comfortable interface for the patient, which adjusts appropriately to minimize possible leaks and achieve maximum comfort and, therefore, adaptability of the patient; and continuous reassessments by the physician, both at the clinical level of the patient, as well as the pressure, flow and volume curves offered by the NIMV devices, as well as the laboratory data [2].

The use of NIMV is usually safe and most of the complications that appear are local and are usually related to the mask.

The most frequent are detailed below:

- Skin complications: skin lesions may appear due to pressure from the masks and straps on the skin, with the bridge of the nose and forehead being the most affected areas. Their appearance has been reduced with the use of new masks that have padded reinforcements incorporated in these locations [2].
- Digestive complications: gastric bloating is a frequent complication that usually has no clinical relevance. However, vomiting and/or aspiration are more dangerous and their frequency of appearance increases with the use of facial or oronasal masks. However, the widespread use of a nasogastric tube is not recommended [2]. Cook and collaborators described in 2019 a case of pneumoperitoneum and percutaneous endoscopic gastrostomy (PEG) tube displacement associated with NIMV [7].
- Complications in the mucosa: due to the dryness caused by positive pressure in the mucosa, eye irritation, sinus pain, congestion and/or epistaxis may appear. They usually improve by reducing inspiratory pressure or using humidifiers [2]. It is a complication related to air pressure or flow [13].
- Psychological complications: during NIMV the patient may experience claustrophobia, anxiety or fear, which can be prevented with correct information and with accompaniment [2].

- Other complications: Barotrauma and hemodynamic instability are exceptional compared to the possibility of appearance during invasive mechanical ventilation [2]. Alava et al. described a case of mumps associated with prolonged use of NIMV in an elderly patient with acute lung edema, who was treated with antibiotic therapy, corticosteroid therapy, and mask repositioning [8].

2. Nasal Complications

2.1. Anatomical, Histological and Physiological Memory

Before delving into the study of nasal complications, let's make a reminder of the anatomy, histology and physiology of the respiratory system.

The respiratory system is made up of a conductive part or airways, a respiratory part and a ventilation mechanism. The first part is divided into upper airways, made up of the nostrils, oral cavity, and pharynx, and it is the larynx, trachea, and bronchi that make up the lower airways. The respiratory part is the continuation of the conductor and includes the regions where the gas exchange takes place (bronchioles and alveoli). Finally, the ventilation mechanism is in charge of mobilizing the air towards the respiratory part and is made up of the thorax, the diaphragm and the elastic connective tissue of the lungs [9, 12].

We will focus on the nose and paranasal sinuses as they are the structures affected in the complications that we treat in this chapter.

- Nose: we can divide it into external nose and internal nose:

    - The external nose extends from the nostrils (anterior openings of the nasal cavities, formed by the junction of the inferior lateral cartilages, columella and nasal vestibule) to the front of the face. It has a pyramidal shape with an anterior vertex consisting of the medial and lateral crura and the columella. It is made up of skin, own bones and superior and inferior lateral cartilage. The lobby is lined with fur with vibrissa, terminal hairs that filter the air inspired by dust and bacteria.
    - The internal nose or nasal cavity is made up of the nasal septum, the lateral nasal wall and the posterior nostrils. The nasal septum is made up of a bony part, a cartilaginous part and a membranous part, and it divides the internal nose into two nostrils. With the union of the septum and the superior lateral cartilage, the choanas (posterior nostrils) are formed. The lateral nasal wall is made up of the turbinates (upper, middle and lower), even structures composed of spongy bone with irregular walls that increase the surface of air

exposure and favor the appearance of turbulence. In the inner nose, the stratified flat epithelium of the outer nose becomes thinner, and a transition zone with mucocutaneous epithelium appears in the vestibule, giving rise to mucosa in the turbinates. Already in the nasal cavity itself, a ciliated pseudostratified cylindrical epithelium appears with numerous goblet cells, which rests on a lamina of connective tissue with numerous mixed mucosacretory glands. This own sheet finally sits on bone tissue. In addition, at the top of the septum and the upper turbinates is the human olfactory mucosa, responsible for detecting odors.

– Paranasal sinuses: they are even structures that develop as excrescences from the nasal cavities with which they communicate through an ostium, eroding the interior of the adjacent bones. Although they are not academic nasal airway structures, they are included here because diseases that lead to inflammation and obstruction, such as sinusitis, can cause nasal congestion and obstructive symptoms.

There are four paranasal sinuses: the ethmoid cells and the sphenoid, maxillary and frontal sinuses:

- Ethmoid cells: inflammation of these cells can cause pain between the eyes, since they are behind the bridge of the nose. In addition, sensitivity to both sides of the nose, anosmia, nasal congestion and swelling of the periocular tissues may also appear.
- Sphenoid sinuses: they are located behind the eyes and nasal structures, so problems in this location are manifested with earache, neckache and headache.
- Maxillary sinuses: with a triangular shape, they are the largest breasts and are located behind the cheeks. When they become inflamed, pain appears in the upper dental arch, upper jaw or cheeks.
- Frontal sinuses: they have a variable size and are located in the most cranial position of the four sinuses, above the eyes. Pain when touching the forehead in the head area of the eyebrows is characteristic of inflammation of the frontal sinuses.

They are connected to each other and to the nose through the ostiomeatal complex. It is a series of openings and bony indentations in the lateral wall of the nose, which allows drainage of mucus and ventilation of the sinuses.

Inflammation of this area can also manifest as nasal congestion, even when the sinuses are free.

An epithelium similar to but thinner than that of the nasal cavity lines the paranasal sinuses; however, the lamina propria is very thin and has almost no mucocretory glands.

- Nasopharynx: The nasopharynx is the most cranial part of the pharynx, posterior to the nasal cavity, superior to the soft palate and the oropharynx, from which it is separated by the pharyngeal isthmus. The anterior border of the nasopharynx is formed by the choanae and the roof is the lower wall of the sphenoid sinus. In this region we also find ciliated pseudostratified epithelium. Both in the nasal cavity, in the paranasal sinuses and in the nasopharynx, a thin layer of mucus covers the entire epithelium [9, 10, 11].

Air enters through the carinae into the nasal cavity and passes to the choanae, to cross the larynx and continue through the trachea and bronchi to the bronchioles and alveoli where the gas exchange will take place. The air flow presents turbulence when passing through these structures in a physiological way and any alteration in them can lead to an anomaly in the perception of air. There is also air flow around the turbinates and sinus ostia, so airborne particles can cause inflammation of the upper airway [10].

During respiration, the air is heated, humidified and released from harmful substances (bacteria, dust, allergens ...) by the mucous membranes of the airways. Specifically, during inspiration the air is heated so that it reaches the lungs in optimal conditions: 37ºC temperature and 44mg/l humidity (internal body environment conditions). This is achieved through the nasal mucosa, so this process dries and cools the mucosa. On expiration much of this heat and moisture added to the air on inspiration are lost. The expired air returns to the mucosa some heat and humidity [18].

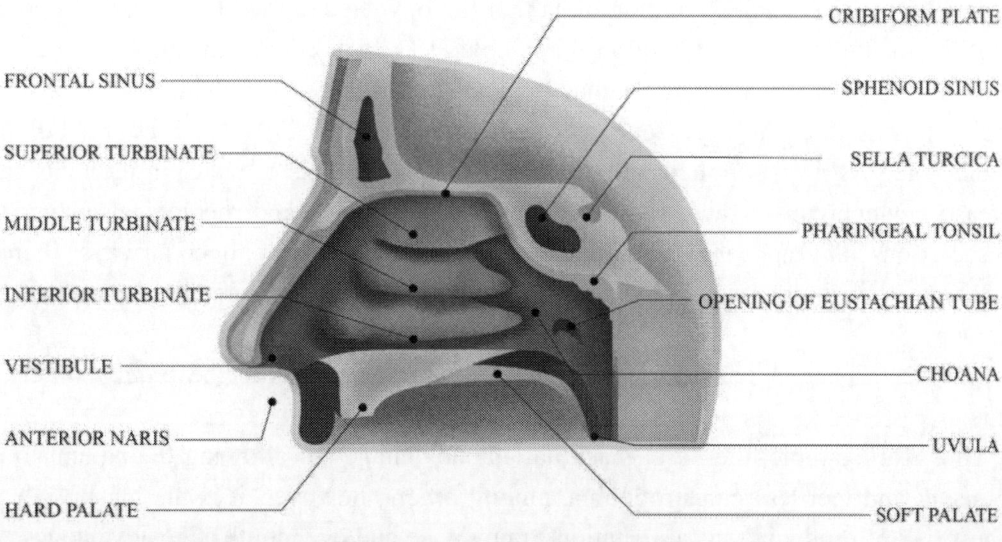

Figure 1. (Image made by Román Urrutia for this chapter).

2.2. Nasal Symptoms: Nasal Congestion and Oronasal Dryness

As explained in previous sections in this chapter, the use of non-invasive mechanical ventilation is not without potential complications. Among them we find nasal symptoms, among which nasal congestion and oronasal dryness stand out.

Both symptoms are relatively frequent during the use of non-invasive mechanical ventilation, being present in 20 - 50% of patients according to some authors [13]. So much so, that in many occasions both symptoms appear together during the use of this therapy [3].

Nasal congestion occurs when the tissues that make up the nose are puffed up by numerous stimuli: allergens, nasal polyps, high-pressure air ... It can be accompanied by a runny nose [14].

On the other hand, nasal dryness is the expression of loss of moisture in the nasal cavity that the patient experiences as a sensation of a dry nose, and epistaxis and nasal crusts may appear [15].

Nasal congestion may be a pre-existing problem in the patient or may be precipitated by treatment with non-invasive mechanical ventilation. Nasal congestion is capable of increasing resistance to air flow with the risk of reducing the benefit of ventilatory therapy and, in addition, can cause discomfort in the patient with the risk of decreasing therapeutic adherence [5].

These symptoms are usually seasonal and usually appear in winter [3].

Some researchers have even detected histological changes in the nasal mucosa in patients in whom positive pressure has been administered without humidifying; we are referring specifically to keratinization and metaplasia of said mucosa [16].

An important aspect to understand the appearance of these symptoms during the use of non-invasive mechanical ventilation is that the oxygen supplied to the patients comes out of the intakes dry (0mg/l humidity) and cold (10 - 15ºC), being the airways in charge of humidifying and heating it so that they reach the alveoli with the same physical conditions in which they are found: 44mg/l humidity and 37ºC temperature. For this reason, when NIMV is applied without humification, the loss of water in the mucosa is increased, which causes them to become dry and congested and rheological changes in the secretions may appear. All of this can occlude the small-caliber airways, thereby increasing respiratory work and decreasing the patient's tolerability compared to treatment [18].

Another aspect to consider regarding these complications is the type of interface used.

Thus, for example, the nasal mask has the advantages of allowing the patient to eat and speak and feel less claustrophobia, among others; however, it is the mask with the highest risk of producing nasal irritation, runny nose and dry mouth. The advantages and disadvantages of each mask are detailed below [13].

Table 1. Different types of masks: advantages and disadvantages [17]

Type of mask	Advantages	Disadvantages
Nasal	Allows to speak, eat, expectorate Less claustrophobia Less dead space Easy to place and fix Less risk of aspiration	Mouth leaks Greater resistance to air flow Back nasal pressure Runny nose and nasal obstruction Dry mouth
Oronasal	Oral leak control More effective in acute failure	Greater dead space Claustrophobia Risk of aspiration Inability to eat or expectorate
Mouth piece	Little dead space May not require harness	Hipersalivation Nasal leaks Dental deformities
Total face	Lower risk of skin ulcer One size	Greater dead space Dry eyes
Helmet	More comfortable for some patients One size Lower risk of facial ulcers	CO2 rebreathing Worse patient-ventilator shynchrony Reduced discharge of respiratory muscles Choking hazard if ventilator fails

Age is also considered an influential factor in the appearance of nasal congestion and dryness. The elderly, physiologically, have some of their abilities reduced. Regarding the issue that concerns us, they have a decreased ability to eliminate secretions, mucociliary mobility, cough reflex and lung elasticity. Therefore, the use of humidifiers in these patients is essential, especially if they have thick secretions and/or are to be administered for more than 8 hours [16]. Trauma to the nasal mucosa has also been observed in children, associated with the use of non-invasive mechanical ventilation, with the use of nasal masks and nasal olives. The use of humidifiers and air heaters is also recommended in these cases to avoid nasal dryness on the one hand and mucous hypersecretion that can obstruct the tubing on the other hand [4].

2.3. Treatment

There are several treatments to avoid or minimize the effect of continuous positive pressure on the upper airways.

The use of humidifiers is the most widely accepted treatment by the scientific community. Heating and humidifying the air reduces both nasal congestion and dryness since the air that enters the airways reaches a temperature of 37ºC and 44mg/l humidity with the use of this device. The heater and humidifier should be adjusted according to local environmental conditions and patient preferences. In general, there are two types of humidifiers: in the first, the gas passes over the surface of the water (pass-over humidifiers) and in the second, the gas passes into the water and bubbles (pass-through humidifiers). Pass-over is normally used with limited pressure fans to avoid pressure drop that could occur in seconds. Insulation of the branch is also useful to reduce the condensation that occurs in it, known as "rain" [3].

Topical nasal corticosteroids, nasal or oral antihistamines, and even ipratropium can improve nasal congestion and rhinorrhea [5]. Saline sera [3, 13] and nasal gels composed mainly of water can also be used. Such gels are also useful in the treatment of skin ulcers [3]. The use of a face mask, which covers both the nose and the mouth, can be useful in cases of nasal congestion, since positive pressure enters through the mouth instead of the nose [5]. Sometimes it is necessary to reduce the inspiratory pressure to alleviate these symptoms [2].

Conclusion

The use of non-invasive mechanical ventilation in selected patients allows clinical improvement, avoiding in many cases endotracheal intubation with its corresponding complications. However, as has been described throughout the chapter, it is a technique not without complications. Most of them are mild, but in many cases they cause discomfort in patients, which limits their tolerability and adherence.

These include nasal congestion and oronasal dryness, present in almost 50% of patients, derived from the entry of an air flow at a certain pressure in the airways at conditions of humidity and temperature lower than those of the human body, which produces an exchange of heat and moisture from the mucosa to the inhaled air, with the consequent resection of the same. This problem is mainly mitigated by the use of humidifiers, which provide the inhaled air with the necessary temperature and humidity. Other treatments described are the decrease in inspiratory pressure, the use of oral and topical antihistamines, topical corticosteroids, ipratropium, nasal gel and gel solutions, and the use of a face mask.

References

[1] Robert, C. H., Kakob, M. C. *Noninvasive Ventilation in Adults with Acute Respiratory Failure: Benefits and Contraindications* [UpToDate] [2020]. Available in: https://www.uptodate.com/contents/noninvasive-ventilation-in-adults-with-

acute-respiratory-failure-benefits-and-contraindications?csi=30e5f08f-d980-4af6-8a8a-ad1d7640ed31andsource=contentShare.

[2] Robert, C. H., Kakob, M. C. *Uptodate: Noninvasive Ventilation in Adults with Acute Respiratory Failure: Practical Aspects of Initiation* [UpToDate] [2020]. Available in: https://www.uptodate.com/contents/noninvasive-ventilation-in-adults-with-acute-respiratory-failure-practical-aspects-of-initiation?csi=1d806427-a226-4540-9ab9-748be61ec21candsource=contentShare.

[3] Nicholas, S. H., Naomi, R. K. *Troubleshooting Problemas with Nonivasive Positive Pressure Ventilation* [UpToDate] [2020]. Available in: https://www.uptodate.com/contents/troubleshooting-problems-with-noninvasive-positive-pressure-ventilation?csi=d4377824-d005-4361-8540-f5b84441cacbandsource=contentShare.

[4] Joshua, N., Ira, M. C. *NIV for Acute and Impending Respiratory Failure in Children* [UpToDate] [2020]. Available in: https://www.uptodate.com/contents/noninvasive-ventilation-for-acute-and-impending-respiratory-failure-in-children?csi=f09d78da-55c7-48b5-969c-434fd8607e3candsource=contentShare.

[5] Lee, K. B., Woon, L. *Initiation of Positive Airway Pressure Therapy for Obstructive Sleep Apneas in Adults* [UpToDate] [2020]. Available in: https://www.uptodate.com/ contents/initiation-of-positive-airway-pressure-therapy-for-obstructive-sleep-apnea-in-adults?csi=508d8263-e81b-42e3-a319-851316f465ddandsource=contentShare.

[6] Bono, J. M., Balsera, E. C. and Lopez, J. L. G. (2011). Indicaciones en ventilación mecánica no invasiva. ¿Evidencias en la bibliografía médica? *Medicina Clínica,* 136(3), 116 - 120. [Indications in non-invasive mechanical ventilation. Evidence in the medical literature? *Clinical medicine*]

[7] Cook, D. T., Dahlhausen, C. M., Draper, K. R. and Hilton, L. R. (2019). Pneumoperitoneum and PEG Dislodgement Secondary to Noninvasive Ventilation after PEG Tube Placement. *The American Surgeon*, 85(11), 1308 - 1309.

[8] Alaya, S., Mofredj, A., Tassaioust, K., Bahloul, H. and Mrabet, A. (2016). Acute Parotitis as a Complication of Noninvasive Ventilation. *Journal of Intensive Care Medicine,* 31(8), 561 - 563.

[9] Hermann, B. Aparato Respiratorio. En: Finn, G. *Histología.* Third edition. Ed. Spain. Panamericana; 2000. p. 535 - 553. [Respiratory apparatus. In: *Histology*.]

[10] Marilene, B. W. *Etiologies of Nasal Symptoms: An overview* [UpToDate] [2020]. Available in: https://www.uptodate.com/contents/etiologies-of-nasal-symptoms-an-overview?csi=f529b75c-76eb-4922-80fe-9db0f2f75ce8andsource=contentShare.

[11] Richard, L. D., Wayne, V., Adam, W. M. *Anatomía Para Estudiantes*. First edition. Madrid: Elsevier; 2005. [*Anatomy For Students*]

[12] Arthur, G., John, H. Ventilación Pulmonar. En: Guyton, Hall. *Tratado de Fisiología Médica.* Tenth edition. In Madrid: McGraw-Hill, 2001. p. 525 - 538. [Pulmonary ventilation. In: *Treaty of Medical Physiology*.]

[13] del Castillo Otero, D., Caballero, A. C., Cuesta, A. G. and de la Cruz Castro, N. P. *Ventilación Mecánica no Invasiva (VNI) en pacientes agudos y crónicos.* [*Non-Invasive Mechanical Ventilation (NIV) in acute and chronic patients.*]

[14] Ríos, J. G., Camón, I. S., Parra, E. C. and Rodríguez, T. R. (2011). Enfermedades Inflamatorias Nasales y de Senos Parasales. *Medicine,* 10(91), 6180. [Inflammatory Nasal and Paranasal Sinus Diseases]

[15] Rodríguez, M. A., Hervás, M. J., Porras, E. Patología Inflamatoria de las Fosas Nasales: Rinitis Agudas y Crónicas. Rinitis Específicas. IV Nariz y Senos Paranasales [Internet]. *SEORL PCF* [cited 26 may 2020]. Available in: https://seorl.net/PDF/Nariz%20y%20senos%20paranasales/052%20-%20PATOLOGÍA%20INFLAMATORIA%20DE%20LAS%20FOSAS%20NASALES%20RINITIS%20AGUDAS%20Y%20CRÓNICAS.%20RINITIS%20ESPECÍFICAS.pdf. [Inflammatory Pathology of the Nasal Fossae: Acute and Chronic Rhinitis. Specific rhinitis. IV Nose and Paranasal Sinuses]

[16] Antonio, E. Ventilación Mecánica no Invasiva: Fundamentos Fisiopatológicos. In: Antonio, E. *Fundamentos de Metodología y Organización Hospitalaria en Ventilación Mecánica no Invasiva*. Third edition. Asociación y Escuela Internacional de Ventilación Mecánica no Invasiva, 2016. p. 43 - 49. [*Fundamentals of Methodology and Hospital Organization in Non-Invasive Mechanical Ventilation.* Third edition. Association and International School of Non-Invasive Mechanical Ventilation]

[17] Del Castillo Otero, D., Galán, C. C., Gordillo, M. A. and Mateos, F. V. (2003). *Ventilación Mecánica no Invasiva*, EB04-13 NEUMOSUR. [*Noninvasive mechanical ventilation*]

[18] Antonio, E. Ventilación Mecánica no Invasiva: Fundamentos Fisiopatológicos. in: Antonio, E. *Fundamentos de Metodología y Organización Hospitalaria en Ventilación Mecánica no Invasiva.* Third edition. Asociación y Escuela Internacional de Ventilación Mecánica no Invasiva, 2016. p. 89 - 91. [Non-Invasive Mechanical Ventilation: Physiopathological Fundamentals. In: *Fundamentals of Methodology and Hospital Organization in Non-Invasive Mechanical Ventilation*]

In: Non-Invasive Mechanical Ventilation Complications ISBN: 978-1-53619-515-6
Editor: Antonio M. Esquinas

Chapter 4

Bilateral Parotiditis. Ocular Complications/ Eye Irritation. Other Unusual Complications

LM. Cabrera Pimentel, T. Herrero Jordan and Sara Abad Abad
Pneumology. Defense general hospital, Zaragoza Spain

Abstract

NIV presents complications that are not common but that we should be aware of. One of them is parotitis, which is due to multiple causes, the most defended being the increase in intraoral pressure due to the application of positive airway pressure, and this leads to obstruction of the Stensen's duct. Other complications are ocular, mostly due to persistent leakage from a poorly fitting mask.

Introduction

Non-invasive mechanical ventilation is a treatment for many respiratory diseases that produce acute respiratory failure, so its use is widespread and well known, especially by intensivists, pneumologists, pediatricians and other specialists. It is a technique that has several complications, the most common being pressure ulcers, due to the compression of the mask. Other complications, which are not common but which all of us who perform VMNI should be aware of, are parotitis, eye irritation, epistaxis, gastric distension, among others.

Bilateral Parotitis

Acute parotid gland inflammation remains a poorly understood complication secondary to NIV1. Multiple causes have been described:

1. Increased intraoral pressure due to the application of positive airway pressure may cause air entry into the Stenon's duct and, as a consequence, its obstruction.
2. Patient characteristics: Advanced age, dehydration states, immunosuppression states, poor oral hygiene.
3. Medication: Decreased salivary flow (antidepressants, anticholinergics, diuretics). Morphine reduces parotid amylase secretion. In addition, morphine has the ability to reduce smooth muscle activity, and the parotid ducts are surrounded by myoepithelial cells that closely resemble smooth muscle cells.
4. Loss of muscle tone induced by muscle relaxants may facilitate passage of air into the parotid gland when the positive pressure in the oral cavity is significantly increased causing pneumoparotitis and is characterized by painless swelling of the gland and subcutaneous emphysema with crepitus of the area.
5. The pressure exerted by the interface on the parotid gland, by compression of the artery or venous vasculature can impair the blood supply of the gland, which can lead to ischemia and, consequently, to ischemic sialoadenitis. This is little defended because cases have been described with oronasal mask.

The most common symptoms are painful swelling (Figure l), fever, and it is possible to visualize purulent secretions from Stensen's duct. If pneumopathotitis is present, there will be painless swelling and subcutaneous emphysema in the area.

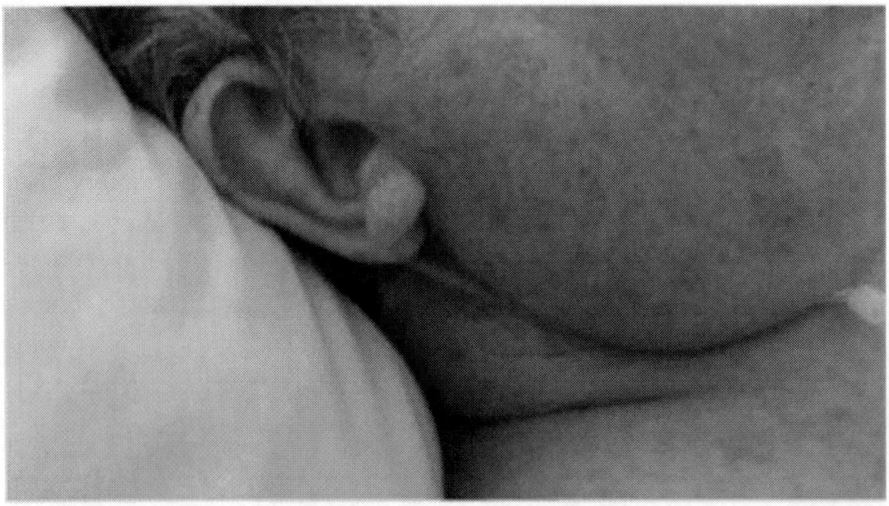

Figure 1. Parotitis in NIV patient with face mask.

Initial treatment should be conservative: hydration, cleaning of the oral cavity, pain control, antibiotics, pressure reduction, and modification of the interface if it supports the gland. Surgical treatment should be exceptional.

Ocular Complications/ Eye Irritation

Patients who are on noninvasive mechanical ventilation often have impaired ocular protective mechanisms as a result of metabolic disorders, mechanical causes and a decrease in the level of awareness. These eye disorders can lead to visual impairment if not prevented.

NIV patients have decreased level of consciousness and are incapable of protecting their eyes and to transmit ophthalmologic complaints.

In a healthy individual, the eyelids provide a mechanical barrier for the eyes against trauma, dryness, and adherence of microorganisms. The lipid layer of the tear film together with the lid closure during sleep prevents evaporation of tears, maintaining corneal moisture. The precorneal tear film maintains the functional integrity of the avascular cornea by providing a moist, oxygenated environment, and nutrients for epithelial cells.

Ocular Surface Disorders

Exposure Keratopathy

Although it is a very prevalent pathology in patients in the ICU with IMV, patients with prolonged use of NIV, decreased level of consciousness, and the use of sedatives, show inhibition of orbicularis oculi muscle contraction, resulting in incomplete eyelid closure (lagophthalmos), corneal exposure, and dryness. Pressure applied to the eyeball reduces choroidal blood flow, resulting in insufficient oxygen to the peripheral cornea, as well as corneal edema and epithelial cell loss.

Exposure keratopathy produces superficial punctuated micro epithelial erosions, most commonly involving the exposed lower third of the cornea, which may join into larger macro epithelial defects.

Chemosis

Chemosis is defined as conjunctival edema. Positive pressure causes an increase in jugular venous pressure, compromising venous return to the ocular structures. This leads to fluid sequestration in the periocular tissues and chemosis. Conjunctival edema leads to ocular surface dryness, inability to close the eyelid with production of exposure keratopathy, and microbial keratitis. Herbert suggested the elevation of the head of the bed and the application of ocular lubricants to prevent corneal exposure and dryness in patients with lagophthalmos.

Eye Irritation/Conjunctivitis

Ocular irritation is produced by direct trauma due to positive pressure leakage from a poorly fitted mask. It is the most common ocular disorder in NIV patients, especially newborns. In addition, these patients may present later with conjunctivitis, caused by bacterial or viral infection.

Prevention and Treatment of Eye Disorders

In the critically ill patient, the main care focuses on the stabilization of vital bodily functions, including cardiovascular and respiratory functions, and neurological status. Both nurses and physicians should be aware of eye disorders and prevent them. Multiple authors recommend:

1. Mask adjustment, avoiding leakage into the eyes.
2. If complications occur, decrease the pressure, if possible.
3. Ocular hygiene regimens to remove any residue with normal saline solution.
4. Prevention of dry eyes by regular instillation of artificial drops, lubricant.
5. Eyelid closure.

Other Unusual Complications

As mentioned above, NIV is a technique that has improved the treatment of respiratory failure and all personnel should be aware of its use and complications. However, there are complications that are not common but that we should be aware of. Among them are:

1. *Acneiform rash* (5-10%). Papulo-pustular injuries. Treatment is with topical steroid solutions or antibiotics.
2. *Arm edema and deep vein thrombosis.* Edema is the result of uncompensated fluid leakage from blood vessels to tissue in the upper extremity that can be

aggravated by lymphatic drainage failure as well as by the use of the Helmet 13 mask. This is a very unusual complication, due to the infrequent use of the Helmet mask.

3. *Claustrophobia:* has a variable incidence ranging from 5% to 20%. Claustrophobia may present as a minor discomfort or, worse, as a feeling of frightening restriction and suffocation, which may prevent initiation or continuation of NIV.
4. *Sleep disruption and impairment of hearing* function (i.e., tinnitus, temporary hearing threshold shift, or permanent hearing loss) caused by device noise. Sleep disruption in the ICU is multifactorial, and such noise is responsible for only a limited proportion of excitation and awakenings.
5. *Gastric insufflation* Aerophagia occurs in most patients with NIV and gastric insufflation in 5%-40% of patients. During NIV, the ventilation volume is distributed between lungs and stomach depending on the respiratory system, resistance and lower esophageal sphincter pressure (20-25 cm H20 in adults). It is adequately managed by placement of a nasogastric probe.
6. *Bronchoaspiration* (< 5%). May happen due to presence of elevated gastric pressures in a patient with an unprotected airway. Perform a proper selection of patients capable of protecting the airway and teaching them to free themselves from the mask in case of vomiting.
7. *Hypotension* (< 5%). Reduce respiratory pressure.
8. *Pneumothorax* (< 5%). Drainage tube placement.

CONCLUSION

In recent years, NIVM has led to the appearance of different complications related to its use, many of them widely described. Others are infrequent, but some may compromise the patient's good evolution or life.

REFERENCES

[1] Alaya S, Mofredj A, Tassaioust K, Bahloul H, Mrabet A. Acute parotitis as a complication of noninvasive ventilation. *J. Intensive Care Med*. 2016; 31:561-3.

[2] Fattahi TT, Lyu PE, van Sickels JE. Management of acute suppurative parotitis. *J. Oral Maxillofac. Surg*. 2002.

[3] Luaces R, Ferreras J, Patín B, García-Rozado A, Vázquez I, López-Cedrún JL. Pneumoparotid: A case report and review of the literature. *J. Oral Maxillofac. Surg*. 2008.

[4] Postaci A, Aytac I, Oztekin CV, Dikmen B. Acute unilateral parotid gland swelling after lateral decubitus position under general anesthesia. *Saudi J. Anaesth.* 2012;6(3):295-297.

[5] Kwon SY, Kang YJ, Seo KH, Kim Y. Acute unilateral anesthesia mumps after hysteroscopic surgery under general anesthesia: a case report. *Korean J. Anesthesiol.* 2015;68(3):300-303.

[6] Andre Grixti, MD, 1 Maziar Sadri, MD, MRCS, DOHNS, FRCA primary, 2 Jonathan Edgar, FRCA, 2 and Amit Vikram Datta, MS (ophthalmol), frcsed, frcophth. *Common Ocular Surface disorders in patients in intensive care units.*

[7] Kirwan J F, Potamitis T, El-Kasaby H, et al. Microbial keratitis in intensive care. *BMJ* 1997;314:433-4.

[8] Parkin B, Cook S. A clear view: the way forward for eye care on ICU. *Intensive Care Med.* 2000;26:155-6.

[9] Rolando M, Zierhut M. The ocular surface and tear film and their dysfunction in dry eye disease. *Surv. Ophthalmol.* 2001;45:203-9.

[10] Herbert L. Ophthalmology in anaesthesia and intensive care. *Anaesthesia Intensive Care Medicine* 2004;5:304-7.

[11] Joyce N. The Joanna Briggs Institute for Evidence-Based Nursing & Midwifery. Eye care for intensive care patients. *Best Practice* 2002;6:1-6.

[12] Neumomadrid.

[13] *Complications of non-invasive ventilation techniques: a comprehensive qualitative review of randomized trials.*

[14] Cavaliere F, Conti G, Costa R, Proietti R, Sciuto A, Masieri S. Noise exposure during noninvasive ventilation with a helmet, a nasal mask, and a facial mask. *Intensive Care Med.* 2004; 30: 1755-60.

[15] *Noninvasive Mechanical Ventilation in Acute Ventilatory Failure Rationale and Current Applications.*

In: Non-Invasive Mechanical Ventilation Complications ISBN: 978-1-53619-515-6
Editor: Antonio M. Esquinas

Chapter 5

COMPLICATIONS DURING NON-INVASIVE MECHANICAL VENTILATION. SKIN BREAKDOWN

Umberto Vincenzi*[*], *MD
Former Head of the Operative Unit of Pneumology and Intermediate Respiratory Intensive Care, "Ospedali Riuniti" Hospital, Foggia, Italy

ABSTRACT

This chapter highlights the side effects of NIMV and in particular the pressure ulcers created by the devices used to ventilate the patient. The need to contain air leaks, which are more commonly encountered during mechanical ventilation at high pressure levels, induces health professionals to increase the tightening of the masks on the patient's face. This tightening, while on the one hand reduces the air leaks, on the other hand increases the contact pressure on the face with the possibility of skin damage. Various severity levels of pressure ulcers are cited and the pathophysiological mechanisms that induce skin damage are explained. The main factors are: pressure and cutting forces, friction on the skin, humidity, time, the characteristics of the mask, the anatomy of the face, the fragility and subtlety of the skin and bacterial pollution. The diagnosis, based on careful visual observation, can also make use of the help of specific instruments to classify the lesions. Prevention is implemented with the identification and removal of possible critical contact points, with the right choice of the best mask, with the possible rotation of the same and with the use of devices to reduce the contact pressure. Lesion treatment involves dressing and applying ointments, creams, alginate or hydrocolloid or protease-based gels. However, a recent and extensive meta-analysis has failed to be an adequate and certain guide for therapeutic choices.

Keywords: Pressure Ulcers (PU), oronasal mask, total face mask, Helmet

[*] Corresponding Author's E-mail: uvincenzi@gmail.com.

Background

Over the past 20 years there has been a progressive increase in the use of non-invasive mechanical ventilation by means of nasal, facial or helmet and today NIMV is considered the first-line treatment in case of acute or chronic exacerbated respiratory failure.

The NIMV is generally applied in E.Rs, in Pneumology, in the Intensive Respiratory Therapy and in Resuscitation Departments, but, in more recent times, also in the Medical departments, in Geriatrics, in the Coronary Intensive Care Units or other Operative Units.

Furthermore, in recent years, there has been a growing diffusion of this ventilation method also at home and in particular on patients suffering from OSAS or on those suffering from chronic respiratory insufficiency who could benefit from intermittent mechanical ventilation.

The advantages of NIMV have been evident for some time and are essentially linked to the possibility of avoiding invasive mechanical ventilation. In fact, the latter involves an increase in morbidity, linked to prolonged sedation, infections of the airways, barotraumas, mortality and costs.

However, disadvantages also exist in the NIMV. These are essentially related to the selection of patients, the choice of the best ventilation mode, the patient's tolerance to adapt to mechanical ventilation, the damage and / or discomfort that the ventilation prosthesis can cause over time including pressure sores, gastric distension and eye irritation.

The pressure sores created by the machine interfacing with the patient assume importance not only for the damage created on the patient's body, but also because, by reducing tolerance and comfort, they can cause patient-ventilator asynchrony, incorrect delivery of lung flows and volumes up to the need to suspend non-invasive mechanical ventilation [1, 2, 3, 4]. Pressure ulcers can affect up to 50% of treated patients [5, 6].

Pressure Ulcers

The main causes of the onset of pressure ulcers are related to the need to increase the tightening of the ventilation prostheses to the head of the patients to avoid air leaks and therefore: pressure losses in the ventilatory circuit, low Tidal Volume, insufficient oxygen fraction inspired (FiO_2), insensitivity of the trigger, and asynchronism with the ventilator. This attempt to check for leaks can cause an overpressure of the interface on the skin areas. The damage is most evident where there is little subcutaneous tissue (chin, cheekbones, nasal bridge, forehead) that predisposes to pressure ulcers (PU).

In the case of the pediatric population, the onset of pressure ulcers can be further favored by the difficult adaptation to the facial anatomy of each child, by incomplete maturation of the skin, by impaired perfusion, reduced mobility, impaired neurological reactivity, fluid retention, humidity and the limited range of masks available for young patients [7, 8].

The increase in pressure in the contact areas determines regional tissue ischemia up to the point it creates deeper damage and affect all layers of the dermis (figure 1).

STAGE OF SKIN PRESSURE INJURIES

As indicated in recent Guidelines on skin lesions, pressure ulcers are classified as follows [9]:

> "A pressure injury is localized damage to the skin and underlying soft tissue usually over a bony prominence or related to a medical or other device. The injury can present as intact skin or an open ulcer and may be painful. The injury occurs as a result of intense and / or prolonged pressure or pressure in combination with shear. The tolerance of soft tissue for pressure and shear may also be affected by microclimate, nutrition, perfusion, comorbid conditions, and condition of the soft tissue."

It is important to note that, in these Guidelines, we speak essentially of "skin lesion" and not only of "ulcer" as the latter does not completely describe the damage caused by the pressure at stage I or that created on the deeper tissues.

Definitions:

- *Stage I* indicates the presence of intact skin, in which there is a non-blanchable erythema which may be painful. Aspects such as a bleaching erythema with acupressure (or with a diascopy) and the increase in local temperature can anticipate clinical objectivity, while the presence of purple or brown complexion suggests deeper tissue damage (DTPI).
- *Stage II* is the loss of epidermis with exposed dermis. The wound has a lively appearance and a color between pink and red and can be covered with a serous exudation. It can also present itself as an intact and serum-filled or burst blister. The lower layers, including the adipose tissue, are not visible and there is no granulation tissue as the healing capacity occurs by re-epithelialization.
- *Stage III* presents a loss of full thickness tissue in which sub-dermal elements are exposed. The underlying fatty tissue and granulation tissue are visible. There are no visible damages to: fascia, muscle, tendon, ligament, cartilage and bone. The wound can burrow under parts of the epithelium, create tunnels or form an "epiboly" which is a migration of the epidermal over the dermal component.
- *Stage IV* presents a pressure injury characterized by a loss of full-thickness tissue that can affect all layers. Included are: fascia, muscle, tendon, ligament, cartilage and bone.
- *Unstageable Full-Tickness Pressure Injury*: the loss of tissue, in this pressure injury, can also affect all the layers, but it cannot be quantified by simple

observation as it is hidden by the presence of eschar and slough. Only after the removal of both is it possible to reach the bottom of the lesion and quantify its damage.

- *Deep Tissue Pressure Injury (DTPI): Persistent Nonblanchable Deep Red, Maroon or Purple Discoloration.* This injury is the result of intense and prolonged pressure or of a cutting force that has had an impact on the muscle-bone interface. In this case the skin may be intact or not intact, but it is evident that the damage is underlying and affects the deep tissues with a color that may vary from an intense non-blanchable red to purple, up to a dark brown. The purple complexion recalls the presence of bruises or ecchymosis.
- *Medical Device-Related Pressure Injury.* These injuries are consequent to the use of medical devices applied to the patient's body for diagnostic or therapeutic purposes. Typically, the devices are made of plastic, although many other materials can be used. The lesions generally follow the shape of the applied device and must be framed according to the aforesaid staging.
- *Mucosal Membrane Pressure Injury.* When the pressure of a medical device affects the surface of a mucosa, lesions ensue and they are different from those found on the skin. The mucous membranes, by their nature, are more fragile than the skin and are more easily affected by the damage created by medical devices. In the evaluation of pressure damage on the mucous membranes, the same classification used for skin damage cannot be used. The nonblanchable erythema cannot be seen. Naked-eye observation of the mucous membranes, devoid of keratinized epithelium and on which open ulcers settle, does not offer a clear distinction between superficial and deeper lesions. The damaged mucosa is inflamed, edematous and soft and a tender consistency clot may be present.

PHYSIOPATOLOGY

From the pathophysiological point of view, the persistence of high pressure on the skin leads, in succession, to: reduction of capillary flow, ischemia, thrombosis of capillaries, occlusion of lymphatic vessels, increase of capillary permeability, leakage of fluids into the extracellular space, edema and cell death.

This is aggravated by ischemia / reperfusion cycles with the formation of cytotoxic free radicals such as malondialdehyde (MDA), superoxide dismutase (SOD), nitric oxide (NO), and also endothelin-1 (ET-1). Ischemic damage may occur even only after a single cycle of a few hours of treatment [10].

Pressure injuries are conditioned at the onset and during their evolution by numerous factors, among them, the most important are:

1) The *pressure* applied by the mask on the face is closely linked to the tension of the straps used to anchor it in a stable position. The tension of the belts, however,

is directly proportional to the ventilation pressures used and the presence of air leaks. The latter are avoided to increase the sensitivity of the trigger, ensure a sufficient amount of volumes and pressures in the airways, and greater stability in the delivery of FiO2. In fact, in the presence of air leaks, which are more noticeable with high pressures, the healthcare personnel, in an attempt to contain them, tend to tighten the belts even more. But, if on one hand the air leaks are reduced and the ventilation is improved, on the other hand, by increasing the pressure on the face, the risks of skin damage increase inexorably. When short-term pressure is relieved, the tissues show reactive hyperemia, which leads to an increase in blood flow to the area. On the other hand, if prolonged high pressure is applied, a reduction in capillary blood flow occurs as well as an occlusion of blood vessels and lymphatic vessels and, therefore, ischemia of the tissues. The pressure detected on the bridge of the nose can be decidedly higher than that measured on the cheeks. In fact, some authors [11] have shown that average pressures of 65.8 mmHg can be reached on the nasal bridge, while average pressures on the cheeks were 15.4 mmHg. They also noted that the pressure on the nose increases not only with the tightening of the mask on the face, but also with the increase in the volume of the air cushion of the facial mask. Finally, it was found that the pressure on the nose decreases with the increase in pressure in the CPAP, while there are no substantial differences with the increase in IPAP pressure in the two-pressure ventilatory mode (BiPAP).

The reduction in skin pressure detected on the nasal bridge during CPAP could be explained by the fact that a constant increase in ventilatory pressure tends to lift the mask from the face and, therefore, to reduce the pressure on the face. While the reasons for a failure to reduce the contact pressure following the increase in IPAP are not clear.

2) The *cutting force* is generated by the displacement of the epidermis with respect to the underlying subcutaneous tissue and bone. The greater is the displacement force, the lesser is the thickness of the subcutaneous layer and, therefore, the smaller is the distance between the bone and the surface, the greater will be the possibility of the onset of the skin lesion. In elderly patients, a reduced amount of elastin in the skin predisposes to the adverse effects of cutting.
3) The *friction* generated by the movement of the mask on the face during mechanical ventilation is dependent on the characteristics of the surface of the epidermis and the humidity present. Stress and mechanical friction occur especially when strong inspiratory air flows are used, delivered to quickly reach a high-pressure level which may lead to a visible movement of the mask on the face on inspiration and a subsequent opposite movement on expiration.

For the reasons listed above, one of the points most at risk of injury is the bridge of the nose.

4) *Humidity*, for the most part, is caused by the occlusive and non-breathable material of the masks, usually made of plastic. This humidity can easily lead to the onset of tissue maceration and infectious overlaps. Furthermore, skin with high humidity has a higher friction coefficient [12]. This greater friction, added to the damage created by mechanical trauma, favors a greater frequency and severity of ulcers (stage II).
5) The *duration of ventilation* or the time in which the skin pressure is exerted on the patient's face, is directly proportional to the extent of the skin damage.
6) The *type of mask* to choose is linked to the ventilation mode, the number of hours per day to be administered, the necessary pressures, the shape of the face and the characteristics of the skin. For example, the use of a CPAP in an OSAS subject does not involve particular ventilator commitments and the pressure delivered is generally low, but since ventilation must affect all the nights of a future life, it is important that the mask is the softest and the most comfortable. On the other hand, in the case of an exacerbated COPD subject who requires ventilation in Pressur Support + PEEP, it is necessary to evaluate above all the adherence of the mask on the face and the correct distance between the nose and the interface. This, in consideration of the fact that it is necessary to deliver much higher pressures than the CPAP and to reduce the consequent air leaks. In this case, therefore, we must not only think of patient comfort, but also of reaching those pressure levels indicated for correct treatment. We also consider that once the acute period has passed, the subject can also reduce the pressures delivered or stop mechanical ventilation. The possibility of having prostheses that have a softer and wider contact area (mask - skin) reduces any pressure peaks in risky skin areas. The oronasal mask, compared to the total-face mask, presents greater possibilities of generating unpleasant air leaks around the mouth and pain at the bridge of the nose, while the total-face mask is more often associated with claustrophobia, eye irritation and dryness of the upper airways [13].
7) The *study of the conformation of the face* is important not only when the patient is a newborn or a child, given the variability of their faces, but also when it is necessary to ventilate people of different ethnicities in which the line of the nose, forehead or cheekbones can vary considerably.

   The characteristics of the skin, its location on the body and its thickness are very important factors in the development of pressure skin lesions. In fact, "*tissue tolerance*" is largely dependent on these factors, even if the oxygenation capacity of the fabric subjected to mechanical pressure must not be overlooked. Tissue oxygenation may still be sufficient if external compression is not greater than diastolic blood pressure, if it is exerted on a tissue that has good elasticity and distribution of pressure forces, and has abundant subcutaneous tissue and sufficient distance from the bone below.

8) The *fragility and subtlety of the skin* is an extremely important problem when we have to ventilate babies or children. Mistakes in the choice of interface or particular carelessness in the periodic control of their skin, can easily lead to the onset of ulcers that, if deep, can disfigure the shape of the face for the entire life. However, we cannot neglect that even older people, given the loss of a large part of the subcutaneous tissue and the higher frequency in the use of anticoagulant drugs, have particularly fragile and easily bleeding skin.
9) Skin mistreated by mechanical stress, with the presence of II-degree ulcers, moist and sometimes with maceration phenomena, may be easily subject to *infections*. The presence of Staphylococci or Gram positive germs is frequently detected, but, in the case of patients already carriers of chronic pathologies of the respiratory system, characterized by a rich bacterial flora, it is not uncommon to find Gram negative germs including: Pseudomonas, Klebsiella, Acinetobacter.

DIAGNOSIS

The diagnosis is based on the frequent control of the skin subjected to contact with the ventilation prostheses. In fact, injuries can occur even only a few hours after the start of the ventilatory treatment and a delayed recognition of the extent of the damage can inexorably worsen the injury.

Identification of the first change from normal skin conditions is essential and this, in particular, is important for patients with dark skin who risk more serious injuries. This is because skin pigmentation can mask an underlying erythema or pressure ulcers with suspected deep tissue injury [14].

In fact, the lesions of the deep tissues are already difficult to confirm by visual inspection, but even more so in dark-skinned subjects.

A finding of a non-blanchable erythema, of an initial edema of the epidermal surface, accompanied or not by pain, may already indicate the presence of a grade I lesion. A Maroon or Purple Discoloration may also be associated with it, which would also indicate a lesion affecting the deeper tissues (DTPI).

For correct observation, good lighting of the injured area is essential.

The objective evaluation of the injury, for a correct classification, must be based on the severity levels indicated by the international guidelines.

In the presence of eschar and slough, mere observation is not enough. Therefore, it is necessary to clean the wound, so that all the layers of tissue involved are clearly visible, including the bottom of the ulcer.

Only when the bottom of the ulcer is clearly visible is it possible to quantify the damage and classify the lesion. In view of a correct treatment, it is also necessary to evaluate whether, in the ulcer, there are tunnels dug under the surface of the epidermis or "epiboly".

Sometimes, in the ulcer, there may be a blood collection that is still fresh and soft on palpation and which does not recommend immediate removal. In this case, in assessing the severity of the injury, it is better to assume a higher degree of injury than the apparent one.

PREVENTION

One of the first things to consider is the study of the conformation of the patient's face and the contact surfaces of the mask. Important is the visual inspection of the skin surface in contact with the mask in order to identify, in time, initial damage to the skin. The check, according to some authors, should be done at least every 8 hours (at every shift change in hospital), while according to others [15] even every 2-4 hours since some clinical studies have shown that pressure ulcers can develop in 4-6 hours under continuous load.

In addition to the simple visual analysis of the skin, you can use a cross polarization dermoscope that has the ability to highlight the dilated capillaries, possibly integrated with high resolution digital photography [16].

A contribution to the analysis of initial skin damage may be given by the use of a phase meter that analyzes the surface electrical capacity of the skin; this is a biophysical measure used to represent the epidermal barrier function of the skin [17, 18, 19]. This device, particularly useful in the study of dark-skinned subjects, is able to detect early the amount of water in the skin and tissues (sub-epidermal moisture, SEM) and, therefore, the initial damage, resulting from compressive trauma.

Knowing that stage II and III pressure ulcers are often open wounds, it is easy to find that the hydration values of the skin are clearly higher than those of intact skin.

The type, material, conformation and method of application of the interface have a significant impact on the success of the NIV and on the patient's tolerance of the device. The literature indicates that there are 6 types of interfaces available: mouthpiece, nasal mask, nasal pillow, oronasal mask, total-face mask, and helmet.

The choice of the mask must be based on the number of hours of application of mechanical ventilation, on the pressures necessary to implement it, on the type of pathology that determines the ventilation insufficiency, on the level of comfort encountered by the patient and on adaptability.

In the case of non-invasive mechanical ventilation at night (for example patients with OSAS), a nasal mask or the nasal olives, which has soft rubber or silicone pledgets that insert directly into the nares, may also suffice. The choice is based on the fact that the interface is more comfortable, as it affects only the nose, allows the patient to communicate and the pressures delivered by the ventilator are relatively low. These devices may be associated with a chin guard that facilitates the closing of the mouth and reduces air leaks.

Recently, to improve adaptability during sleep, particularly comfortable masks have been put on the market built in soft fabric, with good moisture wicking and with a wide fit.

In the case of ventilation at higher pressures, when the patient is unable to keep his mouth closed (e.g., in the presence of nasal obstruction, even partial) or in the event of easy air leaks, an oronasal mask can be used. In this case, the administration of air to the patient takes place both orally and nasally.

When the hours of ventilation take up most or the whole day, the use of a full-face mask or helmet is recommended. In the latter case, tolerability is greater as the areas of the nasal bridge, cheekbones and periorbital areas are generally preserved. The sense of claustrophobia can be increased, but comfort and adaptability are better.

Once the best interface has been chosen, it is necessary to follow the patient in his evolution.

In preventing any damage, many factors must be taken into consideration, including: products to be applied on the face (creams, patches, protective films ...), creation of prostheses with soft and elastic bearing, at low pressure and with an extended surface to distribute the load pressure of the mask, computerized studies of the conformation of the face and of the possible overpressure points with the creation of custom-modeled masks [20] (e.g., with 3-dimensional printers). With the latter method, although still not easily applicable to a large extent today, it has been found that the incidence of nonblanchable erythema and standardized redness intensity values were significantly lower for subjects who used the adaptation device for 30 minutes ($P < .001$). But also, the levels of discomfort on the forehead, on the nasal bridge and on both cheeks, as well as the losses, have been significantly reduced.

As for the patches or the bearings, these are placed between the face and the mask to implement the so-called "meniscus" effect, that is to imitate the physiological action that the meniscus performs in the knee [21].

In recent years, numerous works have been carried out to evaluate which are the most effective and least expensive skin aids to be applied to the face in the prevention of ulcers.

Bishopp A et Al. [22] have shown that applying an early prophylactic hydrocolloid nasal dressing applied in patients requiring acute NIV can relieve pressure on the skin and reduce the risk of developing stage II ulcers.

In reality, albeit in a different way, many medical devices have shown to have a preventive beneficial effect in the course of NIMV.

Products based on transparent polyurethane films with others based on hydrocolloid have often been compared, but the conclusions are not unanimous. It has thus been seen that, according to some authors (Dutra RA et al. [23]), transparent polyurethane films were more effective and less expensive, according to other authors (Pott FS et al. [24]) the advantages were not very evident, while, still, according to others (Guillén-Solà M et Al. [25]), after an 8-week observation, hydrocolloid dressings performed better, as they treated at least 10% more than stage II pressure ulcers and were more convenient than polyurethane foam dressings.

It can be considered, however, that these studies cannot be compared with each other as they are based on non-identical medical aids, with different timelines and data analyzes.

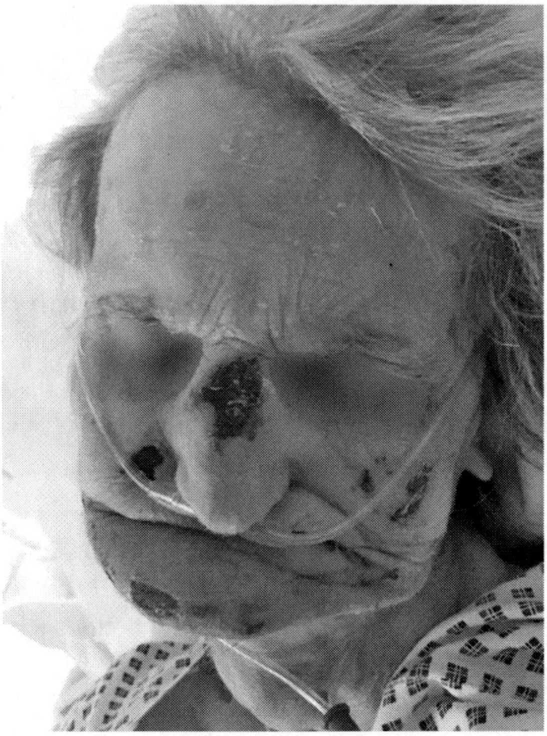

Figure 1. Elderly woman, with large pressure ulcers, favored by a conformation of the face in which the lack of teeth and a more prominent nose are noted.

Solutions of hyperoxygenated fatty acids (HOFA) that seem to have given good results in the preventive field have also been studied [26].

TREATMENT

The first rule to be applied in the treatment of pressure lesions is to remove the source of pressure itself. For this reason, it is necessary to resort to the rotation of the interfaces to be applied on the patient's face. In this way the points of support on the face will be different. An example is the difference between an oronasal mask and a facial mask (Figure 2).

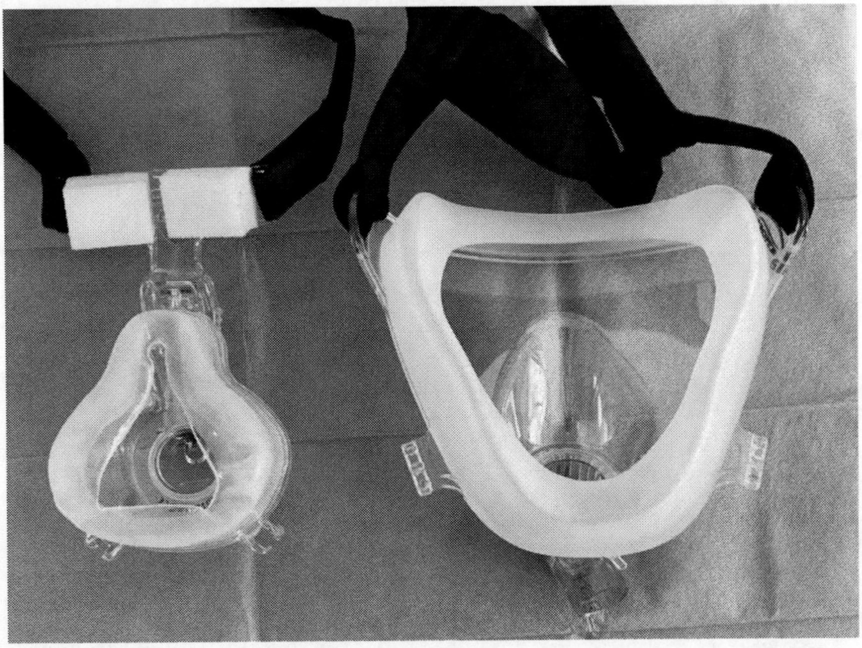

Figure 2. Oronasal mask and total-face in comparison. Note how the contact area on the face is completely different between the two masks.

Or it is possible to resort to masks that rest on the face in a different way. For example, some masks have adjustable front supports and are equipped with large foam or silicone pads which, adapting better to the face line, are able to discharge a good part of the pressure forces on the forehead and, therefore, reduce those that are concentrated on the nasal bridge (Figure 3).

We have already talked about customized masks based on a computerized analysis of the surface of the patient's face, although this is an option, for now, difficult to do.

Alternatively, a helmet may be used.

However, when we are faced with large and deep skin lesions that require the total removal of the masks, frequent checks and medications of the lesions, invasive mechanical ventilation or negative external non-invasive mechanical ventilation may be used.

Pressure sores can affect all layers of the skin based on their severity. Their treatment must be addressed specifically to the type and degree of injury that occurs.

The greatest attention, of course, must be paid when there is a more or less profound ulceration. In the presence of eschar, it must be considered that if it is stable, in a poorly perfused area, its removal causes an open wound that can compromise its healing.

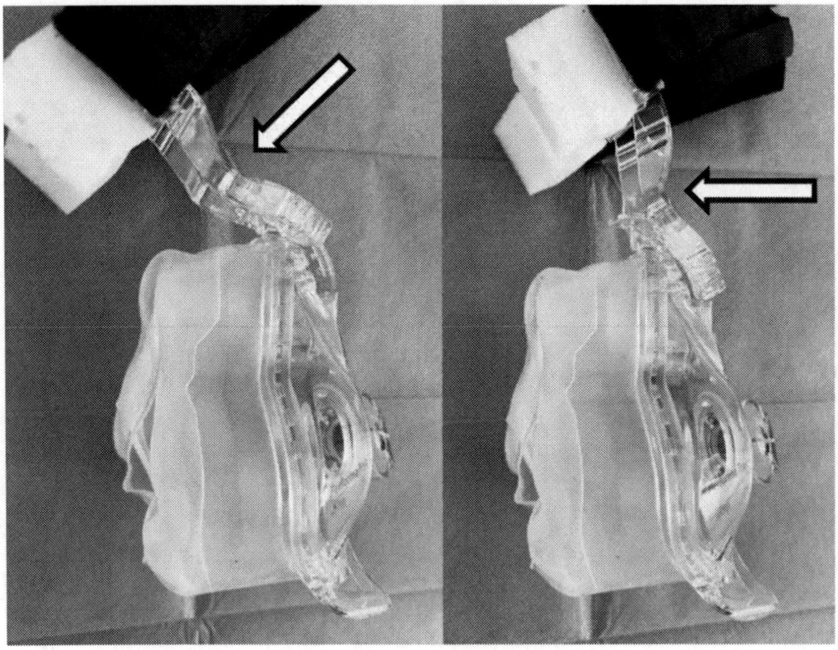

Figure 3. Orofacial masks seen from the side. Note the possibility of tilting the nasal support to relieve pressure on the nasal bridge.

The most important intervention in the management of non-unstageable lesions is the redistribution of pressure rather than the removal of the eschar. When the eschar loosens from the wound bed, it is necessary to cut the edges to avoid inadvertent removal.

Once the ulcer has been cleansed and the deeper layer has been uncovered, in addition to disinfecting the wound, substances can be applied that improve the state of the lesion and promote healing. If tunnels or epiboly are present, the treatment involves reopening the lesion margins by restarting the healing process.

Among the various substances used to improve the state of the lesion we mention the ointments, creams and gels that are applied on unhealed pressure ulcers and left in place to treat the wound. These substances may be covered with a dressing.

In various treatments, alginate, hydrocolloid and protease based products are often used.

A large review study, based on a network meta-analysis (NMA) of data from 39 studies, was recently done by Westby MJ et al. [27] with the aim of identifying the best treatments for pressure ulcer treatment.

Compared to the saline gauze, regimens involving protease-modulating dressings have been found to increase the likelihood of pressure ulcer healing (Risk Ratio or RR = 1.65), albeit with evidence of moderate certainty.

But also, the effect of other medicines, compared with the saline gauze, was uncertain about the probability of recovery. These include collagenase ointment (RR =

2.12), foam dressings (RR = 1.52), basic dressings in contact with the wound (RR = 1.30) and polyvinylpyrrolidone plus zinc oxide (RR = 1.31).

The authors conclude that this meta-analysis network, being subject to a risk of partiality and inaccuracy, is poor and the degree of evidence is of low certainty.

Therefore, they claim that protease-modulating dressings, foam dressings or collagenase ointment may be more effective in healing than gauze, but that the evidence from the NMA is not certain enough to be an adequate guide for therapeutic choices.

REFERENCES

[1] Antonelli M, Conti G, Pelosi P, Gregoretti C, Pennisi MA, Costa R, et al. New treatment of acute hypoxemic respiratory failure: noninvasive pressure support ventilation delivered by helmet - a pilot controlled trial. *Crit Care Med* 2002; 30: 602-608.

[2] Schettino GP, Tucci MR, Sousa R, Valente Barbas CS, Passos Amato MB, Carvalho CR. Mask mechanics and leak dynamics during noninvasive pressure support ventilation: a bench study. *Intensive Care Med* 2001; 27: 1887-1891.

[3] Gay PC. Complications of noninvasive ventilation in acute care. *Respir Care* 2009; 54: 246-257.

[4] Schönhofer B, Sortor-Leger S. Equipment needs for noninvasive mechanical ventilation. *Eur Respir J* 2002; 20:1029-36.

[5] Carron M, Freo U, BaHammam AS, et al. Complications of non-invasive ventilation techniques: a comprehensive qualitative review of randomized trials. *Br J Anaesth* 2013; 110:896-914.

[6] Maruccia M, Ruggieri M, Onesti MG. Facial skin breakdown in patients with non-invasive ventilation devices: report of two cases and indications for treatment and prevention. *Int Wound J* 2015;12(4):451-5.

[7] Schindler CA, Mikhailov TA, Fischer K, et al. Skin integrity in critically ill and injured children. *Am J Crit Care* 2007; 16:568-74.

[8] Visscher MO, White CC, Jones JM, et al. Face masks for noninvasive ventilation: fit, excess skin hydration, and pressure ulcers. *Respir Care* 2015; 60(11):1536-47.

[9] Edsberg LE, Black JM, Goldberg M, McNichol L, Moore L, Sieggreen M. Revised National Pressure Ulcer Advisory Panel Pressure Injury Staging System. *J Wound Ostomy Continence Nurs*. 2016;43(6):585-597.

[10] Li-ping Jiang, Qian Tu, Yanyan Wang, En Zhang. Ischemia-reperfusion injury-induced histological changes affecting early stage pressure ulcer development in a rat model. *Ostomy Wound Manage* 2011 Feb;57(2):55-60.

[11] Munckton K, Ho KM, Dobb GJ, Das-Gupta M, Webb SA. The pressure effects of facemasks during noninvasive ventilation: a volunteer study. *Anaestesia* 2007; 62: 1126-1131.

[12] Sivamani RK, Goodman J, Gitis NV, Maibach HI. Friction Coefficient of Skin in Real-Time. *Skin Res Technol* 2003;9(3): 235-239

[13] Holanda AM., Reis RC., Winkeler GFP., Fortaleza SCB., Oliveira Lima JW., Pereira ED. Influence of total face, facial and nasal masks on short-term adverse effects during noninvasive ventilation. *J Bras Pneumol.* 2009;35(2):164-173

[14] Sullivan R. A 5-Year Retrospective Study of Descriptors Associated With Identification of Stage I and Suspected Deep Tissue Pressure Ulcers in Persons with Darkly Pigmented Skin. *Wounds*. 2014 Dec;26(12):351-9.

[15] Bambi S, Peris A, Esquinas AM. Pressure ulcers caused by mask during noninvasive ventilation. Am J Crit Care. 206 Jan; 25(1): 6

[16] Canning J, Barford B, Sullivan D, Wickett R, Visscher M. Use of digital photography and image analysis techniques to quantify erythema in health care workers. *Skin Res Tecnol.* 2009 Feb; 15(1): 24-34

[17] Palenske J, Morhenn VB. Changes in the skin's capacitance after damage to the stratum corneum in humans. *J Cutan Med Surg.* 1999 Jan; 3(3): 127-31

[18] Miettinen M, Mönkkönen J, Lahtinen MR, Nuutinen J, Lahtinen T. *Measurement of oedema in irritant-exposed skin by a dielectric technique.*

[19] Bates-Jensen BM, McCreath HE, Pongquan V, Apeles NCR. Subepidermal moisture differentiates erythema and stage I pressure ulcers in nursing home residents. *Wound Rep Reg* Mar-Apr 2008;16(2):189-97

[20] Shikama M, Nakagami G, Noguchi H. Development of Personalized Fitting Device With 3-Dimensional Solution for Prevention of NIV Oronasal Mask-Related Pressure Ulcers. *Respir Care* 2018;63(8):1024 –1032.

[21] Weng MH. The effect of protective treatment in reducing pressure ulcers for non-invasive ventilation patients. *Intensive Crit Care Nurs* 2008;24: 295-9.

[22] Bishopp A, Oakes A, Antoine-Pitterson P, Chakraborty B, Comer D, Mukherjee R. The Preventative Effect of Hydrocolloid Dressings on Nasal Bridge Pressure Ulceration in Acute Non-Invasive Ventilation. *Ulster Med J* 2019;88(1):17-20

[23] Dutra RA, Salomé GM, Leal LM, Alves MG, Moura JP, Silva AT, Pereira VO, de Brito MJ, Ferreira LM. Cost Comparison of Pressure Ulcer Preventive Dressings: Hydrocolloid Dressing Versus Transparent Polyurethane Film. *J Wound Care.* 2016 Nov 2;25(11):635-640.

[24] Pott FS, Meier MJ, Stocco JG, Crozeta K, Ribas JD. The effectiveness of hydrocolloid dressings versus other dressings in the healing of pressure ulcers in adults and older adults: a systematic review and meta-analysis. *Rev Lat Am Enfermagem*. 2014 May-Jun;22(3):511-20.

[25] Guillén-Solà M, Soler Mieras A, Tomàs-Vidal AM; GAUPP-Expert Panel. A multi-center, randomized, clinical trial comparing adhesive polyurethane foam dressing and adhesive hydrocolloid dressing in patients with grade II pressure ulcers in primary care and nursing homes. *BMC Fam Pract*. 2013 Dec 21;14:196.

[26] Otero DP, Dominguez DV, Fernandez LH, Magarino AS, Gonzalez VJ, Klepzing JVG, Montesinos JVB. Preventing facial pressure ulcers in patients under non-invasive ventilation: a randomised control trial. *J Wound Care*. 2017 Mar 2; 26(3): 128-136.

[27] Westby M, Dumville JC, Soares MO, Stubbs N, Norman G. Dressings and topical agents for treating pressure ulcers. *Cochrane Database of Systematic Reviews* 2017, Issue 6.

In: Non-Invasive Mechanical Ventilation Complications ISBN: 978-1-53619-515-6
Editor: Antonio M. Esquinas

Chapter 6

Complications During Non-Invasive Mechanical Ventilation. Interface-Specific Complications of Helmet (Arm Oedema and Deep-Vein Thrombosis) and Other Interfaces

***Stefano Bambi*[1,*], *Alberto Lucchini*[2] *and Pasquale Iozzo*[3]**
[1]Medical and Surgical Intensive Care Unit,
Careggi University Hospital, Florence, Italy
[2]General Intensive Care, San Gerardo Hospital, Monza, Italy
[3]Anesthesia and Intensive Care Department, Paolo Giaccone Hospital, Palermo, Italy

Abstract

The strengths and the weaknesses of non-invasive ventilation (NIV) are all located at the same point: the patient-ventilator interface. On the one hand, the interface avoids the need for intubation and all the mechanical or infective complications of invasive ventilation. On the other hand, NIV interfaces cause many problems and risks of complications. Interface-related complications can be the main reason for NIV failure, by making patients unable to endure the process.

The main NIV interface complications reported in scientific literature are discomfort, pressure ulcers on the face, skin rashes, claustrophobia, noise, CO_2 re-breathing, and dyssynchrony with ventilators.

* Corresponding Author's E-mail: stefano.bambi@unifi.it.

The aim of this chapter is to describe and discuss the complications caused by the most common NIV interfaces in adult patients during their stay in hospital (helmet, full-face masks, oro-nasal masks, nasal masks), and suggest the most reasonable solutions to prevent and overcome their adverse effects.

Given that the perfect interface has yet to be developed, healthcare professionals should acquire in-depth knowledge of the characteristics of every available NIV interface, with its potential advantages and disadvantages. This is the only way to optimize the management of patients on NIV support and achieve the desired outcomes.

Keywords: non-invasive ventilation; complication; interface; helmet; mask

INTRODUCTION

When non-invasive ventilation (NIV) has been appropriately started, the three key elements to its success are: checking of the interface-breathing circuit system; dynamic adjusting of ventilation settings; and monitoring the patient for development of discomfort and asynchronies with the ventilator.

The ventilator-patient interfaces play a crucial role in this ideal triangle. In fact, they represent an obvious problem in NIV, because interface-related complications can be one of the main reasons for NIV failure, by making patients unable to endure the NIV process.

The "perfect NIV interface" has yet to be developed and tested, although its features are clear to NIV operators (Table 1). Physicians and nurses should have in-depth knowledge of the potential complications caused by every single type of interface, and make the wisest choice possible for each case, balancing the patient's actual clinical needs, the setting in which they operate, the degree of interface adaptability to the patient's anatomical characteristics, and the potential effect of complications on the patient's NIV endurance.

The main NIV-interface complications reported in scientific literature are discomfort, pressure ulcers on the face, skin rashes, claustrophobia, noise, CO_2 re-breathing, and dyssynchrony with ventilators (Carron et al., 2013, 896–914; Gay 2009, 246–57).

The aim of this chapter is to describe and discuss the potential complications caused by the most common NIV interfaces in adult patients during their stay in hospital (helmets, full-face masks, oro-nasal masks, nasal masks), and suggest the most reasonable solutions to prevent and overcome their adverse effects. Airleaks, patient-ventilator dyssynchronies, and CO_2 re-breathing will be addressed in the other chapters of this book.

Table 1. Characteristics of the "perfect interface" (Nava et al., 2009, 71–82; Alqahtani and Alahmari 2018, 443–52)

Interface
Inexpensive
Available in different sizes
Lightweight
Long-lasting
Non-deformable
Non-allergenic
Airtight
High degree of steadiness
Minimal resistance to airflow
Low dead space
Non-traumatic
Securing device
Rapid and simple application and removal
Single-patient use
Soft
Permeable
Available in different sizes
Adaptable to diverse types of interface
Non-traumatic

MASK-RELATED COMPLICATIONS

There are three currently available mask-type NIV interfaces: oro-nasal masks, full-face masks and nasal masks. All these masks are made of a main rigid plastic external structure, with an internal frame of soft cushion (filled with air or gel) that comes in contact with the patient's skin in order to prevent device-related pressure ulcers and improve his/her comfort and tolerance to Continuous Positive Airways Pressure (CPAP)/NIV. All the types of masks are secured to the patients by quick-release headstraps. This system prevents asphyxia in the event of problems with the ventilator or the breathing circuit.

Complications related to NIV masks can be discomfort (30%-50%), claustrophobia (5%-20%), pressure ulcers on the face/head, especially on the nasal bridge (2%-50%), facial skin erythema (20%-34%), nasal congestion (20%-50%), nasal or oral mucosal dryness (10%-20%). Pain to nose, sinus or ears (10%-30%), and gastric insufflation (10%-50%) are mainly related to the pressures and flows delivered by the ventilators, although the type of interface or headstrap can partially contribute to these problems. The occurrence of aerophagia is frequent, while vomiting is rarely reported (Carron et al., 2013, 896–914; Gay 2009, 246–57).

According to one literature review, headstraps cause patients' discomfort in 10%-30% of cases, and instability of masks is common (Gay 2009, 246–57); the risk of pressure ulcers on the occipital area and ears cannot be altogether excluded.

Discomfort

Interfaces greatly affect patients' levels of comfort during NIV. Discomfort can be one of the main causes of NIV failure (12%-33%) (Carron et al., 2013, 896–914; Nava et al., 2009, 71–82). Therefore, healthcare workers usually take special account of patients' comfort in selecting the type of NIV interface (Crimi et al. 2010, 362–69; Carron et al., 2013, 896–914).

Discomfort causes the highest rates of complications in the use of every type of NIV mask and headstraps (Gay 2009, 246–57).

Beyond the interface issues, discomfort can also be caused by high CPAP or pressure support levels (Gay 2009, 246–57).

A study on healthy volunteers comparing nasal masks, oro-nasal masks and full-face masks did not reveal statistically significant differences in terms of comfort. However, moderate to high NIV pressure settings were less comfortable than low pressures (Holanda et al., 2009, 164–73). By contrast, a randomized trial performed on 60 Chronic Obstructive Pulmonary Disease patients showed higher levels of tolerance for NIV using a full-face mask than an oro-nasal one (compliance with the interface 87% and 46% of patients, respectively; $p = 0.0010$), and longer NIV endurance times (288 and 178 min, respectively; $p = 0.0017$) (Chacur et al., 2011, 426–30).

Symptoms of discomfort can be addressed by careful adjustment of the mask, and with an interface rotation strategy (Gay 2009, 246–57).

General interventions to prevent patient discomfort due to NIV masks include care in selecting patients for NIV, choice of a mask with adequate size and fitting for the face shape, prompt adjustment or changing of headstraps, adequate emotional support for the patient, light sedation levels where necessary, and, overall, the adoption of an interface rotation strategy (Carron et al., 2013, 896–914). The role of the helmet option in obviating mask-related discomfort is unclear, given the contradictory results in literature. In fact, some authors have highlighted similar levels of discomfort between masks and the helmets (Carron et al., 2013, 896–914).

CLAUSTROPHOBIA

Claustrophobia can be a complication related to some NIV interfaces, especially oro-nasal masks, and nasal masks to a lower degree (Carron et al., 2013, 896–914; Gay 2009, 246–57; Nava et al., 2009, 71–82).

The situation of full-face masks in connection with this kind of complication is not completely clear. Some authors propose them as a possible alternative to oro-nasal masks (Gay, 2009, 246–57; Chacur et al., 2011, 426–30), while others have found higher levels of claustrophobia associated with full-face masks than with oro-nasal and nasal masks (Holanda et al., 2009, 164–73).

Furthermore, many authors identify pre-existing claustrophobia as an absolute contraindication to begin NIV or CPAP, because claustrophobia would make it difficult to obtain an adequate level of compliance (Carron et al., 2013, 896–914; Nava et al., 2009, 71–82).

The main interventions to overcome claustrophobia during NIV are: collecting patients' anamnestic information; selecting a suitable interface; familiarization with the mask; allowing a space of two fingers between the headstraps and the patient's skin; increasing the pressure support levels gradually, and reducing them if not tolerated; considering a change to a different type of interface (eg. helmet, nasal mask) (Carron et al., 2013, 896–914). Even though helmets are considered a potential alternative to face masks in patients who complain of claustrophobia, because they do not impede the patient's view and are not directly in contact with their face (Gay, 2009, 246–57), the occurrence of claustrophobia cannot be excluded in the long term (Carron et al., 2013, 896–914). Lastly, it can be appropriate to evaluate the need for light sedation levels to overcome moderate symptoms of claustrophobia (Carron et al., 2013, 896–914).

MASK-RELATED PRESSURE ULCERS

This kind of device-related pressure ulcer mainly develops on the nasal bridge, due to the pressure exerted by the cushions of oro-nasal or nasal masks (Carron et al., 2013, 896–914) that often surpasses the threshold of capillary flow closure (tissue-interface pressures of 30 - 37 mmHg) (Bambi, Peris, and Esquinas 2016, 6). Furthermore, the presence of shear forces and the humidity of the skin can easily cause lesions (Bambi, Peris, and Esquinas 2016, 6).

Almost 100% of patients in NIV develop a pressure ulcer on the nose after 48 hours (Carron et al., 2013, 896–914). Nasal bridge pressure ulcers can rapidly develop into full lesions because of the lack of adipose tissue between the skin and the nasal bones. However, mask-related pressure ulcers can also develop on the upper lip, the chin, the forehead, and the ears. The presence of a nasogastric tube passing under the cushion of the mask can foster the development of skin lesions (Nava et al., 2009, 71–82).

Occasionally, skin grafts are required to repair extremely severe lesions (Gay, 2009, 246–57).

These lesions are mainly due to the cushion of the mask being filled with an increasing volume of air, excessive tightening of headstraps and augmentation of the pressure support levels (Carron et al., 2013, 896–914; Gay, 2009, 246–57). Moreover, the presence of other risk factors should be assessed in NIV patients, such as "body mass index, diabetes, inotropic / vasoactive agents, edema, vascular disease, nutritional status, chronic skin condition, history of previous pressure damage, steroid therapy treatment, and cytotoxic drugs" (Bambi, Peris, and Esquinas 2016, 6). Active humidification, although beneficial for patients' airways during NIV, can be an additional risk factor for development of mask-related pressure ulcers. In fact, humidity and heat can contribute to skin maceration and the friction forces exerted by masks (Alqahtani and Alahmari 2018, 443–52)

An observational study performed on 375 patients undergoing CPAP or NIV support, found that 54 (14.4%) developed at least one pressure ulcer related to masks (Yamaguti et al., 2014, 1530–36). Among those patients 49 (13.1%) developed Stage I pressure ulcers, while 5 (1.3%) had Stage II pressure ulcers. No Stage III or IV pressure ulcers were recorded. Pressure ulcers developed more frequently in patients with oro-nasal masks (50; 42%) than those with full-face masks (4; 1.6%) (Yamaguti et al., 2014, 1530–36). The multivariate analysis showed 2 independent risk factors for the development of pressure ulcers during NIV: the presence of oro-nasal masks (adjusted OR 80.8; 95% CI: 19.6–332.6; $p < 0.001$) and the NIV duration > 26 hours (adjusted OR 8.62; 95% CI: 2.3–32.1; $p = 0.001$) (Yamaguti et al., 2014, 1530–36).

Obviously, the occurrence of mask-related pressure ulcers is often accompanied by pain. Pain is reported on the forehead, at the bridge of the nose, on the cheeks and on the chin. The exceptions are full-face masks because of the low or absent impact on the bridge of the nose, and the nasal mask, which has no contact point on patient's chin (Holanda et al., 2009, 164–73). Understandably, mask-related pressure ulcers and the consequent pain levels, deeply affect patients' NIV compliance and endurance (Carron et al., 2013, 896–914).

Prevention measures for mask-related pressure ulcers include: correctly sized masks for every single patient; choice of masks with wide cushions; preferring masks with gel cushions (or filled with water instead of air); using forehead spacers; timely readjustment of headstraps and allowing a space of two fingers between these and the patient's skin; routine performance of skin and mask hygiene to prevent skin maceration; adopting an interface rotation strategy; lowering the levels of inspiratory pressures on the ventilator whenever possible (Alqahtani and Alahmari 2018, 443–52; Carron et al., 2013, 896–914; Nava et al., 2009, 71–82). The routine application of wound dressings to prevent interface-related pressure ulcers has been extensively discussed in a recent literature review (Alqahtani and Alahmari 2018, 443–52). The authors concluded by recommending the regular use of protective dressings both for prevention and for treatment of skin lesions. Among the studies reviewed, hydrocolloids and silicone pads seem to be more effective than other kinds of wound dressing to prevent pressure ulcers. Furthermore, the application of a solution of hyperoxygenated fatty acids (HOFA) has shown greater effectiveness in reducing the incidence of mask-related pressure ulcers, compared to other strategies (Alqahtani and Alahmari 2018, 443–52).

It is reasonable to assess the condition of the skin under the NIV masks at fixed intervals of 2-4 hours because pressure ulcers can develop in 4-6 hours on skin undergoing prolonged load (Bambi, Peris, and Esquinas 2016, 6). However, for "NIV-dependent" patients (those who cannot clinically tolerate frequent intervals without respiratory support) it is recommended to stop ventilation at least every 11 hours of continuous NIV and to rest the skin for not less than 4 consecutive hours (Alqahtani and AlAhmari 2018, 443–52).

Nasal Congestion; Nasal or Oral Mucosal Dryness; Pain to Nose, Sinus, Ears; Gastric Insufflation

Nasal congestion is a complication mainly, but not only, related to NIV nasal interfaces, such as nasal masks. In fact, this complaint is reported in 20% of NIV patients with oro-nasal masks and 30% of those with total face masks, when the ventilator delivers moderate-high pressures (Holanda et al., 2009, 164–73). This complication can be minimized by the choice of a nasal mask of the correct size for the patient, decreasing ventilator inspiratory pressure, the use of decongestant medication such as local emollients and saline solution, or systemic corticosteroids and antihistaminergics; and lastly, considering a change to a helmet or face mask (Carron et al., 2013, 896–914; Gay 2009, 246–57).

Nasal or oral mucosal dryness are due to air-leaks from the mouth during NIV. The lack of gas passage through the nose causes dryness and inflammation with consequent congestion, increased resistance to airflow and lowering of tidal volume. All these problems cause high levels of discomfort to the patient (Carron et al., 2013, 896–914; Nava et al., 2009, 71–82). Dryness of mouth and throat are reported in 70% of patients with full-face masks and 60% with oro-nasal masks, versus 20%-30% of patients with nasal masks (Holanda et al., 2009, 164–73). Interventions to reduce these problems are similar to those to counteract nasal congestion: careful choice of the interface, use of emollients or saline solution for the nose, checking and minimizing airleaks, decreasing ventilator pressure, and active humidification of the inspired gas (Carron et al., 2013, 896–914; Gay 2009, 246–57).

Just as the congestion or dryness of oral and nasal mucosa are mainly due to flow-related problems, the pain to nose, sinus or ears is probably more related to ventilator pressure than the type of NIV interface. Pain to nose, sinus or ears during NIV can be prevented with the 3 basic interventions before starting NIV: choosing the right interface and size for every single patient; optimizing the mask fitting and readjusting the headstraps when needed; and decreasing the inspiratory pressure levels on the ventilator (Carron et al., 2013, 896–914; Gay 2009, 246–57).

Gastric insufflation is a potentially dangerous condition because it can foster the occurrence of vomiting with the risk of patient aspiration of gastric content (5%) and consequent NIV failure. Gastric insufflation is caused by ventilator setting of peak pressure higher than 20-25 cm H_2O (Carron et al., 2013, 896–914; Gay 2009, 246–57). This value corresponds to the pressure threshold of the lower esophageal sphincter opening with consequent ingestion of the gas insufflation. This condition could be prevented by avoiding NIV with high pressure (Carron et al., 2013, 896–914; Gay 2009, 246–57). The insertion of a nasogastric tube in all patients cannot be a wise choice, because "one size does not fit all". In our opinion nasogastric tube insertion should be required only in patients with a reduced level of consciousness and with impaired protective reflexes. All other patients should be monitored for the occurrence of gastric distension and receive a nasogastric tube only if necessary. This conservative approach will save the patient from the pain of gastric tube insertion, the risk of gastric reflux due to presence of the tube altering the functionality of the lower esophageal sphincter, the risk of pressure ulcers on the nose due to the gastric tube; additionally, airleaks from the mask can be controlled better.

Helmet-Related Complications

Helmets are interfaces first created in Italy, which have been used in critical care settings, emergency departments, and general wards. Helmets are widely employed in interface rotation strategies as an alternative to face masks, especially in Italy and Spain, to gain higher levels of patient NIV endurance (Crimi et al., 2010, 362–69). In fact, they were designed to reduce the rates of mask-related pressure ulcers and improve overall patient comfort despite the difference among face shapes (Liu et al., 2016). Furthermore, like the full-face mask, helmets can prevent symptoms related to claustrophobia since they do not obstruct the patient's view, and there is no contact point with forehead, ears, nose, or chin (Gay 2009, 246–57).

A recent systematic review has highlighted the reduced probability of complications from the use of helmets as compared with other interfaces (OR 0.60; 95% CI:0.40-0.92, $p = 0.02$) (Liu et al., 2016).

Helmets are made of a transparent plastic hood and a soft rubber collar connected by a rigid plastic collar, with inlet and outlet gas ports (Nava et al., 2009, 71–82). Additional ports to allow the passage of a nasogastric tube or a straw can be available according to the different manufacturers. Padded armpit straps keep the helmet fastened to the patients (Nava et al., 2009, 71–82). CPAP-helmets usually have a greater amount of dead space than NIV-helmets (15 lt versus 5 lt, respectively). This element probably represents the major disadvantage of these interfaces since NIV or CPAP must be performed with systems able to deliver flow rates higher than 40 lt/min (Lucchini et al., 2018, 369–74).

Beyond the positive characteristics of this unique interface, some specific disadvantages and complications are reported in literature, such as CO2 re-breathing, discomfort, noise, fog effects during heated humidification, asynchronies with ventilator, axillary skin lesions, arm edema, pain, and risk of deep-vein thrombosis (Carron et al. 2013, 896–914; Lucchini et al., 2018, 369–74; Lucchini et al., 2019, 65–71; Lucchini et al., 2020a).

NOISE

Concerning the ICU environment, the World Health Organization recommends maximum noise thresholds between 45 and 60 dB during the hours of day, and not higher than 35 dB at night (Lucchini et al., 2020b, 194–202).

Noise levels recorded inside helmets during NIV by Cavaliere et al., were 105 ± 6 dB with PSV/PEEP (pressure support ventilation / positive end expiratory pressure) set at 10/5 cm H_2O, and 108 ± 6 dB with 15/5 cm H_2O. When an HME (heat and moisture exchanger) filter was applied before the helmet inlet port during PSV, the level of noise did not drop below the threshold of 100 dB (Cavaliere et al., 2004, 1755–60). Therefore, helmets are much noisier than nasal masks and facial masks, which produce average levels of 62-65 dB with analogous NIV settings (Cavaliere et al., 2004, 1755–60).

Lucchini et al., have recently shown that average noise levels inside the helmet with 5 cm H_2O CPAP at gas flow rates of 60 and 80 lt/min reached 99.56 ± 13.30 Decibel A (dBA). However, the application of an HME filter on the inlet port reduces this mean level to 92.26 ± 10.72 dBA ($p < 0.001$) (Lucchini et al., 2020b, 194–202). The same study reported a significant change in patients' perception of noise measured on an 11-point visual analog scale (from 0 = absence of noise to 10 = noise completely impeding human interactions): median 6 (IQR 4–7) with HME filter, versus 7 (IQR 5–8), without it ($p < 0.001$) (Lucchini et al., 2020b, 194–202).

The use of earplugs has been suggested, although this can impair communication between patient and healthcare workers or significant others.

Armpit Edema and Axillary Vein Thrombosis

In order to prevent armpit edema and axillary vein thrombosis due to helmet armpit straps, some authors have suggested some measures such as not using helmets in cases of severe malnutrition, using elastic bands to fix the helmet to the bedrails, decreasing the NIV/CPAP pressures, and, lastly, changing to a different type of interface (Carron et al., 2013, 896–914). The point of this last intervention is to avoid the decreasing of the pressure support or CPAP levels to reduce the patient's discomfort and prevent the arm edema, as previously suggested by some authors (Carron et al., 2013, 896–914)

However, Lucchini et al., have studied and implemented an alternative method of fixing the helmet in order to prevent that complication and improve patients' overall tolerance (Lucchini et al., 2020a) (Figure 1). The authors used a counterweights system aiming to keep the armpits free (Lucchini et al., 2020a). The system includes counterweights of 2 kg (e.g., skeletal traction counterweights) attached to both the helmet straps that are placed over the patient's shoulders. It has been reckoned that 5 kg is a weight sufficient to counterbalance the upward push caused by PEEP levels of 5-15 cm H2O (with a gas flow rate of 60 lt/min) and maintain the helmet firmly in place over the patient's head (Lucchini et al., 2020a).

When compared to the armpit straps option, the counterweight system seems not to increase the pain levels recorded by patients. In fact, with the use of counterweights the mean scores of pain recorded on a numerical rating scale (0-10 points) were 0.3 ± 0.6 at T0 (baseline), 0.3 ± 0.2 at T1 (1 hour after the beginning of CPAP) and 0.5 ± 0.7 at T2 (end of the cycle of CPAP) ($p = 0.069$) (Lucchini et al., 2018, 369–74). Conversely, the use of armpit straps showed increased pain levels: 0.5 ± 1.4 at T0, 1.5 ± 2.0 at T1, and 2.6 ± 2.5 at T2 ($p = 0.023$). Moreover, the counterweights system was associated with higher average lengths of CPAP cycles: 3.9 ± 2.3 versus 3.0 ± 1.0 hours ($p < 0.001$). After 1 hour of therapy with the counterweight option and armpit straps, the mean increase of the vein section was 0.27 ± 0.21 ($p = 0.099$) and 0.30 ± 0.25 cm^2 ($p = 0.080$), respectively (Lucchini et al., 2018, 369–74). Therefore, the armpits strap application exerted a higher influence on venous drainage of the upper limbs when compared with counterweights fixing system. (Lucchini et al., 2018, 369–74).

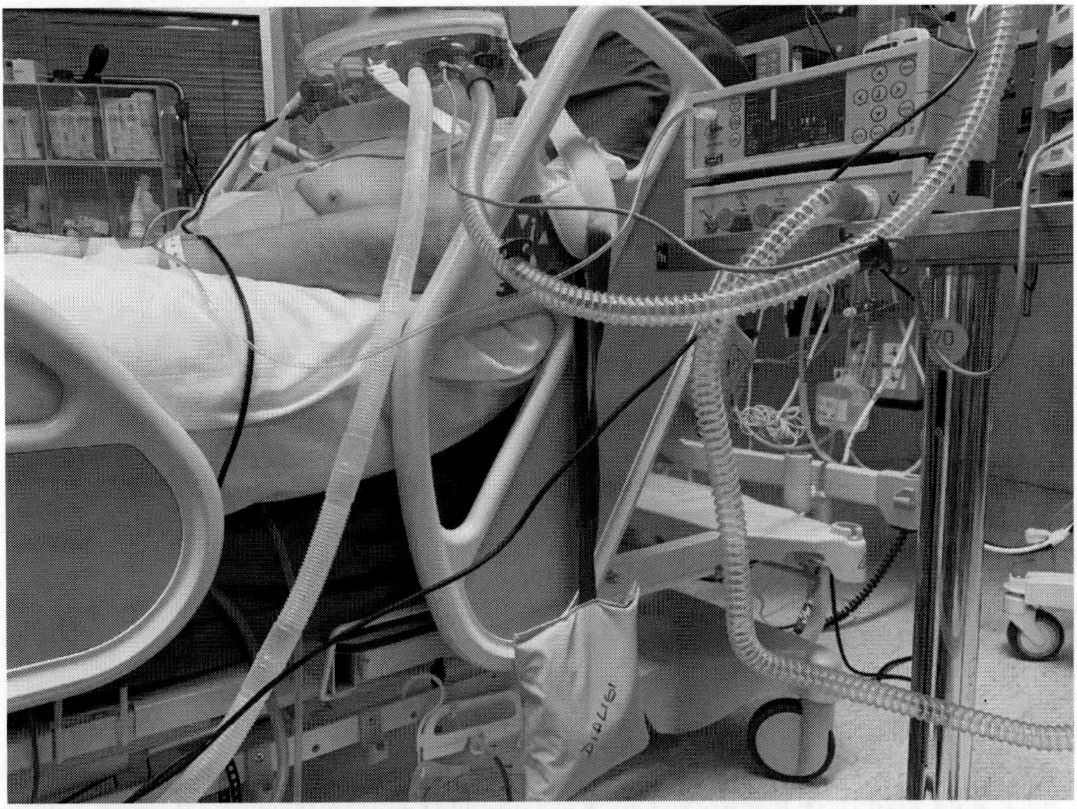

Figure 1. Helmet CPAP with counterweights system.

HUMIDIFICATION

A really challenging issue is humidification during CPAP and NIV with a helmet interface. Some authors have stated that active humidification is difficult or virtually impossible to implement because of the occurrence of condensation inside the helmet with a "fog effect" (Nava et al., 2009).

The lowest threshold of absolute humidity (AH) needed to prevent and reduce the risks of damage to the airways has been set at 10 mg H_2O/lt by the American National Standards Institute (Lucchini et al., 2019, 65–71). Considering that standard, the AH obtained inside the helmet during CPAP delivered by a Venturi system in an environment with 22.0 °C - 22.7 °C and RH of 40% is insufficient; in fact, the hygrometric values inside the helmet are AH between 6.79 and 7.0 mg H20/lt and RH = 35-36% (Lucchini et al., 2019, 65–71).

A crossover study was performed on 6 healthy persons using helmet-CPAP with different gas flow rates (60 lt/min, 80 lt/min) and FiO_2 (0.35, 0.5, 0.7, 1) and with active humidification set at 26 °C (chamber) to reach 28 °C at the helmet inlet port (Lucchini et al., 2019, 65–71). Inside the helmet without any humidification system, the authors recorded an average AH of 5.9 ± 2.1 mg H_2O/lt, and an average temperature of 25.8 ± 0.9 °C. With active humidification, the average AH and temperature inside the helmet were 15.0 ± 3.5 mg H_2O/lt and 29.0 ± 0.1 °C, respectively. Also, patients' comfort levels were recorded on an 11-point analog scale (0-10); median comfort values without and with active humidification were 6 (IQR: 5.25-6.75) and 8 (IQR: 7.25-8.0) ($p < 0.01$), respectively (Lucchini et al., 2019, 65–71). No "fog effect" was recorded. Even though there are not yet any published studies about the use of active humidification systems during helmet-interface NIV, we could hypothesize that similar settings could be used for those patients, to obtain the same results in terms of humidification and comfort levels, because the gas flow rates to maintain the PSV levels are usually between 30 lt/min and 70 lt/min (Chiumello et al., 2001).

A Bundle to Prevent Helmet-Related Complications

With the aim of overcoming all the potential complications occurring during the helmet CPAP, Lucchini et al., recently collected all the above effective interventions in a "Helmet CPAP Bundle" (Lucchini et al., 2020a). The helmet bundle includes noise reduction through an HME filter on the helmet gas inspiratory limb, preferably using "single box high-flow flowmeters, new-generation Venturi systems, and tubes with a smooth inner surface" (Lucchini et al., 2020a); counterweights fixing system with 2 kg for each armpit strap; and heated wire tube with active humidification set at 26 °C, to reach 28 °C at the inlet port of the helmet (+2 °C temperature gradient) (Lucchini et al., 2020a).

Conclusion

The strengths and weaknesses of non-invasive ventilation are all located at the same point: the interface. On one hand the interfaces obviate the need for intubation and all the mechanical and infective complications of invasive ventilation. On the other, NIV interfaces have many problems and cause many risks of complications, as described in this chapter. Currently, the perfect interface has yet to be conceived and developed. In the meantime, healthcare professionals should acquire in-depth knowledge of the characteristics of every available interface, with all its potential advantages, disadvantages, and complications. This is the only way to optimize the management of patients on NIV support in order to reach the desired outcomes and, moreover, provide in-depth observations and reflections that could be used to devise innovative features to improve NIV interfaces, offer patients greater NIV treatment endurance and optimize safety during their clinical management.

REFERENCES

Alqahtani, Jaber, and Mohammed Alahmari. 2018. "Evidence Based Synthesis for Prevention of Noninvasive Ventilation Related Facial Pressure Ulcers." *Saudi Medical Journal* 39 (5): 443–52. https://doi.org/10.15537/smj.2018.5.22058.

Bambi, Stefano, Adriano Peris, and Antonio M. Esquinas. 2016. "Pressure Ulcers Caused by Masks During Noninvasive Ventilation." *American Journal of Critical Care* 25 (1): 6–6. https://doi.org/10.4037/ajcc2016906.

Carron, M., U. Freo, A.S. Bahammam, D. Dellweg, F. Guarracino, R. Cosentini, P. Feltracco, A. Vianello, C. Ori, and A. Esquinas. 2013. "Complications of Non-Invasive Ventilation Techniques: a Comprehensive Qualitative Review of Randomized Trials." *British Journal of Anaesthesia* 110 (6): 896–914. https://doi.org/10.1093/bja/aet070.

Cavaliere, Franco, Giorgio Conti, Roberta Costa, Rodolfo Proietti, Antonino Sciuto, and Simonetta Masieri. 2004. "Noise Exposure during Noninvasive Ventilation with a Helmet, a Nasal Mask, and a Facial Mask." *Intensive Care Medicine* 30 (9): 1755–60. https://doi.org/10.1007/s00134-004-2347-9.

Chacur, Fernando Hauaji, Luis Marcelo Vilella Felipe, Cintia Gonçalves Fernandes, and Luiz Claudio Oliveira Lazzarini. 2011. "The Total Face Mask Is More Comfortable than the Oronasal Mask in Noninvasive Ventilation but Is Not Associated with Improved Outcome." *Respiration* 82 (5): 426–30. https://doi.org/10.1159/000324441.

Crimi, C., A. Noto, P. Princi, A. Esquinas, and S. Nava. 2010. "A European Survey of Noninvasive Ventilation Practices." *European Respiratory Journal* 36 (2): 362–69. https://doi.org/10.1183/09031936.00123509.

Gay, Peter C. 2009. "Complications of Noninvasive Ventilation in Acute Care." *Respiratory Care* 54 (2): 246–57.

Holanda, Marcelo Alcantara, Ricardo Coelho Reis, Georgia Freire Paiva Winkeler, Simone Castelo Branco Fortaleza, José Wellington De Oliveira Lima, and Eanes Delgado Barros Pereira. 2009. "Influence of Total Face, Facial and Nasal Masks on Short-Term Adverse Effects during Noninvasive Ventilation." *Jornal Brasileiro De Pneumologia* 35 (2): 164–73. https://doi.org/10.1590/s1806-37132009000200010.

Liu, Qi, Yonghua Gao, Rongchang Chen, and Zhe Cheng. 2016. "Noninvasive Ventilation with Helmet versus Control Strategy in Patients with Acute Respiratory Failure: a Systematic Review and Meta-Analysis of Controlled Studies." *Critical Care* 20 (1). https://doi.org/10.1186/s13054-016-1449-4.

Lucchini, Alberto, Stefano Elli, Stefano Bambi, Christian De Felippis, Simona Vimercati, Dario Minotti, Sara Pasquali, Luigi Cannizzo, Roberto Fumagalli, and Giuseppe Foti. 2018. "How Different Helmet Fixing Options Could Affect Patients' Pain Experience during Helmet-Continuous Positive Airway Pressure." *Nursing in Critical Care* 24 (6): 369–74.

Lucchini, Alberto, Stefano Bambi, Stefano Elli, Martina Bruno, Roberto Dallari, Pamela Puccio, Silvia Villa, et al., 2019. "Water Content of Delivered Gases during Helmet Continuous Positive Airway Pressure in Healthy Subjects." *Acta Biomedica Health Professions* 90 (S.11): 65–71.

Lucchini, Alberto, Marco Giani, Stefano Isgrò, Roberto Rona, and Giuseppe Foti. 2020a. "The 'Helmet Bundle' in COVID-19 Patients Undergoing Non Invasive Ventilation." *Intensive and Critical Care Nursing* 58: 102859. https://doi.org/10.1016/j.iccn.2020.102859.

Lucchini, Alberto, Stefano Bambi, Silvia Gurini, Enrico Di Francesco, Luigino Pace, Roberto Rona, Roberto Fumagalli, Giuseppe Foti, and Stefano Elli. 2020b. "Noise Level and Comfort in Healthy Subjects Undergoing High-Flow Helmet Continuous Positive Airway Pressure." *Dimensions of Critical Care Nursing* 39 (4): 194–202. https://doi.org/10.1097/dcc.0000000000000430.

Nava, Stefano, Paolo Navalesi, and Cesare Gregoretti. 2009. "Interfaces and Humidification for Noninvasive Mechanical Ventilation". *Respiratory Care* 54 (1): 71–82.

Yamaguti, W. P., E. V. Moderno, S. Y. Yamashita, T. G. Gomes, A. L. V. Maida, C. S. Kondo, I. C. De Salles, and C. M. De Brito. 2014. "Treatment-Related Risk Factors for Development of Skin Breakdown in Subjects With Acute Respiratory Failure Undergoing Noninvasive Ventilation or CPAP." *Respiratory Care* 59 (10): 1530–36.

In: Non-Invasive Mechanical Ventilation Complications ISBN: 978-1-53619-515-6
Editor: Antonio M. Esquinas

Chapter 7

Complications during Non-Invasive Mechanical Ventilation. Barotrauma: Pneumothorax. Pneumomediastinum/Subcutaneous Emphysema Pneumocephalus

Carolina Dantas* and David Silva
Pulmonology Department,
Hospital de Santa Marta - Centro Hospitalar Universitário Lisboa Central (CHULC),
Lisboa, Portugal

Abstract

One of the most recognized complications of mechanical ventilation is barotrauma, referring to the manifestations of extra-alveolar air, such as subcutaneous emphysema, pneumopericardium, pneumomediastinum, pneumoperitoneum and even pneumocephalus.

Barotrauma results from positive pressure mechanical ventilation and is caused by alveolar rupture due to overdistension. This allows the passage of air into the perivascular sheath and tissue dissection into the mediastinum and subcutaneous tissue. Increased pressures can also lead to pleural rupture and subsequently a pneumothorax. Clinical manifestations range from absent symptoms and subtle radiographic signs, as in interstitial emphysema, to respiratory distress and cardiac arrest caused by a tension pneumothorax.

The occurrence of barotrauma in non-invasive mechanical ventilation (NIV) is much lower when compared to invasive mechanical ventilation. Nonetheless any patient can develop barotrauma, especially in the presence of predisposing lung disease such as acute

* Corresponding Author's E-mail: carolinadantas91@gmail.com.

respiratory distress syndrome (ARDS), obstructive pulmonary disorders and interstitial lung disease.

Keywords: barotrauma, non-invasive ventilation, pneumothorax, pneumomediastinum, subcutaneous emphysema, pneumocephalus

Understanding of the pathophysiological mechanisms related to barotrauma allows its prevention and its management. Any ventilated patient can develop barotrauma, however certain ventilator settings, as well as underlying diseases, may increase the risk significantly.

Patients with pulmonary conditions associated with either dynamic hyperinflation or poor lung compliance, as chronic obstructive pulmonary disease (COPD), asthma, interstitial lung disease (ILD), pneumocystis jirovecii pneumonia and acute respiratory distress syndrome (ARDS), have higher predisposition to pulmonary barotrauma [1, 2].

Alveolar overdistension is the key element in the development of barotrauma [3]. Positive pressure ventilation seems to increase the transalveolar pressure, which is the pressure gradient between the alveoli and the perivascular sheath. This pressure elevation can result in alveolar disruption, allowing leakage of air into the extra-alveolar tissue and proximal dissection into the mediastinum.

High plateau pressure, peak inspiratory pressure and positive end-expiratory pressure (PEEP) have been implicated as risk factors for barotrauma [3].

The plateau pressure (pressure applied to the alveoli and small airways during ventilation) seems to be the best estimator of the transalveolar pressure, and therefore is one of the key elements to monitor. Elevated plateau pressures, particularly higher than 35 cmH2O, have been associated with an elevated risk for barotrauma [4]. Although the exact value of the optimal plateau pressure is still debated, the consensus is that a plateau pressure of less than 30 cm H2O is protective and recommended in patients on mechanical ventilation for ARDS by the ARDSnet protocol [5].

The peak pressure is the plateau pressure in addition to the pressure needed to overcome flow resistance and the elastic recoil of the lungs and chest wall. The risk for barotrauma increases when the peak pressures and plateau pressures become elevated to the same degree [1].

Elevated positive end-expiratory pressure (PEEP; or EPAP in NIV) may theoretically lead to over distention of alveoli and ultimately barotrauma. However, clinical data has not associated increased PEEP with increased risk of barotrauma when used in conjunction with lung protective strategies, such as low tidal volume and target plateau pressure under 30 cmH2O [1].

On the other hand, high tidal-volume ventilation also produces overdistended alveoli and therefore seems to represent a higher risk of barotrauma [3], particularly in ARDS.

Current data show that barotrauma has been associated with high peak inspiratory airway pressures (>40 cm H2O) and plateau pressures (>35 cm H2O); however, its association with high tidal volumes has not been confirmed. The ARDS Network trial to compare high and low tidal volumes demonstrated a mortality benefit with low tidal volumes, but incidences of barotrauma did not differ between the groups [5]. Currently, clinicians have recognized the hazards of alveolar over distention in all patients, not only in ARDS, and lower tidal volumes (in the range of 8-10 mL/kg) have generally been adopted in general [3].

Another important current concept is ventilator induced injury (VILI), which designates different types of lung damage related mechanical ventilation according to its pathophysiological mechanism, and includes barotrauma, volutrauma, atelectotrauma and biotrauma (cytokine- and chemokine mediated) [6]. Improved understanding of the mechanisms of VILI and barotrauma allows the adjustment of the ventilator settings to prevent alveolar overdistention. Controversy remains regarding the optimal approach for lung protective ventilation, but consistent benefit has been noted with low tidal volume, whereas no increased risk with varying levels of positive end-expiratory pressure (PEEP/EPAP) has been described. Low-tidal-volume ventilation is strongly advocated as well as limiting plateau pressure to less than 30 cm H2O seems an effective approach to reduce barotrauma risk in these patients [3].

Using a pressure-set and pressure-limited ventilator reduces peak airway pressure, as well as aiming for the lowest IPAP and EPAP settings compatible with arterial blood gas and symptoms control. A permissive hypercapnia sometimes can be tolerated [7].

The clinical manifestations of barotrauma can vary from absent symptoms with the subtle radiographic findings of pulmonary or perivascular interstitial emphysema to respiratory distress or cardiac arrest due to a large tension pneumothorax. Other manifestations include subcutaneous emphysema, pneumopericardium, pneumomediastinum, pneumoperitoneum and even pneumocephalus, singly or in combination. The severity of the presentation depends on the amount of extra-alveolar air present, and occasionally the diagnosis is made only through chest radiographic findings or CT-scan. In general barotrauma complications do not require major interventions besides ventilator adjustments, targeting low-volume ventilation and limiting pressures. The exception is a tension pneumothorax, a medical emergency, that demands immediate needle thoracostomy or chest drain for decompression. Patients with pneumothorax (caused or not by ventilation) require drainage before applying positive pressure ventilation.

Despite being more frequently described as a complication of invasive mechanical ventilation, it is important to recognize that barotrauma can also be associated with NIV. The difference probably consists in a drop of pressure across the upper airway related to the leaks surrounding the mask used in NIV. The risk of barotrauma in NIV is low, with pneumothorax being reported in less than 5% [8, 9].

Data available about barotrauma in NIV comes from single case reports or case series with pneumonia [10], asthma, COPD, neuromuscular or cystic fibrosis patients. In a series [11] of 334 cystic fibrosis (CF) patients, 16% developed a pneumothorax over 17 years. Within the subgroup of 23 patients which received NIV, only 3 had a pneumothorax, but in one case this iatrogenic in origin. In conclusion Haworth et al., suggest that the occurrence of pneumothorax in CF in patients receiving NIV is rare.

Regarding specialized units providing NIV for neuromuscular patients, Simmonds describes the experience of The Royal Brompton Hospital, reporting 1 or 2 cases of pneumothorax in approximately 80 Duchenne muscular disease patients over the last decade, and none was a life-threatening event [12]. There are some reported cases of pneumocephalus after NIV in patients with cranial trauma or neurosurgery [13, 14]. A case reported by Ruggeroni et al., describes a fatal pneumomediastinum in a patient with several risk factors for barotrauma. This patient presented with acute respiratory failure caused by an exacerbation of COPD and interstitial lung disease, aggravated by noninvasive mechanical ventilation. Initial pressures were not high, but the patient's cough attacks during NIV rapidly increased the peak inspiratory pressure, contributing to worsening of the pneumomediastinum [15]. A similar case of pneumomediastinum, in an asthmatic pediatric patient was also published, reinforcing the need to monitor the occurrence of barotrauma in high risk patients under NIV [16].

In conclusion, regarding barotrauma the clinical consequences range from almost innocuous, as subcutaneous emphysema, to potentially fatal in the case of a hypertensive pneumothorax. Despite the rarity of barotrauma in NIV its importance must be recognized and they should be prevented. The deleterious effects of alveolar over distention, limiting plateau pressures to less than 30 cm H2O while balancing other ventilator settings (tidal volume and PEEP) against oxygenation and metabolic parameters may be an effective approach for all patients, irrespective of the cause of their respiratory failure.

REFERENCES

[1] Diaz R., Heller D. Barotrauma and Mechanical Ventilation. *Treasure Island,* FL: StatPearls; 2019.

[2] Anzueto A., Frutos-Vivar F., Esteban A., Alía I., Brochard L., Stewart T., Benito S., Tobin M. J., Elizalde J., Palizas F., David C. M., Pimentel J., González M., Soto L., D'Empaire G., Pelosi P. Incidence, risk factors and outcome of barotrauma in mechanically ventilated patients. *Intensive Care Med.* 2004 Apr;30(4):612-9.

[3] Soo Hoo G. W., Francisco Talavera, Zab Mosenifar, Barotrauma and Mechanical Ventilation, *Medscape.* Accessed 22 of April 2020.

[4] Esteban A., Anzueto A., Frutos F., Alía I., Brochard L., Stewart T. E., Benito S., Epstein S. K., Apezteguía C., Nightingale P., Arroliga A. C., Tobin M. J., Mechanical Ventilation International Study Group. Characteristics and outcomes in adult patients receiving mechanical ventilation: a 28-day international study. *JAMA.* 2002 Jan 16;287(3):345-55.

[5] The Acute Respiratory Distress Syndrome Network: Ventilation with lower tidal volumes as compared with traditional tidal volumes for acute lung injury and the acute respiratory distress syndrome. *N Engl J Med.* 2000; 342:1301-1308.

[6] Ferreira Cruz F., Lorenzo Ball, Patricia Rieken Macedo Rocco & Paolo Pelosi. 2018. "Ventilator-induced lung injury during controlled ventilation in patients with acute respiratory distress syndrome: less is probably better." *Expert Review of Respiratory Medicine*. doi: https://10.1080/17476348.2018.1457954.

[7] Simonds A. 2015. ERS practical handbook - Noninvasive ventilation. *European Respiratory Society*.

[8] Mehta S., Hill N. S. Noninvasive ventilation. *Am J Respir Crit Care Med* 2001; 163: 540-77.

[9] Gay P. C. Complications of noninvasive ventilation in acute care. *Respir Care* 2009; 54: 246-57.

[10] Carron M., Gagliardi G., Michielan F., Freo U., Ori C. Occurrence of pneumothorax during noninvasive positive pressure ventilation through a helmet. *Journal of Clinical Anesthesia* (2007) 19, 632-635.

[11] Haworth C. S., Dodd M. E., Atkins M., Woodcock A. A., Webb A. K. Pneumothorax in adults with cystic fibrosis dependent on nasal intermittent positive pressure ventilation (NIPPV): a management dilemma. *Thorax* 2000;55:620-2.

[12] Simonds A. K. Pneumothorax: An Important Complication of Non-Invasive Ventilation in Neuromuscular Disease. *Neuromuscul Disord.* 2004 Jun;14(6):351-2.

[13] Andreu-Ruiz A. et al., Tension pneumocephalus secondary to non-invasive mechanical ventilation in a patient with severe traumatic brain injury, *Neurocirugia* (Astur) May-Jun 2018;29(3):157-160. Epub 2017 Sep 28.

[14] Nair S., Henry M., Pneumocephalus induced by non-invasive ventilation: A case report, *Respiratory Medicine Extra Volume* 1, Issue 3, 2005, Pages 75-77.

[15] Ruggeroni P., Girbino G., Fatal pneumomediastinum associated with use of noninvasive mechanical ventilation, *Respirology Case Reports* 2014; 2(4):126-128.

[16] Gonzalez Garcia L. et al., Severe subcutaneous emphysema and pneumomediastinum secondary to noninvasive ventilation support in status asthmaticus, *Indian J Crit Care Med.* 2016 Apr; 20(4): 242-244.

In: Non-Invasive Mechanical Ventilation Complications
Editor: Antonio M. Esquinas
ISBN: 978-1-53619-515-6

Chapter 8

COMPLICATIONS DURING NON-INVASIVE MECHANICAL VENTILATION. SECRETIONS MANAGEMENT

Ana Raquel Magalhães*, MD and Inês Moreira, MD
Serviço de Pneumologia, Hospital Santa Marta - Centro Hospitalar e Universitário Lisboa Central, Lisboa, Portugal

ABSTRACT

Secretion accumulation may cause atelectasis, increased work of breathing, ventilation/perfusion mismatch and can lead to infection. Various factors may contribute for retained secretions on the mechanically ventilated patient such as immobility, altered state of consciousness, secretion viscosity and increased production of sputum. To avoid the failure of NIV, airway clearance techniques and secretion management measures should be carried out.

Manual techniques, via chest percussion and the application of vibration, and postural drainage are of greatest importance on the patient that is unable to cooperate. The active cycle of breathing and autogenic drainage technique can be modified for use during NIV treatment. High-frequency chest wall oscillation involves compression of the thorax at a high frequency and, in intrapulmonary percussive ventilation, a pneumatic device delivers small volumes of air at high frequencies, both promoting the vibration and mobilization of secretions. Heated humidification may also aid the clearance of thick and viscous sputum.

The state of hydration of the patient should always be kept in mind, as it can influence the viscosity of the secretions. The use of mucolytic agents, bronchodilators, and antibiotics, when necessary, should be considered. Finally, flexible bronchoscopy may play a role in the setting of large amounts of secretions.

* Corresponding Author's E-mail: ana.magalhaes91@gmail.com.

Keywords: non-invasive ventilation, secretions, airway clearance, respiratory physiotherapy

INTRODUCTION

The constant clearance of airway secretions is essential for pulmonary hygiene and is sustained by the mucociliary system and the ability to cough [1]. Secretion accumulation may cause atelectasis, increased work of breathing, ventilation/perfusion mismatch and can lead to infection. Various factors may contribute to retained secretions on the mechanically ventilated patient such as immobility, altered state of consciousness, secretion viscosity and increased production of sputum in diseases like COPD, bronchiectasis and pneumonia [2]. Contrary to invasive mechanical ventilation, non-invasive mechanical ventilation (NIV) does not allow direct access to the airway. Additionally, the unidirectional flow of air, low humidity and trauma of nasotracheal suctioning can contribute to thickened secretions in NIV. Conversely, the preservation of the cough reflex is an advantage over invasive ventilation, and thus the incapacity of the patient to spontaneously remove secretions has been associated with early NIV failure and is considered a relative contraindication for NIV [3, 4]. To avoid the lack of success of NIV, airway clearance techniques and secretion management measures should be carried out.

MANUAL TECHNIQUES AND POSTURAL DRAINAGE

Manual techniques are of greatest importance on the patient that is unable to cooperate with therapy. They consist of chest percussion and the application of vibration. The therapist uses his hands to deliver force at the beginning of expiration followed by oscillatory compressions until all the air is exhaled [5].

Postural drainage is one of the oldest techniques for bronchial hygiene and still remains widely used. Its purpose is to aid in the clearance of secretions through gravity assisted positioning. These techniques can easily be applied during the delivery of NIV [6].

ACTIVE CYCLE OF BREATHING AND AUTOGENIC DRAINAGE

The active cycle of breathing technique has three main phases: 1) breathing control (the patient should be instructed to breathe in and out gently according to his own respiratory rate. This technique allows for relaxation of the airways and it can relieve dyspnea and anxiety); 2) thoracic expansion exercises (deep breathing exercises focused on the inspiratory phase of the breathing cycle that help loosen peripheral secretions. The patient takes a deep breath in and holds the air for a few seconds before exhaling) and 3) the forced expiration technique (used to move the secretions that were mobilized in the previous steps. It consists of a fast exhalation maneuver through an open glottis) [5-7]. This technique depends on the patient cooperation, so it may not be possible if the patient has weak respiratory muscles or if he is highly dependent on the ventilator. However, it can be modified for use during NIV treatment. The breathing control phase, with a few respiratory cycles with the patient's normal tidal volume, should be followed by three to four thoracic expansions achieved by increasing the pressure support or volume delivered by the ventilator. The cycle ends with a forced expiration using the abdominal and chest muscles to force the air out [8].

The autogenic drainage technique also aims to transport peripheral secretions to more central airways by breathing exercises at different lung volumes. This effect can also be achieved by changing the settings of the ventilator to deliver different tidal volumes at each breathing cycle [7, 8].

Instrumental Techniques

High-frequency chest wall oscillation involves an air pulse generator that delivers intermittent airflow to an inflatable vest. This causes compression of the thorax at a high frequency (typically adjusted between 5-20 Hz, according to patient tolerance) promoting the vibration and mobilization of secretions towards more central airways. This treatment can be applied during NIV, commonly in five-minute sessions [5, 8].

In intrapulmonary percussive ventilation, a pneumatic device intermittently delivers small volumes of air at high frequencies (100-300 cycles per minute), creating an effect of vibration in the lungs. The interface to the patient could be a face mask, endotracheal tube, or tracheostomy [5, 9]. The device can simultaneously provide ventilatory support so it can be used on patients highly dependent on NIV [8].

The patient will probably still need the aid of proximal airway clearance techniques or suctioning to eliminate secretions from the mouth and central airways. When mobilizing large amounts of secretions there is a risk of airway obstruction, therefore these techniques should always be implemented by an experienced team and under close surveillance of the patient [5].

Humidification

Heated humidification may be an important factor to consider in the setting of thick and viscous sputum [10]. This topic will be reviewed in another chapter.

Hydration, Bronchodilators, Antibiotic Therapy and Bronchoscopy

The patient's state of systemic hydration can influence the viscosity of the secretions, making them more fluid and easy to expel. It is not uncommon for the ventilated patient to be dehydrated due to fluid intake restriction, and so proper attention to this matter should be taken into consideration [1, 2]. The use of mucolytic agents has been well established for COPD patients and should be considered for other patients as well [8, 11].

In the setting of a patient with obstructive lung disease or bronchospasm, bronchodilator therapy should be administered, either in the form of nebulization or pressurized. Both these forms can be administered without discontinuation of NIV therapy [8, 11].

When pneumonia or respiratory infection is suspected, appropriate antibiotic therapy is key in reducing the purulence and thickness of the sputum. In cystic fibrosis and bronchiectasis, inhaled antibiotic therapy may play a major role in the reduction of the number of exacerbations and in decreasing sputum volume [12].

Even though it is not routinely recommended, when dealing with a large volume of secretions, flexible bronchoscopy could be a tool for performing effective bronchial hygiene. Considering it is an invasive procedure, various factors should be taken into consideration including potential risks but also the experience of the team. There are a number of interfaces that allow the maintenance of non-invasive ventilatory support during bronchoscopy [13].

Key Messages

- Airway clearance techniques and secretion management measures are of upmost importance to avoid the failure of NIV;
- Conventional techniques like the active cycle of breathing and autogenic drainage can be adapted to the mechanically ventilated patient;
- High-frequency chest wall oscillation and intrapulmonary percussive ventilation can be used to loosen peripheral secretions during NIV treatment;
- Other factors may contribute to the management of secretions like proper hydration of the patient and the need for antibiotic or bronchodilator therapy.

REFERENCES

[1] Marcelo B. Antunes NAC. Mucociliary clearance - a critical upper airway host defense mechanism and methods of assessment. *Curr. Opin. Allergy Clin. Immunol.* 2007;(10):2573-2576.

[2] Branson RD. Secretion management in the mechanically ventilated patient. *Respir. Care*. 2007;52(10):1328-1342.

[3] Vandenberghe N, Vallet AE, Petitjean T, et al. Absence of airway secretion accumulation predicts tolerance of noninvasive ventilation in subjects with amyotrophic lateral sclerosis. *Respir. Care*. 2013;58(9):1424-1432.

[4] Ozyilmaz E, Ugurlu AO, Nava S. Timing of noninvasive ventilation failure: Causes, risk factors, and potential remedies. *BMC Pulm. Med*. 2014;14(1).

[5] Michelle Chatwin, Michel Toussaint, Miguel R Gonçalves, Nicole Sheers, Uwe Mellies, Jesus Gonzales-Bermejo, Jesus Sancho, Brigitte Fauroux, Tiina Andersen, Brit Hov, Malin Nygren-Bonnier, Matthieu Lacombe, Kurt Pernet, Mike Kampelmacher, Christian Devaux, BMM. Airway Clearance Techniques in Neuromuscular Disorders: A State of the Art Review. *Respir Med*. 2018;136:98-110.

[6] Bott J, Blumenthal S, Buxton M, et al. Guidelines for the physiotherapy management of the adult, medical, spontaneously breathing patient. *Thorax*. 2009;64(Suppl I).

[7] Rodriguez Hortal MC, Nygren-Bonnier M, Hjelte L. Non-invasive Ventilation as Airway Clearance Technique in Cystic Fibrosis. *Physiother. Res. Int*. 2017;22(3).

[8] Michelle Chatwin. 2015. "Airway clearance methods and nebulised therapy in acute NIV" In: *ERS Practical Handbook Noninvasive Ventilation*, edited by Anita K. Simonds, 86-91.

[9] Reychler, Gregory, Emilie Debier, Olivier Contal NA. *Intrapulmonary Percussive Ventilation as an Airway Clearance Technique in Subjects With Chronic Obstructive Airway Diseases*. 2018:620-631.

[10] Cerpa F, Cáceres D, Romero-Dapueto C, et al. Humidification on Ventilated Patients: Heated Humidifications or Heat and Moisture Exchangers? *Open Respir. Med. J*. 2015;9(1):104-111.

[11] Ides K, Vissers D, De Backer L, Leemans G, De Backer W. Airway clearance in COPD: Need for a breath of fresh air? A systematic review. *COPD J. Chronic Obstr. Pulm. Dis*. 2011;8(3):196-205.

[12] Hill AT, Sullivan AL, Chalmers JD, et al. *British Thoracic Society Guideline for bronchiectasis in adults*. 2019;74(Suppl 1).

[13] Scala R, Naldi M, Maccari U. Early fiberoptic bronchoscopy during non-invasive ventilation in patients with decompensated chronic obstructive pulmonary disease due to community-acquired-pneumonia. *Crit. Care*. 2010;14(2).

In: Non-Invasive Mechanical Ventilation Complications ISBN: 978-1-53619-515-6
Editor: Antonio M. Esquinas

Chapter 9

Complications during Non-Invasive Mechanical Ventilation Digestive Alterations

Catarina Cascais Costa*[1,*], *MD and João Cravo*[1], *MD
[1]Pulmonology Department, Centro Hospitalar Baixo Vouga – Hospital Infante D. Pedro, Aveiro, Portugal

Abstract

Secretion accumulation may cause atelectasis, increased work of breathing, ventilation/perfusion mismatch and can lead to infection. Various factors may contribute for retained secretions on the mechanically ventilated patient such as immobility, altered state of consciousness, secretion viscosity and increased production of sputum. To avoid the failure of NIV, airway clearance techniques and secretion management measures should be carried out.

Manual techniques, via chest percussion and the application of vibration, and postural drainage are of greatest importance on the patient that is unable to cooperate. The active cycle of breathing and autogenic drainage technique can be modified for use during NIV treatment.

High-frequency chest wall oscillation involves compression of the thorax at a high frequency and, in intrapulmonary percussive ventilation, a pneumatic device delivers small volumes of air at high frequencies, both promoting the vibration and mobilization of secretions. Heated humidification may also aid the clearance of thick and viscous sputum.

The state of hydration of the patient should always be kept in mind, as it can influence the viscosity of the secretions. The use of mucolytic agents, bronchodilators, and antibiotics, when necessary, should be considered. Finally, flexible bronchoscopy may play a role in the setting of large amounts of secretions.

---

* Corresponding Author's E-mail: catarinacascaisc@gmail.com.

Keywords: Digestive complications, Non-invasive ventilation, Gastric insufflation, fistulae, Colonic pseudo-obstruction

Introduction

Purpose of Review

Noninvasive ventilation (NIV) is a method of ventilatory support which may help avoid endotracheal intubation in critically ill patients, as well as its potential complications.

The benefits of this technique strongly outweigh its challenges. Its negative consequences and adverse effects are generally uncommon and relatively innocuous. Complications associated with NIV may be localized, such as rash or skin ulcers, dry mouth, irritant conjunctivitis [2], or may be associated with difficulty adapting to NIV and serious and life-threatening systemic complications [3].

In critically ill patients, the gastrointestinal complications of ventilation may overlap with systemic complications of the underlying disease, and the true cause of the gastrointestinal complaints can be difficult to pinpoint [4]. Mechanical ventilation may potentiate adverse effects and worsen the gastrointestinal disorder, namely in terms of splanchnic blood flow, both as a result of decreased mean blood pressure and increased vascular resistance [4].

Throughout this chapter, we will discuss digestive complications associated with the use of noninvasive ventilation.

Esophagitis

Esophageal mucosal injury and erosive esophagitis occurs in 50% of patients requiring mechanical ventilation [4]. This prevalence is associated with multiple mechanisms which may promote mucosal changes, such as the use of nasogastric tubes, gastroesophageal reflux or even bile reflux [4].

The severity of esophagitis depends on the gastric residual volume and gut microbiota of each individual [4].

Nasogastric tubes cause mucosal irritation due to mechanical trauma and interference with esophageal and sphincter motility [4]. To prevent lesions caused by nasogastric tubes, the head of the bed should be raised, tubes should be used only if strictly necessary, and strategies that promote gastric emptying and reflux should be used [4]. Any risk factor for lower esophageal sphincter disorder, such as the presence of hiatal hernia, must be identified and promptly treated as needed to prevent complications of a potentially life-saving treatment [5].

Gastric Distension

Ventilation volume is distributed to both lungs and also to the stomach. This is physiologically regulated by airway resistance and lower esophageal sphincter pressure. The pressure exerted on the digestive tract may be altered by NIV [6].

Gastric distension is one of the most frequently described digestive complications and may occur in association with stomach hypomotility [4] in 5 to 40% of patients on NIV [6]. It is generally considered a minor complication as NIV pressure rarely exceeds 25 cmH2O [7].

The increase in positive pressure as a result of the procedure may generate greater cricopharyngeal pressure, leading to an increase in gastric pressure and consequent distension [6, 8, 9]. It may have serious consequences, such as regurgitation and pulmonary aspiration [10] in 5% of patients [11], gastric perforation [12], compartmental syndromes and even death [6].

Gastric distension may also develop as a result of aerophagia [9, 11], which may occur in up to 50% of patients on NIV [13]. Gastric inflation compresses the lungs, reducing patient compliance and increasing airway ventilation pressure [10] and parasympathetic tone, which may cause bradycardia, bronchoconstriction and bronchial hyperreactivity [9].

Therapeutic options for gastrointestinal motility are limited and are based on the correction of electrolyte imbalance and avoidance of medications that promote changes in motility [14].

Abdominal compartment syndrome is characterized by an intra-abdominal pressure higher than 20–25 mmHg resulting in organ damage [6]. A higher intra-abdominal pressure also increases intrathoracic pressure, which can lead to restriction, altered gas exchange, and reduced capillary blood flow [9].

The increase in pressure caused by NIV may damage the digestive mucosa, allowing air to pass through the layers of the gastrointestinal tract wall, a condition known as pneumatosis intestinalis [2]. Although rare, this has also been shown to occur in the stomach and is known as gastric emphysema [15].

Put simply, it may be essential to accelerate bowel transit time, change certain ventilation parameters, specifically, decreasing the inflation pressure, or adjust respiratory rate in these clinical settings. However, the presence of organic disease cannot be ruled out [13].

Gastric Perforation and Fistulas

The benefits of NIV strongly outweigh the potential risks of gastrointestinal tract perforation, and the treatment of chronic respiratory failure should not be called into question. However, it may be necessary to lower the pressure as much as possible while still allowing the management of the patient's respiratory function [5].

Increased intrathoracic pressure caused by ventilation may also decrease venous return, which reduces cardiac output and induces hypotension in individuals with predisposing factors. This effect will significantly reduce gastrointestinal tract blood flow as a consequence of local hypoperfusion [4]. Hypoperfusion may be worsened by the activation of the renin-angiotensin-aldosterone system, with neurohormonal changes intended to redistribute blood flow away from the vascular beds [4]. These vascular changes may lead to the development of pressure ulcers [4], which may originate fistulas with adjacent organs.

Gastric perforation is a serious yet uncommon complication of NIV [5] and is usually associated with intra-abdominal surgical interventions or tube placement, namely gastroesophageal tubes, especially in obese patients [5]. However, gastric perforation may also occur as a consequence of vascular and metabolic imbalance in critically ill patients [4].

Within a few hours of clinical worsening, macroscopic changes to the mucosa become evident as subepithelial petechiae lesions appear which may progress to ulcerated lesions over time [4]. These lesions are usually multiple and superficial and tend to develop predominantly in the stomach [4]. The distal digestive tract is generally affected at a later stage and is associated with deeper perforations which are more susceptible to bleeding [4].

Bleeding

The main causes of gastrointestinal bleeding in patients on mechanical ventilation are bleeding from stress-related mucosal damage and erosive esophagitis [14].

Most critically ill patients admitted to a specialized care unit exhibit mucosal changes with bleeding potential within the first 24 hours of admission [4]. These are generally asymptomatic and may lead to microscopic blood loss [4].

Gastric mucosal changes in a critically ill patient are the result of a complex interaction between intraluminal mechanisms, reduced blood flow, activation of inflammatory metabolic cascades, medications (particularly antibiotics) which alter local microbiota, reduced intraluminal pH, and altered gastric intrinsic defense mechanisms [4]. All of these mechanisms cause gastric mucosal changes which may result in local bleeding due to the presence of erosions, ulcers or perforated lesions [4]. However, a ventilator-induced increase in pressure in critically ill patients may contribute to the loss of integrity of an already frail mucosal barrier, and it may be difficult to recognize the true cause of the bleeding [4].

The lesions described can be prevented with appropriate and timely hemodynamic support and use of medication which neutralizes luminal acids [4]. Given its cytoprotective effect, enteric feeding should be started as soon as possible [4].

Colonic Pseudo-Obstruction

The abovementioned changes in blood flow, followed by periods of reperfusion, may be responsible for episodes of nonocclusive mesenteric ischemia in critically ill patients [4].

Metabolic, neurological and chemical changes associated with serious disease promote episodes of bacterial translocation, which occur more frequently in the presence of high pressure induced by mechanical ventilation. These changes induce altered gastrointestinal motility and gut barrier function as a result of changes in the local microbiota, which may lead to pseudo-obstruction [4].

Gastric Content Aspiration

A potential complication of the use of NIV is an increased risk of gastric acid aspiration due to a rise in intra-abdominal pressure.

The use of NIV in patients with intractable vomiting or hematemesis should ideally be avoided whenever possible [1].

Summary

Gastrointestinal complications in critically ill patients are complex, dynamic [14], and diverse yet uncommon. However, it remains unclear if these complications are a direct effect of ventilation or whether ventilation may contribute to physiologic changes which induce gastrointestinal disorders [4]. The impact of these disorders on mortality is not yet fully understood, but they have an unmistakable influence on morbidity and affect patient recovery [4]. However, an appropriate use of NIV, namely the pressure used, and special attention to the early identification of these complications, allow a positive outcome in most cases.

Key Messages

- Digestive complications associated with the use of non-invasive ventilation are uncommon.
- Nevertheless, abdominal distension (gastric and intestine distension) is more common than other complications.
- Should digestive complications occur, they can be managed with ventilatory parameter readjustment and symptomatic treatment.

References

[1] Guy, W., Soo Hoo. *Noninvasive Ventilation. Medscape*. https://emedicine.medscape.com/article/304235-overview. Updated: Oct. 22, 2018. Accessed April 2, 2020.

[2] Bakkali, H. et al. Complication inhabituelle de la ventilation non invasive: la pneumatose œsogas- trique associée à un emphysème sous-cutané. *Rev. Pneumol. Clin.*, (2014), http://dx.doi.org/10.1016/j.pneumo.2013.10.003. [Unusual complication of non-invasive ventilation: esogastric pneumatosis associated with subcutaneous emphysema]

[3] Hamadziripi Ngandu, Gale, Nichola, Hopkinson, Jane B. Experiences of noninvasive ventilation in adults with hypercapnic respiratory failure: A review of evidence. *European Respiratory Review*, Dec. 2016, 25 (142) 451 - 471; DOI: 10.1183/16000617.0002-2016.

[4] Mutlu, G. M., Mutlu, E. A., Factor, P. GI complications in patients receiving mechanical ventilation. *Chest,* 2001; 119(4):1222 - 1241. doi:10.1378/chest.119.4.1222.

[5] Jean-Lavaleur, M. et al. Rupture gastrique au de´cours d'une se´ance de ventilation non invasive. *Annales Franc¸aises d'Anesthesie et de Reanimation*, 28 (2009) 588 - 591. doi:10.1016/j.annfar.2009.04.012. [Gastric rupture during a non-invasive ventilation session. *French Annals of Anesthesia and Reanimation*]

[6] Carron, M., Freo, U., BaHammam, A. S., Dellweg, D., Guarracino, F., Cosentini, R., Feltracco, P., Vianello, A., Ori, C., Esquinas, A. Complications of non-invasive ventilation techniques: a comprehensive qualitative review of randomized trials. *Br. J. Anaesth.,* 2013 Jun.; 110(6): 896 - 914. Published online 2013 Apr. 5. doi: 10.1093/bja/aet070.

[7] Hill, Nicholas S., Kramer, Naomi R. Troubleshooting problems with noninvasive positive pressure ventilation. *Uptodate,* Published Jun. 21, 2018. Accessed March 3, 2020.

[8] Takeshi Nishimura, Kunihoro Shirai, Atsunori Nakao and Joji Kotani. Gastric Perforation Because of Non-Invasive Positive-Pressure Ventilation: Review of Complications. *Surgical Infections Case Reports,* Dec. 2016.41 - 43. http://doi.org/10.1089/crsi.2016.29008.tn.

[9] De Keulenaer, B. L., De Backer, A., Schepens, D. R., Daelemans, R., Wilmer, A., Malbrain, M. L. Abdominal compartment syndrome related to noninvasive ventilation. *Intensive Care Med.,* 2003; 29: 1177 - 81.

[10] Luria, O., Reshef, L., Barnea, O. Analysis of non-invasive ventilation effects on gastric inflation using a non-linear mathematical model. *Resuscitation,* 2006; 71: 358 - 64.

[11] Gay Peter, C. Complications of Noninvasive Ventilation in Acute Care. *Respiratory Care,* February 2009, 54 (2) 246 - 258.

[12] Nishimura, T., Shirai, K., Nakao, A. and Kotani, J. (2016). Gastric Perforation Because of Non-Invasive Positive-Pressure Ventilation: Review of Complications. *Surgical Infections Case Reports,* 1(1), 41 - 43. doi:10.1089/crsi.2016.29008.tn.

[13] Mayoralas Alises, S., Gómez Mendieta, M. A., Díaz Lobato, S. Aerophagia due to noninvasive mechanical ventilation: a first manifestation of silent gastric carcinoma. *Archivos de Bronconeumologia,* 2003 Jul.; 39(7):321 - 323. DOI: 10.1016/s0300-2896(03)75393-9. [*Bronconeumology Archives*]

[14] Mutlu, G. M., Mutlu, E. A., Factor, P. Prevention and treatment of gastrointestinal complications in patients on mechanical ventilation. *Am. J. Respir. Med.,* 2003; 2(5):395 - 411. doi:10.1007/BF03256667.

[15] Malik, Fahad, Lattanzio, Natalia, Veloso, Karen and Nfonoyim, Jay. (2019). A case report of gastric emphysema induced by noninvasive positive airway pressure. *Journal of Community Hospital Internal Medicine Perspectives*, 9:3, 244 - 246. DOI: 10.1080/20009666.2019.1618669.

In: Non-Invasive Mechanical Ventilation Complications
Editor: Antonio M. Esquinas
ISBN: 978-1-53619-515-6

Chapter 10

COMPLICATIONS DURING NON-INVASIVE MECHANICAL VENTILATION. ASPIRATION PNEUMONIA. PHYSIOPATHOLOGY, RISK FACTORS

Biljana Lazovic - Popovic[1,*], Radmila Dmitrovic[1], Isidora Simonovic[1] and Antonio M. Esquinas[2]

[1]Department of Pulmonology, University Clinical Center, "Zemun," Belgrade, Serbia
[2]Intensive Care Unit, Hospital Morales Meseguer, Murcia, Spain

ABSTRACT

Aspiration pneumonia is a major, serious and life-threatening complication of NIV. The incidence of aspiration pneumonia in patients with NIV has been reported in about 5% of cases, and the mortality rate has been very high. Developed aspiration pneumonia is very difficult to treat, so it is necessary, before applying NIV, to consider all risk factors that could lead to its development.

Keywords: non-invasive ventilation, aspiration, pneumonia, life-threatening

ABBREVIATIONS

ACPO	acute cardiogenic pulmonary edema
ARF	acute respiratory failure
BiPAP	bilevel positive airway pressure

* Correspondence Author's E-mail: lazovic.biljana@gmail.com.

COPD	chronic obstructive pulmonary disease
CPAP	continuous positive airway pressure
EPAP	expiratory positive airway pressure
FRC	functional residual lung capacity
IDS	Infectious Diseases Society
IPAP	inspiratory positive airway pressure
NG	nasogastric
NIV	non-invasive ventilation
NIVPS	non-invasive pressure-assisted ventilation

NON-INVASIVE MECHANICAL VENTILATION, MAIN CHARACTERISTICS

Non-invasive mechanical ventilation (NIV) is defined as ventilatory support that is achieved by creating positive airway pressure, with no endotracheal tube, laryngeal mask, or endotracheal cannula used to secure the airway [1]. According to some researchers, the history of NIV dates back to more than 100 years, but the development of "modern" NIV is related to 1987 when Delaubier and Rideau successfully ventilated a patient with Duchenne's disease [2]. The choice of the appropriate NIV mode is the most important for improving the clinical status of patients where this type of ventilatory support is necessary. The application of the appropriate NIV mode is reduced respiratory work and dyspnea and improves gas exchange in the lungs. NIV can be achieved through standard mechanical ventilation fans used in intensive care units (ICU) and portable fans constructed exclusively for NIV. For which type of fan would clinicians decide upon, depends on the experience of the clinician, patients status, therapeutic requirements, and NIV sites. It should be considered that appliances used in ICU do not have the possibility of correcting potential one's losses if they occur, while small portable appliances exclusively designed for NIV have this possibility due to the microprocessor which notes the differences between the inspiratory and the expiratory tidal volume (TV). The main topic of this chapter is aspiration pneumonia, as one of the major complications of NIV application but foremost our objective is to delineate the main characters and modalities of NIV, indications and contraindications for its use.

NIV Modalities

Continuous positive airway pressure (CPAP) was introduced to clinical practice in the 1980s and represented the simplest mode of NIV. During the application of CPAP, airway pressure is maintained continuously (in inspiration and expiration) above atmospheric pressure value which allows the alveoli to open in the inspiration and at the same time prevent their collapse in expiration, the end effect is a correction of hypoxemia. Bilevel positive airway pressure (BiPAP) was introduced to clinical practice in 1989. Positive pressure during ventilation is realized in two different levels: upper and lower, during inspiration (inspiratory positive airway pressure-IPAP) and expiratory (expiratory positive airway pressure-EPAP i.e., CPAP). The difference between IPAP and EPAP represent pressure supported lung ventilation. This mode of NIV can contribute to a reduction in inspiration breathing work to a greater extent than CPAP. Non-invasive pressure-assisted ventilation (NIVPS) is limited by pressure and the patients' effort at inspiration while expiration is passive. The duration of inspiration and expiration is determined by the patient himself. The device delivers a predetermined inspiratory pressure to assist the patient's spontaneous respiratory attempts. This type of ventilatory support is flow-cycled which means that expiration begins when the flow falls below the values previously set on the device. In this way, it helps respiratory muscles operate, improves the efficiency of the patient's respiratory efforts, and reduces respiratory work [1].

Indications and Contraindications

According to some authors, NIV is indicated in patients with acute and chronic respiratory failure (moderate and severe dyspnea, tachypnea, paradoxical abdominal breathing, the partial pressure of oxygen (PaO2) < 60 mmHg, the partial pressure of carbon dioxide (PaCO2) > 45 mmHg, pH $< 7{,}35$ and PaO2/FiO2 < 200 [3]. NIV can be used in respiratory tract insufficiency caused by an acute exacerbation of chronic obstructive pulmonary disease (COPD), neuromuscular diseases, acute cardiogenic pulmonary edema, in immunocompromised patients, postoperative respiratory failure, after extubation, in patients with diffuse pneumonia that are hypoxic despite using all other therapeutic measures [4, 5]. For example, in patients with acute cardiogenic pulmonary edema and consequent respiratory insufficiency, NIV could be applied only in absence of acute cardiogenic shock. By applying NIV in acute cardiogenic pulmonary edema there will be an increase in the functional residual lung capacity (FRC) thus opening collapsed alveoli and improving oxygenation, increasing lung compliance, and reducing respiratory work [3]. Contraindications for clinical use of NIV and CPAPs are numerous, and the list continues to expand (Table 1). It is important to note that there are no absolute contraindications for the use of the NIV, however, to avoid these complications, a clinical assessment of each patient is necessary, a good knowledge of the potential risks from the unsuccessful implementation of NIV, and creating our own NIV protocol in each institution where this ventilation technique will be applied [1].

Table 1. Contraindications for NIV [1]

Facial injuries/ facial burns	**Cardiac arrest**
Anatomical or functional airway obstruction	Absence of spontaneous breathing
Inability to protect the upper respiratory tract	Severe hypoxemia or acidosis (Ph < 7.1)
Disorder of consciousness	Cardiogenic shock, myocardial infarction
Severe encephalopathy	The presence of severe comorbidities
Epilepsy	Pregnancy
Vomiting	Abundant secretion from the respiratory tract
Ileus	Presence of focal consolidation on chest X-ray
Bleeding from the gastrointestinal tract	Undrained pneumothorax

Aspiration Pneumonia-Like Complication of NIV

According to some researchers, complications of NIV are divided into two groups: major and minor. Major complications are prospective life-threatening and they lead to a rise of morbidity while minor complications are defined as bland and passable linked with a characteristic of modality (Table 2). According to the data collected by the group of authors, aspiration pneumonia is considered a major complication of NIV [6].

The term aspiration pneumonia is defined as an infectious pulmonary process that occurs after an abnormal entry of fluid into the lower parts of the respiratory tract. The aspirated fluid can be gastric content, particulate matter, or oropharyngeal secretions. In the case of aspiration of sterile gastric contents, aspiration pneumonitis can develop, which is described as an acute inhalation injury of the lungs. According to some researchers, the risk of developing aspiration pneumonia in hospitalized patients is 13.8%, and the mortality rate, which largely depends on the volume and content, is around 70%. The literature lists some conditions that may lead to an increased risk of developing aspiration pneumonia such as stroke, drug overdose, alcohol use disorders, seizure, intracranial masses, head trauma, general anesthesia, dementia, Parkinson disease, esophageal stricture, gastroesophageal reflux disease, pseudobulbar pulses, tracheostomy, bronchoscopy, NG tube, and protracted vomiting.

The pathophysiological mechanism of aspiration pneumonia is related to the entry of fluid into the bronchi and alveolar spaces, which triggers an inflammatory reaction accompanied by the release of pro-inflammatory factors such as cytokines, tumor necrosis factor-alpha, and interleukins. Inoculation of normal oropharyngeal flora in the aspirate results in the infectious process and results in aspiration pneumonia. If the bacterial load of aspirate is low normal host defenses will clear the secretions and prevent infection [7]. According to others, the development of aspiration pneumonia is also influenced by a compromise in the usual defenses that protect the lower airways including glottic closure, cough reflex, and other clearing mechanisms [8].

The diagnosis is made based on a physical examination that often describes symptoms such as fever, sudden onset dyspnea, hypoxemia, and crackles on lung auscultation. On chest radiography, the lower lobe on the right is most often affected. Patients who aspirated the contents in an upright position generally have affected lower lobes on both sides. The involvement of the right upper lobe is more common in patients who aspirate in the supine position. The indication for bronchoscopy is the aspiration of food particles during which the contents could be taken for the culture of microorganisms [7].

Treatment is supportive, including supplemental oxygen and mechanical ventilation. Antibiotics such as beta-lactamase inhibitors or clindamycin are given to patients with witnessed or known gastric aspiration due to the difficulty of excluding bacterial infections. If no infiltrates develop within 48-72 hours, antibiotics may be ruled out. According to the protocols of the Infectious Diseases Society of America (IDS), the most commonly used antibiotics are beta-lactams, carbapenems, or clindamycin. For example, some researchers treated aspiration pneumonia with a combination of clindamycin 600 mg intravenously every eight hours and then 300 mg orally four times a day and amoxicillin and clavulanic acid 875 mg intravenously every 12 hours. The duration of therapy will be around 7-14 days. It is not uncommon for aspiration pneumonia to be accompanied by complications such as ARDS, empyema, lung abscess, parapneumonic effusion, and respiratory failure [7, 9].

Table 2. Complications of NIV [6]

Major complications	**Minor complications**
Failure (hypoxemia): COPD exacerbation, ACPO, hypoxaemic ARF, hypercapnic-hypoxaemic ARF, post-extubation ARF, and weaning	CO2 rebreathing
Aspiration pneumonia	claustrophobia
Barotrauma	Arm oedema
Hypotension	Nasal skin lesion
	Discomfort, noise
	Patient ventilatory dyssynchrony

Searching the literature, we noticed that there was barely any research on the topic of aspiration pneumonia as a complication of NIV application. One group of researchers found that the incidence of aspiration pneumonia in patients with NIV is about 5%, which requires caution regarding the risk of aspiration. Pneumonia is a possible occurrence during the use of NIV and is the result of inhalation of the aforementioned substances or most often aspiration of gastric contents. To reduce the possibility of aspiration pneumonia, it is necessary to exclude patients with severe impairment of the function of the upper parts of the respiratory tract or those with excessive production and accumulation of secretions. They are prohibited to eat or drink until they are stabilized and are advised to take a sitting position during the application of NIV. The focus should be on all patients with gastric distension, ileus, nausea, vomiting, and gastroesophageal reflux disease. In such patients, the placement of a nasogastric tube is advised, however, it can be an interfering factor for the placement of the mask, because there is often an additional air leak, while discomfort is something that patients often complain about [6]. That aspiration pneumonia carries a high mortality rate is shown by the data of one cohort study monitored in two periods, from 2001 to 2003 and from 2004 to 2006 before and after adopting an "NIV-trial" strategy in which NIV was applied in the emergency department to any non-contraindicated ARF patients needing ventilatory support and was then continued in the intermediate-care-unit. The mortality rate from recurrent aspiration pneumonia for the period from 2001 to 2003. (before introduction "NIV-trial") was 43%, and for the period between 2004 to 2006. ("after introduction NIV trial") was 52%. In the mentioned study, all patients with bronchial asthma, COPD, interstitial lung diseases, etc., after the application of NIV had a lower mortality rate compared to those with recurrent aspiration pneumonia [10].

CONCLUSION

Aspiration pneumonia is a serious and life-threatening complication due to the use of NIV. According to the above data, the mortality rate is high, especially in recurrent aspiration pneumonia. Before applying NIV, it is necessary to evaluate all possible conditions that could potentially lead to its development, and after that, difficulties in its treatment and prolongation of hospitalization.

KEY MESSAGES

- Aspiration pneumonia is a major complication of NIV.
- Its incidence is around 5%, and the rate of mortality is at an increase.
- Before applying NIV, it is necessary to pay attention to the associated conditions which can lead to its development such as gastroesophageal reflux disease, gastric distension, ileus, or vomiting.
- In the future, it is necessary to pay more attention to this complication and the choice of treatment in case of its occurrence.

REFERENCES

[1] Dolinaj, Vladimir, Lončar Tatjana, Božić Teodora, Karišik Mirjana, Marković Dejan and Janjević Dušanka. 2014. *Serbian Journal of Anesthesia and Intensive therapy* Available from: https://scindeks-clanci.ceon.rs/data/pdf/2217-7744/2014/2217-77441402097D.pdf [Review article in Serbian].

[2] Lobato, Salvador Díaz and Alises Sagrario Mayoralas. 2013."Modern Non-invasive mechanical ventilation turns 25". *Archivos de Bronconeumología* 49:475-9 doi: 10.1016/j.arbres.2012.11.008. [*Bronconeumology Archives*]

[3] Hill, Nicholas S, Brenan John, Garpestad Erik, and Nava Stefano. 2007. "Non-invasive ventilation in acute respiratory failure" *Critical Care Medicine* 35:2402-7 doi: 10.1097/01.CCM.0000284587.36541.7F.

[4] Bersten, Andrew D. 2011. "Best practices for non-invasive ventilation." *Canadian Medical Association Journal* 183:293-4 doi: 10.1503/cmaj.110122.

[5] Nava, Stefano, and Hill Nicholas. 2009. "Non-invasive ventilation in acute respiratory failure." *Lancet (London, England)* 374:250-9 doi: 10.1016/S0140-6736(09)60496-7.

[6] Carron, Michaele, Freo Ulderico, BaHammam S Ahmed, Dellweg Dominic, Guarracino Fabio, Cosentini Roberto, Feltracco Paolo, Vianello Andrea, Ori Carlo, and Esquinas Antonio. 2013. "The complication of non-invasive ventilation techniques: a comprehensive qualitative review of randomized trials." *British Journal of Anaesthesia* 110:896-914 doi: 10.1093/bja/aet070.

[7] Raghavendra, R. Sanivarapu, and Gibson Joshua. 2020." Aspiration pneumonia" In: StatPearls [Internet]. Treasure Island (FL): StatPearls Publishing.

[8] Bartlett, John G. 2020. *Aspiration pneumonia in adults.* Available from: https://www.uptodate.com/contents/aspiration-pneumonia-in-adults.

[9] Sanjay, Sethi. 2019. *Aspiration pneumonitis and pneumonia.* Available from: msdmanuals.com/professional/pulmonary-disorders/pneumonia/aspiration-pneumonitis-and-pneumonia.

[10] Keisuke, Tomii, Ryutaro Seo, Ryo Tachikawa, Yuka Harada, Kimihiko Murase, Reiko Kaji, Yoshimi Takeshima, Michio Hayashi, Takashi Nishimura, and Kyosuke Ishihara. 2008. "Impact of noninvasive ventilation (NIV) trial for various types of acute respiratory failure in the emergency department; decreased mortality and use of the ICU" *Respiratory Medicine* 103:67-73 doi:10.1016/j.rmed.2008.08.001.

In: Non-Invasive Mechanical Ventilation Complications ISBN: 978-1-53619-515-6
Editor: Antonio M. Esquinas

Chapter 11

COMPLICATIONS DURING NON-INVASIVE MECHANICAL VENTILATION. VENTILATOR-INDUCED LUNG INJURY AND EFFORT-INDUCED LUNG INJURY; THE IMPORTANCE OF PaO_2/FiO_2 AND TIDAL VOLUME

Ricardo Amaral**, MD, José Miguel Maia, MD and Nelson Barros, MD

Department of Intensive Care Medicine, Centro Hospitalar Trás-os-Montes e Alto Douro, Vila Real, Portugal

ABSTRACT

Non-invasive ventilation (NIV) as supportive therapy in acute respiratory failure has become popular. But concerns exist for potential complications due to ventilator support and patient effort interaction.

Ventilator-induced lung injury (VILI) and effort-induced lung injury (EILI) are two of those complications. They have some common pathophysiologic pathways only with different origin of applied forces to the lung. In fact this two entities co-exist and may aggravate lung injury.

Usually the ratio between PaO_2/FiO_2 is diminished in lung pathology of various aetiologies this possibly correlating with lung heterogeneity with local variability in lung compliance. This heterogeneity exacerbates the negative effects of both positive (ventilator) and negative (patient) intrapleural pressure.

Correlation between higher tidal volume and NIV failure has been established. But although pathophysiologic mechanisms suggest lung injury occurrence with higher tidal volumes, that has not been undoubtedly demonstrated.

* Correspondence Author's E-mail: ricaja@gmail.com.

Reviewing VILI and EILI mechanisms, its differences, and the importance of both tidal volume and PaO_2/FiO_2, may help us optimize monitoring and therapeutic actions to both prevent or minimize lung injury in NIV setting.

Keywords: non-invasive mechanical ventilation; complications; Ventilator-induced lung injury

Ventilator-induced and Effort-induced lung injury are two processes often concurrent that potentiate lung injury in acute pulmonary diseases. These types of lung injury consist of: pulmonary edema with increased alveolo-capillary permeability, surfactant dysfunction, hyaline membranes formation and fibroproliferation. The consequences of this are low compliance, increased dead space and gas exchange impairment with low PaO_2/FiO_2 and increase in $PaCO_2$. Also, these changes lead to a pro-inflammatory state with release of multiple inflammation mediators active both local and systemically such has: Interleukin-8, 6, 1β, Tumor necrosis factor α. The release to systemic circulation of this mediators may increase systemic inflammation ultimately leading to distant organ failure [1].

Ventilator-induced lung injury (VILI) has traditionally been described in invasive mechanical ventilation. But its pathophysiology is easily translated to non-invasive ventilation (NIV) and studies have demonstrated its occurrence in this setting [2, 3, 4].

The pathophysiology of VILI may be divided in the following effects of mechanical ventilation (MV):

- Barotrauma: pressure driven injury – stress, distending pressure applied to lung: transpulmonary pressure (alveolar minus pleural pressure);
- Volutrauma: tidal volume driven injury – strain, lung deformation, it is related to transpulmonary pressure;

As the reader may perceive the author of this chapter adopts a non-classic definition for the barotrauma, using transpulmonary pressure and not airway pressure. This way the barotrauma and volutrauma unify since tidal volume is intrinsically related to transpulmonary pressure.

- Atelectrauma: tidal recruitment and derecruitment of lung units; recruitable areas are inflated during inspiration and collapse during expiration with significant strain;
- Biotrauma: systemic injury led by inflammation.

During NIV there is double contribution for the energy applied to the lung: the ventilator and the patient inspiratory effort. This effort is linked to respiratory drive measured by P0.1. The inspiratory effort consists in negative pressure swings in pleural pressure (oesophageal pressure may be used has a surrogate) and translates in increased trans-pulmonary pressure – alveolar minus pleural pressure. That is the basis for potential deleterious effects resulting in Effort Induced Lung Injury – EILI such has: higher than set tidal volume, atelectrauma, edema [through pulmonary trans-vascular pressure (intra-vascular pressure minus pleural pressure) increase – intra-vascular pressure increase and pleural pressure decrease [1, 5, 6, 7, 8].

Although not associated to EILI it has been demonstrated in an observational study that tidal volumes higher than 8,5mL/kg are associated with NIV failure in patients with PaO2/FiO2 < 200mmHg. However, on the same study authors conclude that tidal volume is impossible to control during NIV [9].

Hyperventilation was proved to cause self-inflicted lung injury in an experimental model that stimulated sheep respiratory drive by Mascheroni 1988: respiratory rate and tidal volume increase were associated with lung injury [10].

The forces applied to the lungs are not homogeneously distributed due to compliance variability across the lungs and the type of pressure applied to the lungs (negative pressure due to diaphragmatic contraction is applied mainly in the posterior lungs and positive pressure due to MV is predominantly applied in the non-dependent lung). This exacerbates volutrauma and atelectrauma in states of diminished regional compliance. In 2013 Yoshida demonstrated the pendelluft mechanism consisting of movements of air from non-dependent to dependent lung units in presence of patient effort [4, 11]. Takishima and Leith in 1970 built mathematical models to predict local stress variation due to lung unit distortion [12].

Take home messages:

- VILI and EILI may co-exist in NIV
- Barotrauma and Volutrauma are linked by the transpulmonary pressure
- EILI occurs in settings of augmented respiratory drive and effort, exacerbating transpulmonary pressure negative effects
- PaO2/FiO2 may be a marker of lung disease severity, heterogeneity and identify at risk patients for both VILI and EILI.
- Tidal volume is tendentially augmented in high respiratory drive and effort; high tidal volume is associated with NIV failure; tidal volumes cannot be controlled in NIV

REFERENCES

[1] Slutsky, Arthur S. and V. Marco Ranieri. "Ventilator-Induced Lung Injury." *New England Journal of Medicine* 2013;369:2126-36; doi: 10.1056/NEJMra1208707.

[2] Brochard Laurent, Arthur Slutsky, and Antonio Pesenti. "Mechanical Ventilation to Minimize Progression of Lung Injury in Acute Respiratory Failure." *American Journal of Respiratory and Critical Care Medicine Volume 195 Number 4* (February 2017): 438–442; doi: 10.1164/rccm.201605-1081CP.

[3] Brochard, Laurent. "Ventilation-induced lung injury exists in spontaneously breathing patients with acute respiratory failure: Yes." *Intensive Care Medicine*, published online: 10 January 2017; doi: 10.1007/s00134-016-4645-4.

[4] Gattinoni, Luciano. "Ventilation-induced lung injury exists in spontaneously breathing patients with acute respiratory failure: We are not sure." *Intensive Care Medicine* (2017) 43:256–258; doi: 10.1007/s00134-016-4483-4.

[5] Madahar, Purnema and Jeremy R. Beitler. *"Emerging concepts in ventilation-induced lung injury"* [version 1; peer review: 4 approved]. F1000Research 2020, 9(F1000 Faculty Rev):222; doi: 10.12688/f1000research.20576.1.

[6] Marini, J. J. "Microvasculature in ventilator-induced lung injury: target or cause?" *Minerva Anestesiologica* 2004;70:167-73.

[7] Katira, Bhushan H. "Ventilator-Induced Lung Injury: Classic and Novel Concepts." *Respiratory Care* 2019;64(6):629–637; doi: 10.4187/respcare.07055.

[8] Goligher, Ewan C. et al. "Lung and Diaphragm-Protective ventilation." *American Journal of Respiratory and Critical Care Medicine*, Published online 9 June 2020; doi: 10.1164/rccm.202003-0655CP.

[9] Carteaux, Guillaume et al. "Failure of Noninvasive Ventilation for De Novo Acute Hypoxemic Respiratory Failure: Role of Tidal Volume." *Critical Care Medicine* (2016) 44:282–290; doi: 10.1097/CCM.0000000000001379.

[10] Mascheroni, D. et al. "Acute respiratory failure following pharmacologically induced hyperventilation: an experimental animal study." *Intensive Care Medicine* (1988) 15:8-14.

[11] Yoshida, Takeshi et al. "Spontaneous Effort Causes Occult Pendelluft during Mechanical Ventilation." *American Journal of Respiratory and Critical Care Medicine* (2013) Vol 188 iss. 12, pp. 1420–1427; doi: 10.1164/rccm.201303-0539OC.

[12] Mead, Jere et al. "Stress distribution in lungs: a model of pulmonary elasticity." *Journal of Applied Physiology* Vol. 28, No. 5, May 1970.

In: Non-Invasive Mechanical Ventilation Complications ISBN: 978-1-53619-515-6
Editor: Antonio M. Esquinas

Chapter 12

MASK INTERFACE LEAKAGES. UNINTENTIONAL LEAK AND DEAD SPACE MASK DISPLACEMENT

Tina Herrero Jordán[1], MD, Luisa Cabrera Pimentel[2], MD and Sara Abad Abad[3], MD

[1]Department of Pneumology, Hospital Reina Sofia, Navarra, Spain
[2]Department of Pneumology, Hospital General de la Defensa, Zaragoza, Spain
[3]Department of Pneumology, Hospital de Alcañiz, Teruel, Spain

ABSTRACT

Non Invasive Ventilation (NIV) has vastly developed and grown in the last decades becoming one of the main treatments used both in acute respiratory failure (ARF) and in chronic respiratory failure (CRF). There are a lot of factors which determine the success or failure of NIV, from a good patient selection to medical expertise and choosing the right interface. Finding a suitable interface for each patient and each situation is essential to the success of the treatment.

Keywords: non-invasive ventilation, interface, acute respiratory failure, leak, dead space

INTERFACE SELECTION

Non Invasive Ventilation (NIV) has became one of the main treatments for patients with both acute and chronic respiratory failure. Its great development in the last decades has allowed the constant improvement of all its elements in order to increase the overall success rates of the treatment.

In recent years a greater variety of interfaces have been developed, being the main ones: oronasal masks, nasal masks, nasal plugs, mouth pieces, total face masks and helmets. Selecting from all the different interface classes the right one for each pacient in each situation is crucial for the success of NIV. We cannot pick the same interface for a patient with a chronic respiratory failure who will be in long-term home NIV than for the same patient during an acute exacerbation.

Although developers are constantly creating new interfaces, even custom made ones, there is not such thing as the perfect interface. As previously said, every patient is different and the same patient will evolve during time so it is important to always assess each case as many times as needed in order to select the right interface, optimizing patient tolerance, and avoiding as much as possible interface-related side effects.

The main characteristics that an ideal interface should meet are:

- Low air leaks
- Small dead space
- Comfortable
- Non claustrophobia inducing
- Easy placement and removal
- Easy maintenance and cleaning
- Stable
- Difficult to deform.

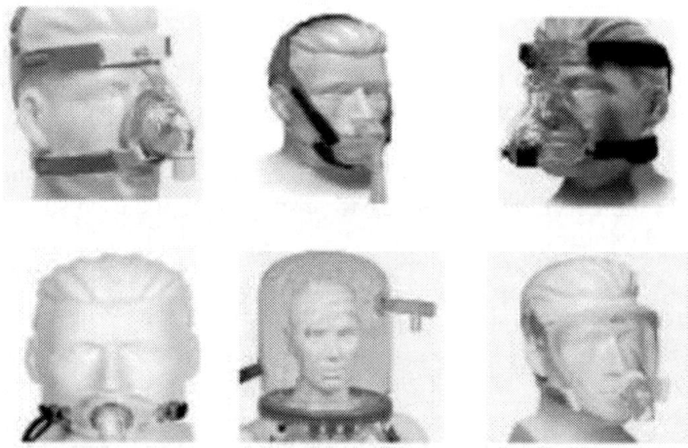

Figure 1. From left to right: 1. Nasal mask, 2. Nasal pillows, 3. Oronasal Mask, 4. Mouth Piece, 5. Helmet, 6. Total Face Mask.

In patients with ARF, who breathe through both the nose and the mouth, it is important to select an interface that covers mouth and nose in order to avoid air leaks. Recent studies have shown that in up to 70% of patients with ARF oronasal mask is the preferred interface, followed by facial masks and nasal masks (Crimi et al., 2010, 362-369).

On the other hand, in patients with CRF achieving patient comfort and preventing interface related complications are key to the long term success and tolerance of NIV. Usually the preferred interfaces for these kind of patients are nasal masks and nasal plugs which are rated as the most comfortable interfaces, are not as claustrophobic, allow expectoration and communication more easily and also are the ones that cause skin problems less often.

INTERFACE LEAKAGES

The presence of air leaks in order to facilitate CO2 removal and avoid patient re-breathing is one of the defining characteristics of NIV. That's the reason why ventilators for NIV are designed to compensate for a variable amount of air leaks. When talking about air leaks we have to differentiate between intentional and unintentional. The former group appear as a result of the use of single limb circuits without an expiratory valve, they are responsible of avoiding the re-breathing phenomenon and that's why they are deliberate and compensated by the ventilator. Usually we find these air leaks points in the interface or in the tubing depending if the circuit is for an acute setting or for a home NIV.

The unintentional air leaks can be found in any point of the circuit, being the most frequent locations: the point of contact between the skin and the mask and the nose or the mouth when the interface does not cover one of them. These leaks, especially the large ones, difficult the success of the treatment, they can create patient-ventilator trigger asynchrony, affect patient-ventilator synchronization, reduce tidal volume and drop the delivered intra-alveolar pressure. But not only unintentional large air leaks are troublesome, small air leaks can cause noise, eye irritation, conjunctivitis, etc. Avoiding all kinds of unintentional leaks is vital to achieve patient comfort and long term tolerance of the treatment.

Not only selecting the right type of interface, also selecting the correct size and material are useful in order to avoid air leaks. There are other strategies that help to minimize the leaks: use of a mask-support ring, changing the type of mask, tightening the mask straps, chinstraps, masks with hydrogel cushions, taping the mouth, etc. Despite the fact that it can be uncomfortable for the patient, the most used intervention to reduce leaks is tightening the mask straps. When doing this we have to be careful because if the pressure on the patient skin increases too much painful skin lesions, even pressure ulcers, can appear.

One of the worst iatrogenic interface-related complications in NIV are facial pressure ulcers. These can develop at any place where the mask, headgear or straps have contact with the skin, being the most common areas the bridge of the nose, the upper lip and the nasal mucosa. The most important strategy to prevent pressure ulcers remains avoiding an excessively tight fit, therefore selecting the appropriate mask size and giving the skin regular breaks from the interface pressure is vital to avoid skin complications.

Another frequent air leak related complication is dryness of oral and nasal mucosa with or without the association of nasal congestion. Despite the fact that it can also occur without an air leak, usually it indicates the existence of an unintentional one. Treatment options include the addition of moisture exchangers or an external heated humidifier to the ventilator, as well as mouth and nasal care, topical nasal application of saline and the use of antihistamines.

Unfortunately air leaks may still exist even with these interventions and the compensation mechanisms of the ventilators. In those situations with unavoidable air leaks multiple studies have shown that a pressure-targeted mode of ventilation is able to better sustain intra-alveolar pressure and tidal volume than a volume-targeted one (Mehta, McCool, and Hill 2001, 259-267). A reduction of peak inspiratory pressure or an increase in tidal volume have also been reported as useful techniques as long as the patient tolerates them (Storre et al., 2009, 1477-1483).

DEAD SPACE

The other main challenge regarding interfaces is the amount of dead space that it adds to the system and its repercussion in the success of the technique.

A crucial distinction that should be made when talking about dead space and CO2 rebreathing is about the circuits. When ventilating a patient with a double-circuit ventilator, which always includes an expiratory valve, the risk of rebreathing disappears. It is in patients who are being ventilated with single-circuit ventilators, which do not include true expiratory valves, that dead space and its influence in the risk of rebreathing is an important concern, this is the case of the vast majority of patients treated with NIV.

In NIV dead space results of the physiological dead space from the air ways, unavoidable, plus the dynamic dead space of the apparatus. The interface, specifically its inner volume, and the circuit, both represent a sizeable addition of dynamic dead space which, as said previously, increases the chances of patient rebreathing in proportion to dead space volume.

Interface manufacturers are constantly developing different types of interfaces. Each type of interface has its own mechanical characteristics and its own internal volume and compliance. In the last 2 decades a large amount of studies have been made in order to evaluate the different interfaces, its dead space, internal volume and compliance and the risk of rebreathing. The main findings show that, despite the heterogeneity of the interfaces in mask internal volume, and despite previous beliefs, the resulting dynamic dead space and clinical efficacy of the interfaces is on average very similar.

Despite being always important, in patients with ARF it is especially significant to select the most adequate interface, the one that is going to be most helpful to the patient and at the same time the one that is going to generate less complications. As previously remarked, for ARF oronasal masks followed by total face masks are the most used ones. When analyzing these types of interfaces there is a big difference in internal volume, despite that, important studies have shown that, in ARF, not only they have the same clinical efficiency but also the ventilator settings do not have to be modified if we decide to interchange interfaces (Cuvelier et al., 2009, 519-526). These results suggest that masks should be selected in terms of functional dead space and that internal volume itself should not be a limiting factor for mask selection.

Mask Displacement

Despite selecting the adequate interface, interface-related complications might still happen. Unless the patient is under sedative medication head movement has to be considered because it can cause mask displacement. Not only movement, also beard, hair, pillows or sweat are elements that can disturb the interface placement and tolerance.

When assessing the interface and its possible related complications it is important to also asses the rest of the components that interact with it, the circuit and its state of cleanliness and repair, and specially the mask straps. Mask straps are really important for the patient tolerance of NVI. If the straps are too tight patient will refer pain and skin lesions may appear. On the other hand if mask straps are too loose the contact between the skin and the interface will lessen and air leaks will appear.

Conclusion

- There is no such thing as an ideal interface. Each patient and each situation should be assessed as many times as needed in order to select the adequate interface.
- In patients with ARF interface efficiency must prevail over patient comfort.
- In patients with CRF comfort and preventing interface related complications is key to long term tolerance of NIV.
- Limiting unintentional air leaks is vital for a successful NIV treatment.
- Masks should be selected in terms of functional dead space. Internal volume should not be a limiting factor for mask selection.

REFERENCES

Cabrini, L., C. Idone, S. Colombo, G. Monti, et al., 2009. "Medical Emergency Team and Non-Invasive Ventilation Outside ICU for Acute Respiratory Failure." *Intensive Care Medicine* 35 (2): 339-343.

Crimi, C., A. Noto, P. Princi, A. Esquinas, and S. Nava. 2010. "A European Survey of Noninvasive Ventilation Practices." *The European Respiratory Journal* 36 (2): 362-369.

Cuvelier, A., W. Pujol, S. Pramil, L. Molano, et al., 2009. "Cephalic Versus Oronasal Mask for Noninvasive Ventilation in Acute Hypercapnic Respiratory Failure." *Intensive Care Medicine* 35 (3): 519-526.

Elliott, M. W. 2004. "The Interface: Crucial for Successful Noninvasive Ventilation." *The European Respiratory Journal* 23 (1): 7-8.

Kysh, L. 2018. *Review Articles.* http://norris.usc.libguides.com/reviewarticles.

Mehta, S., F. D. McCool, and N. S. Hill. 2001. "Leak Compensation in Positive Pressure Ventilators: A Lung Model Study." *European Respiratory Journal* 17 (2): 259-267.

Nava, S., MD and N. Hill MD. 2009. "Non-Invasive Ventilation in Acute Respiratory Failure." *The Lancet,* 374 (9685): 250-259.

Pisani, L., A. Carlucci, and S. Nava. 2012. "Interfaces for Noninvasive Mechanical Ventilation: Technical Aspects and Efficiency." *Minerva Anestesiologica* 78 (10): 1154.

Schettino, G., S. Chatmongkolchart, D. Hess, and R. Kacmarek. 2003. "Position of Exhalation Port and Mask Design Affect CO2 Rebreathing during Noninvasive Positive Pressure Ventilation." *Critical Care Medicine* 31 (8): 2178-2182.

Sferrazza Papa, G. F., F. Di Marco, E. Akoumianaki, and L. Brochard. 2012. "Recent Advances in Interfaces for Non-Invasive Ventilation: From Bench Studies to Practical Issues." *Minerva Anestesiologica* 78 (10): 1146.

Storre, J. H., P. Bohm, M. Dreher, and W. Windisch. 2009. "Clinical Impact of Leak Compensation during Non-Invasive Ventilation." *Respiratory Medicine* 103 (10): 1477-1483.

In: Non-Invasive Mechanical Ventilation Complications ISBN: 978-1-53619-515-6
Editor: Antonio M. Esquinas

Chapter 13

Complications during Non-Invasive Mechanical Ventilation. Response, Carbon Dioxide Rebreathing

***Sara Abad Abad*[1,*], *Tina Herrero Jordan*[2] *and Luisa Cabrera Pimentel*[3]**

[1]Department of Pneumology, Alcañiz Hospital, Alcañiz, Teruel, Spain
[2]Department of Pneumology, Reina Sofía Hospital, Tudela, Navarra, Spain
[3]Department of Pneumology, General de la defensa Hospital, Zaragoza, Spain

Abstract

Non-invasive ventilation (NIV) is a therapy treatment that has been successfully applied for global respiratory failure. A cause of failure of non-invasive mechanical ventilation as therapy is rebreathing. It consists of rebreathing the expired air, which causes a poor removal of the carbon dioxide. It has a direct impact on the clinical worsening of the patient. The rebreathing of carbon dioxide is influenced by a large number of different factors such as the type of mask, the number of branches used in the ventilatory circuit, the level of espiratory positive airway pressure (EPAP), the tidal volume, the use of an expiratory port or an antirebreathing valve, the expiratory time, the respiratory rate of the patient and the degree of adaptation of the patient to non-invasive mechanical ventilation. The use of anti-rebreathing valves is recommended when using low EPAPs. If it is not possible to use an anti-rebreathing valve, EPAP greater than 8 cm H2O should be used to avoid rebreathing.

* Corresponding Author's E-mail: abadsara6@gmail.com.

Keywords: non-invasive ventilation, rebreathing, EPAP, air leak, anti-rebreathing valves

INTRODUCTION

Non-invasive ventilation (NIV) is a therapy that has been successfully applied as a treatment for global respiratory failure. It is a safe therapy but could have complications and side effects. The different possible causes for failure on non-invasive ventilation therapy should always be evaluated. One cause of failure of non-invasive mechanical ventilation is rebreathing.

Rebreaing consists of rebreathing the expired air causing a poor removal of carbon dioxide. It has a direct impact on the clinical worsening of the patient.

There are many factors that influence rebreathing of carbon dioxide (CO_2) such as the type of mask, the number of branches used in the ventilatory circuit, the level of espiratory positive airway pressure (EPAP) used, the tidal volume, the use of an expiratory port or an anti-rebreathing valve, the expiratory time, the respiratory rate of the patient and the degree of adaptation of the patient to non-invasive mechanical ventilation [1-4] (Table 1).

It is important to verify that the patient is well adapted to non-invasive ventilation. Besides, it is also required to verify that the chosen ventilation parameters are correct and that the mask is the best choice to avoid CO_2 rebreathing [4, 5].

Table 1. Factors Related to CO2 Removal

Type of mask used as an interface
Number of branches in the ventilatory circuit
Level of EPAP
Tidal volume
Expiratory port/anti-rebreathing valve
Expiratory time and respiratory rate
Degree of adaptation of the patient to non-invasive ventilation

Table 2. Methods Anti-Rebreathing

Increase EPAP
Expiratory port/antirebreathing valve in the ventilation circuit
Decrease air leakage
Decrease dead space

The most common methods to prevent rebreathing are: decrease air leakage in the ventilation circuit, decrease dead space, use an expiratory port or anti-rebreathing valve in the ventilation circuit or increase EPAP [1-4] (table 2).

Unlike invasive mechanical ventilation, non-invasive mechanical ventilation is not a hermetic ventilation system. The continuity solution between the airway and the ventilator is very important and justifies the ineffectiveness of non-invasive mechanical ventilation in some patients due to the existence of excessive air leaks.

Air leakage through the circuit influences the volume of air provided by the ventilation equipment and, therefore, the pressure levels reached. Excessive air leakage favors carbon dioxide retention, so it is important to control and minimize air leakage [5].

The mask used in non-invasive mechanical ventilation generates a dead space and therefore the rebreathing of CO_2. As such, the choice of mask is of great importance to avoid or minimize rebreathing of CO_2.

The mask should be watertight, non-compliant, with low flow resistance and minimal dead space. In addition to air leakage, rebreathing is one of the main problems posed by non-invasive ventilation [5].

There is an increased risk of rebreathing carbon dioxide if the ventilation equipment is turned off, if low EPAP levels are used, or if the air flow supplied by the ventilation equipment decreases to increase the resistance of the branch or exhalation port [1-5].

The use of anti-rebreathing valves is recommended when using low EPAPs. When it is below 2 cmH2O, 50% of the volume of current air supplied by the ventilation equipment remains stopped in the branch and this air would be re-inhaled. According to Lofaso, an EPAP of 5 cmH2O generates 20% of the rebreathing tidal volume, so lower EPAP values should not be used to ensure the removal of carbon dioxide. The anti-rebreathing valve should be placed as close to the mask as possible in the respiratory circuit. If an anti-rebreathing valve cannot be used, EPAP greater than 8 cmH2O should be used to avoid rebreathing [4].

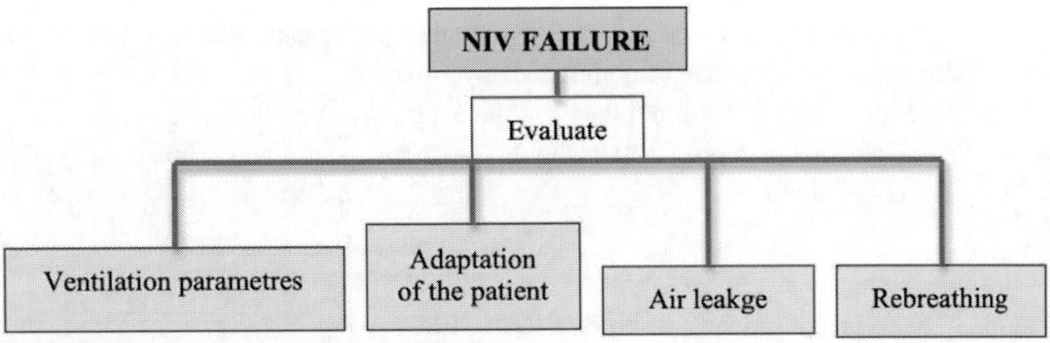

Figure 1.

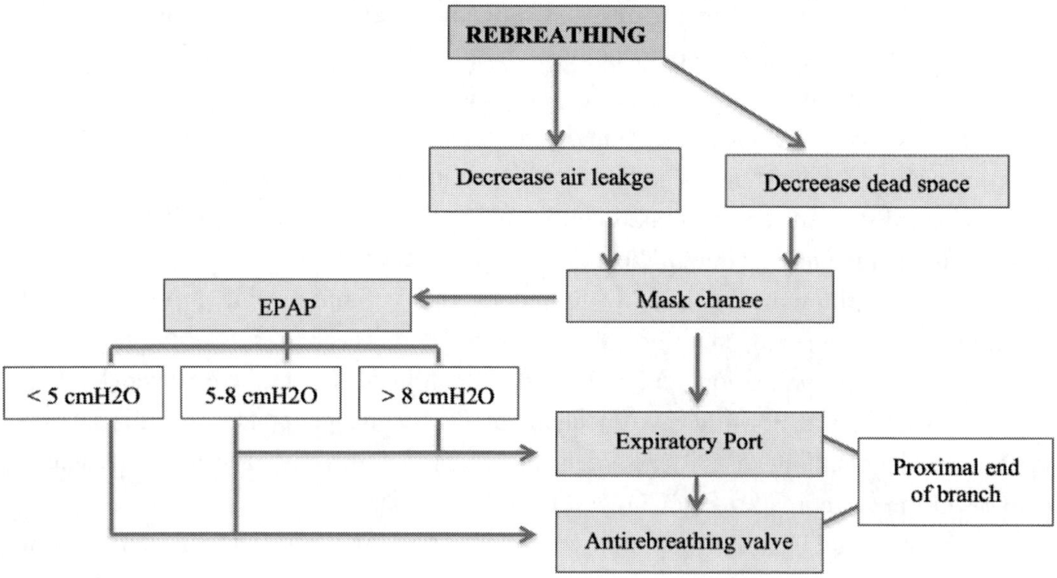

Figure 2.

Rebreathing occurs in ventilation equipment using a single branch in the ventilation circuit. Single branch ventilation equipment is the most widely used in the hospital. Under normal conditions, the pressure generated by the ventilation equipment drives a flow of fresh air through the branch of the ventilation circuit that removes CO2 exhaled through an exhalation port and minimizes rebreathing. Therefore, when using single branch ventilation equipment, you should always insert an exhalation port or an anti-rebreathing valve in the ventilation circuit to prevent rebreathing.

Key Messages

1. Rebreathing is a common cause of failure of non-invasive ventilation.
2. It is important to check: ventilatory parameters, mask used as interface and adaptation of the patient to non-invasive ventilation.
3. Air leakage should be minimized and the expiratory port should be checked.
4. To reduce rebreathing, EPAP should be increased or anti-rebreathing valves should be placed.

References

[1] Barrot Cortés, E., Sánchez Gómez, E., Coords. *Manual SEPAR de Procedimientos: Ventilación Mecánica no Invasiva.* Barcelona: Respira Fundación Española del

Pulmón-SEPAR; 2009. [*SEPAR Procedures Manual: Non-Invasive Mechanical Ventilation.*]

[2] Esquinas Rodríguez, A. M. ed. *Fundamentos de la Organización Hospitalaria en Ventilación Mecánica no Invasiva.* Murcia: Asociación y Escuela Internacional de Ventilación Mecánica no invasiva; 2011. [*Fundamentals of the Hospital Organization in Non-Invasive Mechanical Ventilation.*]

[3] European Respiratory Society. Non-invasive mechanical ventilation. *European Respiratory Monograph,* Vol 6. Monograph 16. Lausanne. European Respiratoy Society; 2001.

[4] Albani Perez, M., Abad Abad, S. Rebreathing en Ventilación Mecánica no Invasiva. En: Esquinas Rodríguez, A. M., coordinador. *Guía esencial de Metodología en Ventilación Mecánica no Invasiva.* 2ª ed. Madrid: Editorial Médica Panamericana; 2018. 144 - 146. [Rebreathing in Non-Invasive Mechanical Ventilation. In: Esquinas Rodríguez, A. M., coordinator. *Essential Guide to Non-Invasive Mechanical Ventilation Methodology*]

[5] Mediano, O., García-Río, F., Villasante, C. Comparación de la reinhalación de anhídrido carbónico originada por 3 mascarillas nasales durante la aplicación de CPAP. *Arch. Bronconeumol.,* 2006; 42(4):189 - 93. [Comparison of carbon dioxide rebreathing caused by 3 nasal masks during CPAP application. *Arch. Bronconeumol*]

In: Non-Invasive Mechanical Ventilation Complications ISBN: 978-1-53619-515-6
Editor: Antonio M. Esquinas

Chapter 14

COMPLICATIONS DURING NON-INVASIVE MECHANICAL VENTILATION. PATIENT–VENTILATOR ASYNCHRONY

Giuseppe Fiorentino[1,*], MD, Anna Annunziata[2], MD and Maurizia Lanza[2], MD
[1]Head of Unit of Respiratory Physiopathology, Monaldi Hospital, Naples, Italy
[2]Unit of Respiratory Physiopathology, Monaldi Hospital, Naples, Italy

ABSTRACT

Assisted mechanical ventilation (MV) is applied early, following the critical stage of the critical disease, to eliminate the injurious consequences of controlled MV, most reputably the rise of ventilator-induced diaphragmatic dysfunction. The development of patient-ventilator asynchrony often counteracts the advantages of assisted MV. Patient-ventilator asynchrony happens when both the beginning and/or finish of mechanical breath is not in time accord with the beginning and finish of neural inspiration, respectively, or if the measurement of mechanical assist does not respond to the patient's respiratory need. As patient-ventilator asynchrony has been correlated with several adverse results and can unfavourably impact patient result, every effort should be performed to identify and change this occurrence at the bedside. Patient-ventilator asynchrony is usual during mechanical ventilation. Asynchrony reduces the comfort, increases mechanical ventilation and intensive care unit stays, and it could lead to worse results. To identify patient-ventilator dyssynchronies, the physician should estimate patient comfort and carefully investigate the pressure and flowtime waveforms, accessible on the ventilator screen of every modern ventilators. Contemporary ventilators give several modifiable settings to promote patient-ventilator synergy. New comparative modes of ventilation are likewise very helpful in enhancing patient-ventilator interaction.

* Corresponding Author's E-mail: giuseppefiorentino1@gmail.com.

Keywords: asynchrony, mechanical ventilation, assisted mechanical ventilation, critical illness

INTRODUCTION

Mechanical ventilation (MV) can be divided in two principal sections: controlled MV, where the act of breathing is completely controlled by the ventilator and assisted MV, where the patients' respiratory mode and the ventilator work concomitantly. Controlled ventilation is principally used for short times, particularly during the critical phase of illness. There are no contraindications to sedation decrease and the patient is able to breathe spontaneously, an assisted ventilator mode is utilised. This practice has been dictated by a excess of evidence affirming the detrimental effects of controlled MV and associated respiratory muscles inactivation, most distinctly the improvement of ventilator-induced diaphragmatic dysfunction [1, 2]. Contrariwise, assisted ventilation is correlated with diminished dose and duration of sedation and reduced used of neuromuscular blockade which have been shown to improve hemodynamic stability, decrease the risk of critical illness polyneuropathy, improve gas exchange and decrease the duration of MV [3]. With the start of assisted MV, two completely different systems are called to cooperate: the respiratory system and the ventilator. The condition of their interaction, temporal and quantitative, is required for MV to be advantageous and is described by the Greek word "synchrony." Patient-ventilator synchrony happens when the ventilator gives flow and pressure as soon as patient effort begins; the magnitude of this pressure and flow meets patient respiratory request; and the ventilator assistance is terminated when patient effort ends. Whenever any of the above is not fulfilled, patient-ventilator asynchrony occurs. Adverse effects of patient-ventilator asynchrony include: increased work of breathing, patient discomfort, alveolar overdistention and lung injury, sleep disturbances, periodic breathing, optional use of sedation and excessive unloading of the diaphragm leading to ventilator-induced diaphragmatic dysfunction [4]. To detect patient-ventilator dyssynchronies, the physician should assess patient comfort and carefully examine the pressure- and flow-time waveforms, accessible on the ventilator screen of all modern ventilators.

BASIC PRINCIPLES OF ASSISTED VENTILATION

To understand the necessary waveforms and subsequently to recognize patient-ventilator dyssynchronies, it is valuable to consider the basic principles recording the operation of assisted ventilator modes. Three variables define the function of a positive pressure ventilator: the triggering variable, the variable that measures the delivered pressure or flow throughout the mechanical inspiration, and the cycling off variable. The triggering variable is the sign that begins the mechanical breath. In assisted ventilation, the most usually used triggering variables are flow and pressure. Mechanical inspiration begins during patient inspiratory effort reduces both the flow (flow triggering) or the pressure (pressure triggering) in the ventilator circuit. It is commonly believed that flow triggering is more favourable to the patient regarding the work of breathing because the pressure triggering requires isometric contraction of the respiratory muscles. Nevertheless, studies have revealed that, in the modern ventilators, there are minimum variations, if any, concerning the work of breathing within the two ways of triggering [5]. Other triggering variables combine flow waveform, volume, transdiaphragmatic pressure (Pdi)-driven servo-ventilation and the electromyographic activity of the diaphragm (neurally adjusted ventilator assist [NAVA]) but their use in clinical application is restricted [6]. The variable that controls the pressure and flow delivery distinguishes the various assisted MV modes [7]. In assist volume control, the ventilator delivers a preset tidal volume with a preset flow-time profile. These are the independent variables, while the airway pressure (Paw) needed to deliver the preset flow and volume depends on the mechanical properties of the respiratory system and is the dependent variable. In pressure control or pressure support, the ventilator delivers a preset pressure (independent variable). The dependent variables on pressure-preset modes are the volume and flow. These variables change according to the mechanical properties of the respiratory system and the pressure delivered. In proportional modes of ventilation, no variable is preset: the ventilator delivers support which is proportional to patient inspiratory effort. The later is expressed either through changes in instantaneous flow and volume (proportional assist ventilation [PAV]) or through changes in the neural activity of the diaphragm (NAVA) [8]. The cycling off variable is defined as the signal of terminating the delivery phase. The frequent cycling off criterion in assisted pressure-preset modes of MV is airway pressure or flow: the ventilator terminates assist and opens the expiratory valve when Paw increases or flow decreases to a preset criterion. Another cycling off criteria is time, volume and the flow-waveform method. Ideally, the cycling off should coincide with the end of neural inspiration. However, this fact rarely, if ever, happens and an expiratory asynchrony is a popular event with all conventional modes of assisted ventilation. With pressure-preset modes, the rise time is a setting that determines how fast the ventilator will reach the selected Paw. It is available in the new generation ventilators during pressure support and pressure control ventilation. Fast-rising time is associated with a sharp increase in inspiratory flow and may cause pressure overshoot and promote dyspnoea. A rounded shaped inspiratory flow may recognize prolonged rising time. Both the low and high rise time may alter the mechanical inspiratory time, and the volume delivered and may provoke dissociation within mechanical and neural inspiration [9]. Considering there are no rules for setting an optimal beginning time, both very rapid and slow rise time should be avoided, and rising time should be adjusted according to patient respiratory drive [9].

Patient-Ventilator Dyssynchronies

Patient-ventilator dyssynchronies can be classified into two major categories: dyssynchronies that happen because neural breath is not in phase with the mechanical breath. This group comprises: triggering delay, ineffective efforts, auto triggering, reverse triggering, delayed opening of the expiratory valve, early opening of the expiratory valve, double triggering, and breath stacking and dyssynchronies compared to a discrepancy within the level of assist that the subject demands and the actual assist that the ventilator provides.

The Causes of Patient-Ventilator Asynchrony

Wasted Effort

Work of breathing increases because:

- The mode is necessary, but the patient is conscious and fighting the ventilator;
  - The effort is wasted if the patient tries to end a breath (straining to exhale against a closed expiratory valve)
  - The effort is wasted when the patient tries to begin a breath (straining to inhale against a closed inspiratory valve)
- The trigger is too high, and the ventilator fails to supply gas when the patient requires it.
- Inadequate level of support: the flow rate is too low, and it does not meet the patient request.
- The auto-PEEP is too high, and the patient spends much effort trying to defeat it

Auto-Triggering

Something other than the patient's respiratory application initiates a breath, e.g., cardiac oscillations

Double-Triggering, Premature Breath Termination

The ventilator delivers an inappropriately short breath, and the patient wants more air.

DELAY OF TRIGGERING AND INEFFECTIVE EFFORTS

Triggering delay is the period within the start of the neural and mechanical inspiration [8]. Ineffective efforts are patient's efforts that fail to activate trigger the ventilator. Although generally defined as a triggering associated asynchrony, ineffective efforts can happen at any time through the mechanical breath, during mechanical inspiration, expiration or at the passage between these two statuses. The gold standard for their classification is the contemporary observation of the patient inspiratory movement. In most significant cases, ineffective efforts can be recognised non-invasively at the bedside, by following the flow-time and Paw-time waveforms at the ventilator screen. Ineffective efforts produce distortions in the Paw and, more positively, in the flow curve: an irregular increase in inspiratory flow and a decrease in expiratory flow show the presence of ineffective efforts through mechanical inspiration and expiration, sequentially [9]. Triggering delay and ineffective efforts share common pathophysiological mechanisms. Their causes can be classified into two main categories: ventilator settings and patients' characteristics [10]. Ventilator settings that predispose to triggering delay and ineffective efforts are the high assist level, the delayed opening of the expiratory valve and the low triggering sensitivity. The physician determines these factors. The primary patients' characteristics include low respiratory drive (i.e., sedation, central nervous diseases, etc.), weak inspiratory muscles (i.e., critical illness polyneuropathy, myasthenia, etc.), and high resistance and compliance that increase the time constant of the respiratory system. The incidence and the magnitude of the delay of triggering and ineffective efforts are not minor in clinical practice. Ineffective efforts are the most prevalent form of patient-ventilator asynchrony. Vaporidi et al. [11] evaluated the role of ineffective efforts, particularly clusters of them, during MV on the outcome of critically ill patients. Events of ineffective efforts were identified in 38% of patients with extended MV, and these events were associated with prolonged MV and increased mortality. Their incidence is higher in patients with obstructive lung disease. In these patients, the low elastic recoil pressure and/or increased resistance increase the time required for the patient to exhale (high time constant), predisposing to air trapping and dynamic hyperinflation. Dynamic hyperinflation is the most significant problem of triggering delay and ineffective efforts. In the presence of dynamic hyperinflation, an elastic threshold load (PEEPi) is imposed on the inspiratory muscles at the beginning of inspiration. The inspiratory muscles must first counterbalance PEEPi to decrease alveolar pressure below external positive end-expiratory pressure (PEEPe) and trigger the ventilator. This creates a delay among the beginning of inspiratory effort and ventilator triggering. In severe cases of dynamic hyperinflation, especially if the effort is weak, the patient may fail to trigger the ventilator (ineffective effort). High airway resistance can be recognized in all ventilator modes by observing the expiratory flowtime curve. Early in expiration, a spike in expiratory flow signifies the dynamic compression of central airways [11]. After that, the expiratory flow decreases but very slowly, if ever, returns to zero lines before the following inspiration (Figures 2).

Delayed or missed triggers represent eccentric contractions of the diaphragm which may be deleterious for its function. They may cause distress, and in their presence, the respiratory rate on the ventilator screen does not reflect the exact respiratory rate of the patient. Strategies, to reduce the triggering delay and the number of ineffective efforts, should be investigated. Firstly, ventilator settings should be revised. Setting the most sensitive triggering that does not cause auto triggering is an option. About triggering sensitivity, it has been shown that the flow-waveform method [6], compared to flow triggering, enhances the sensitivity and thus reduces the incidence of these events. Ventilator settings that decrease dynamic hyperinflation and, hence, triggering delay and ineffective efforts are reduction of minute ventilation by lowering assist (decrease set pressure, set tidal volume) and respiratory rate decrease, lengthening expiratory time through a higher flow. Ventilator settings that decrease dynamic hyperinflation and, hence, triggering delay and ineffective efforts are: reduction of minute ventilation by lowering assist (decrease set pressure, set tidal volume) and respiratory rate decrease, lengthening expiratory time through a higher flow threshold for cycling off and a faster rising time in pressure support or a higher inspiratory flow and a shorter plateau inspiratory pressure in assist volume control mode and application of PEEPe.

The PEEPe narrows the distinction within the alveolar pressure and the threshold of pressure for the beginning of the mechanical inspiration, hence improving the patient to trigger the ventilator. This is particularly helpful in some subjects with severe obstructive lung disease [12]. Secondly, patient-related conditions should be evaluated. Consideration should be provided in respiratory drive and the factors that may reduce it, such as unreasonable sedation and alkalemia. Efforts to minimise the consequence of dynamic hyperinflation also should be made, in instance the use of corticosteroids, bronchodilating treatment and aspiration of secretions may occur in reduced expiratory resistance.

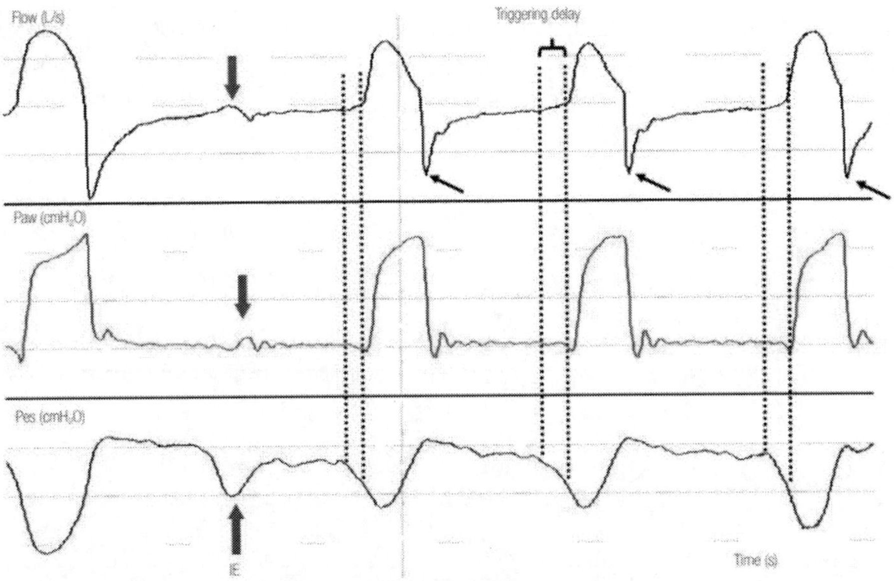

Figure 1. This is ineffective effort (IE) during expiration and is manifested by a slight decrease in Paw associated with a simultaneous decrease in expiratory flow (red arrows).

AUTOTRIGGERING

Autotriggering happens if the ventilator is triggered in the loss of patient effort. This event can also be identified by examination of the ventilator waveforms. The lack of decrease in Pes (if it is monitored) or in Paw before the delivery phase, especially in the presence of a zero flow long just before the mechanical breath, are indications that the patient does not trigger the breath. The flow-time profile of the autotriggered breaths is, usually, different from the corresponding of patient-triggered breaths (Figure 2). If secretions or cardiac oscillations are the event, one might notice the associate flow distortion and suspect the phenomenon. A low threshold may cause autotriggering for triggering and/or artefacts that may cause a drop of Paw or flow, which is misinterpreted by the ventilator as patient effort. Artefacts that commonly cause autotriggering are circuit leaks, presence of water in the circuit, hiccups and stable cardiogenic oscillators [12]. Factors that predispose a patient to increased risk of autotriggering are the low respiratory drive and breathing frequency, the low time constant of the respiratory system (increased elastic recoil, low resistance) and the presence of hyperdynamic circulation (more massive cardiac output and higher ventricular filling pressures). Autotriggering is a common phenomenon during assisted modes of MV (invasive and non-invasive) [13]. When apparent, the respiratory rate is falsely elevated. These additional breaths may lead to hyperventilation, respiratory alkalosis, hyperinflation, and diaphragmatic dysfunction. To eliminate autotriggering, the physician must try to repair the underlying cause:

enhance the respiratory drive by reducing sedation, correct alkalosis by reducing the level of assist, aspirate secretions, and minimize circuit leaks. Moreover, a higher triggering threshold, or change from flow to pressure triggering may abolish autotriggered breaths [12].

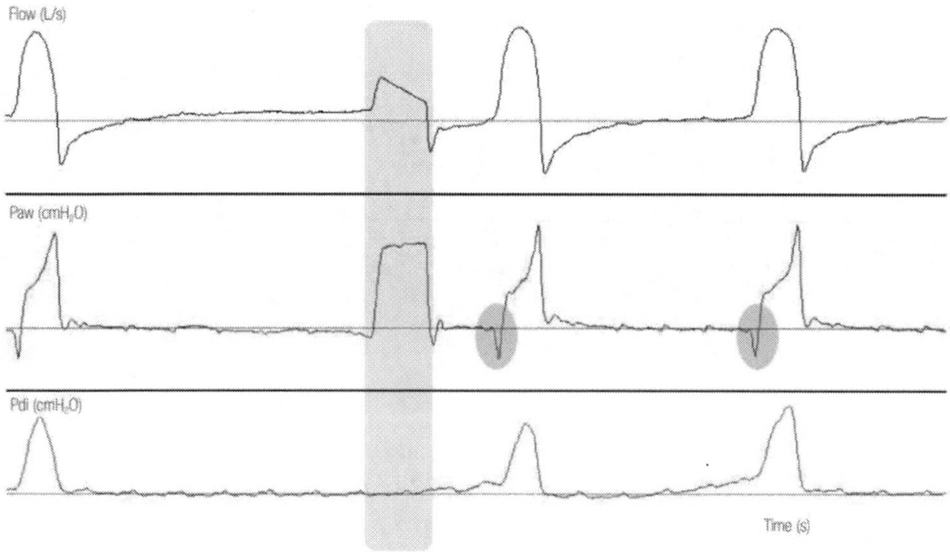

Figure 2. In comparison to patient-triggered breaths, where a decrease in Paw is observed before the start of mechanical inflation (grey shaded areas), there is no distortion in the Paw- (no decrease in Paw) and flow-time curve in the autotriggered breath.

PREMATURE CYCLING OFF

During the exhalation valve of the ventilator opens excessively early, mechanical inspiration lasts more abbreviated than neural inspiration. This kind of asynchrony is usually correlated with insufficient support. Inspiratory muscle effort next the end of ventilator insufflation improves the work of breathing and puts the subject at risk for double triggering. The asynchrony can perform with the following ways [8]. Zero or small inspiratory flow for any time after the opening of the exhalation valve (Paw decreases to zero or PEEP level) means that inspiratory muscles extend to contract following the end of mechanical inspiration. A sharp decrease from the peak expiratory flow which lasts few milliseconds followed by an improvement and then declines gradually to zero toward the end of expiration: this pattern in the flow-time waveform is also a sign that significant inspiratory muscle activity is started after the opening of exhalation valve. When mechanical inspiration ends, end-inspiratory elastic recoil pressure is more significant than inspiratory muscle pressure, creating positive alveolar pressure and, consequently, expiratory flow. Elastic recoil pressure declines while lung volume declines due to inspiratory muscle contraction. Increasing opposing pressure to expiratory flow occurs, causing an abrupt decrease in expiratory flow. This decrease is interrupted by the relaxation of the inspiratory muscles and expiratory flow increases and, therefore, follows the route as determined by the elastic recoil pressure and resistance of the patient and expiratory circuit [8].

Double (or Multiple) Triggering

This refers to the delivery of two (or even more) ventilator insufflations during one single inspiratory effort. The inspiratory muscle contraction is significant sufficient to overcome the elastic recoil pressure of the respiratory system and trigger the ventilator multiple times. Premature cycling is associated with appropriate ventilator settings, such as low level of assist, a comparatively high threshold for cycling off and short inflation time. The short time constant of the respiratory system and long neural inspiration time are influencing factors for this asynchrony. Furthermore, risk factors for multiple triggering are the low elastic recoil at the end of mechanical inflation and the intense inspiratory muscle activity [7-8]. As already mentioned, the early opening of the exhalation valve is related to increased work of breathing. Moreover, double triggering may provoke high tidal volumes (up to twice of the predetermined value) putting the patient at risk of ventilation-induced lung injury and ventilation-induced diaphragmatic dysfunction. Premature opening of the expiratory valve and related various triggering can be minimized either by increasing the mechanical inspiration time and, if possible, by decreasing the neural inspiration time. The latter should be recognised in patients with prolonged inspiratory efforts due to excessive administration of opioids. Actions that increase the mechanical inflation time include the lower flow threshold for cycling, the higher support and the slower rising time with pressure support mode [8]. With control modes, higher duration of mechanical inspiration should be easily achieved by proper regulation of ventilator settings, such as inspiratory time, inspiratory flow or application of end-inspiratory pause [8].

Delayed Cycling Off

While the exhalation valve opens too late, mechanical inspiration increases into neural expiration. This may support rigorous expiratory muscle activity and enhance the work of breathing as the patient struggles to end inspiration. Moreover, it may optionally improve the delivered tidal volume and reduce the possible expiratory time. These results may promote dynamic hyperinflation and associated dyssynchronies (delayed triggering, ineffective efforts), particularly in patients by obstructive lung condition or provoke lung overdistention. Recognition of the limited opening of the exhalation valve is, often, challenging. When pressure support mode, it can be shown by the fast reduction of the inspiratory flow accompanied by an exponential decline towards the end of mechanical inspiration [8]. An abrupt development (spike) of the Paw near the end of mechanical inspiration is both a manifestation of inspiratory muscle relaxation or expiratory muscle contraction [14]. Whichever is the cause, this spike is evidence of delayed cycling off (Figure 3).

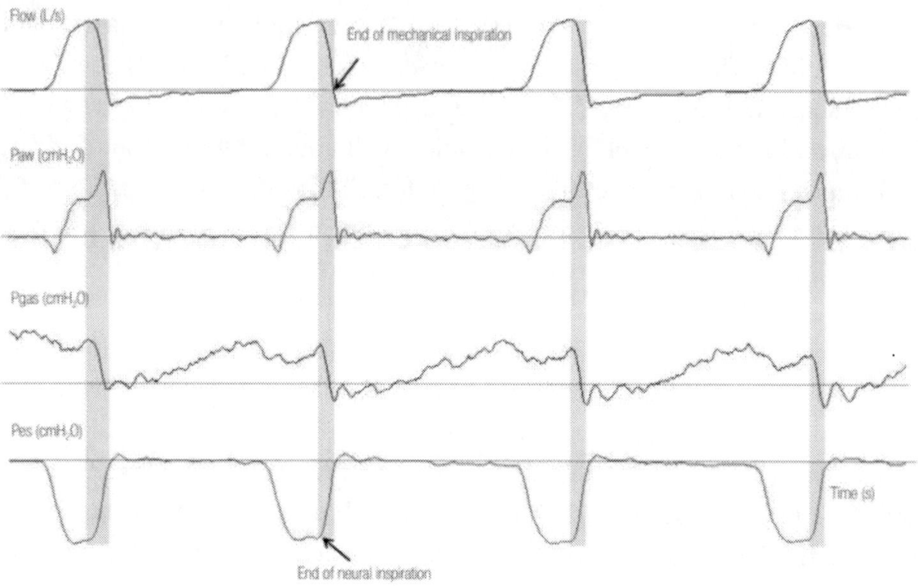

Figure 3. Significant time delay (blue shaded area) between the end of neural inspiration, recognized by a rapid increase in Pes, and the end of mechanical inspiration, signified by the termination of inspiratory flow (inspiratory flow equals zero).

With assist-volume control ventilation, the acute rise of Paw towards the end of mechanical breath means that mechanical inspiration is more extended than neural. Low flow origin for cycling off, great support and quiet rise time are influencing factors for this asynchrony during pressure support ventilation. Among assisted volume control mode, high tidal volume, improved inflation time, low inspiratory flow and application of end-inspiratory stop may cause delayed opening of the exhalation valve. With pressure support mode, delayed availability of the expiratory valve is generally approved in patients with a long time constant of respiratory systems, such as in patients with chronic obstructive lung diseases. Changes of the ventilator settings should be combined by actions that minimize the airway resistance and dynamic hyperinflation (i.e., bronchodilation, steroid therapy, aspiration of secretions).

REVERSE TRIGGERING

Reverse triggering was reported initially by Akoumianaki et al. [45] who recognised, in a group of slowly sedated patients, the episodes of patient inspiratory efforts that were triggered by the ventilator. That event, known as respiratory entrainment, has been earlier reported in animals, healthy subjects and preterm babies. It varies from the different types of dyssynchronies in that the patient completely misses its natural breathing variability and really breaths like a machine, exhibiting a fixed temporary connection (1:1 or, less commonly, 1:2 or 1:3) within the start of his inspiratory efforts and the onset of mechanical breaths. Vagal feedback and cortical influences are implicated in the pathophysiological mechanism of these events. Reverse triggered breaths may happen at any phase of the respiratory cycle and for variable periods. Their attention, when Pes or EAdi recording is unavailable, is often complicated and needs careful inspection of the Paw- and flow-time waveforms. Depending on the phase of the mechanical breath that they occur, they may induce isometric or eccentric contractions of the respiratory muscles, augment the increased tidal volume in pressure targeted modes or even trigger second breaths (breath stacking) producing hyperventilation and improving the risk for lung overdistention (Figure 4).

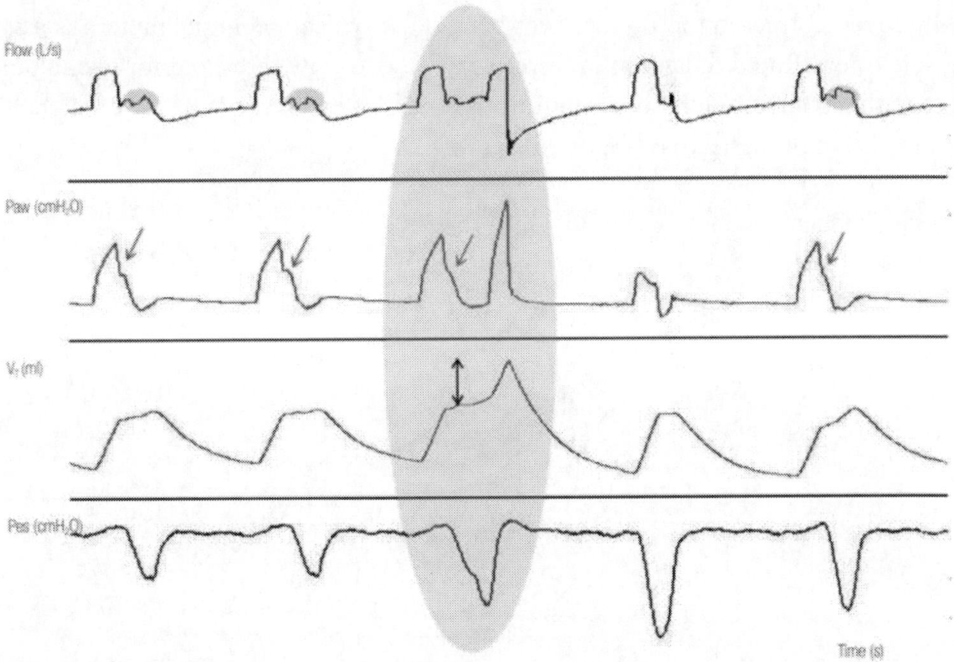

Figure 4. Reverse triggering in a patient ventilated with assist volume control ventilation. Esophageal pressure (Pes) decrease reveals patient inspiratory efforts (blue line) after every mechanical inflation in 1:1 relationship.

DYSYNCHRONIES RELATED TO A DISCREPANCY BETWEEN THE NEEDS OF THE PATIENT AND THE VENTILATOR ASSIST

Inapplicable assist level (inadequate or excessive assist) including regard to patients' ventilator needs is a different cause of patient-ventilator asynchrony [8]. Insufficient assist level is habitually recognised in patients with high requirements and improved respiratory drive (i.e., sepsis and metabolic acidosis). This mistake is connected with enhanced work of breathing, and usually, the clinical status of the patient is indicative (i.e., use of accessory respiratory muscles, high respiratory rate). Excessive assist level is typically an outcome of low respiratory drive and/or improper ventilator settings, yet the conflicting issues of this opposition are essential. Dynamic hyperinflation, respiratory alkalosis, periodic breathing pattern due to a more moderate apnoeic threshold, sleep disorders, ventilator-induced diaphragmatic dysfunction and/or lung damage are possible results of high assist. By examining the waveforms of Paw or flow, the respiratory effort in relationship to assist level can be estimated [8]. Paw reductions during the inspiratory muscles contract and increases when the expiratory muscles contract. Paw is more sensitive in assist-volume control ventilation because it is the dependent variable. Although in pressure targeted methods Paw should remain relatively constant, its shape may modify when the respiratory muscles contract rigorously (Figure 5).

Moreover, correct in the flow pattern behind the typical declining pattern is a symbol of muscle effort. Rapid reduction in inspiratory flow to flow threshold for cycling off in a subject with moderately long time uniform is a sign of expiratory muscle contraction and therefore, a sign of high assist (Figure 6).

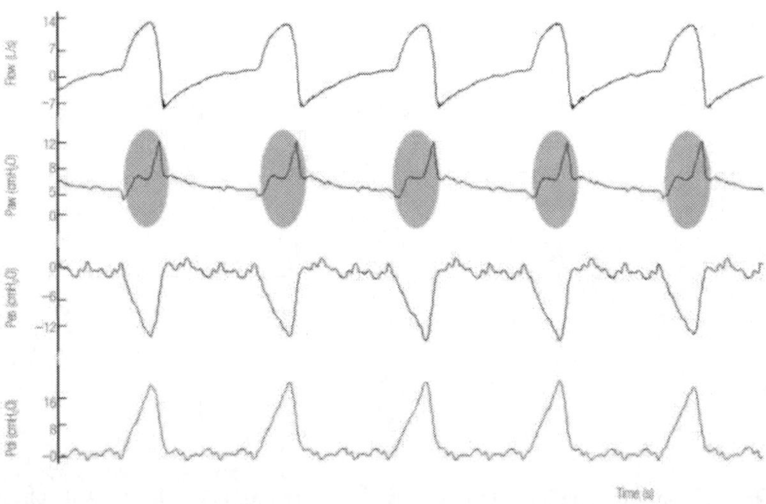

Figure 5. Rounded flow and Paw decrease are signs of low ventilator assist with respect to patients ventilator demands.

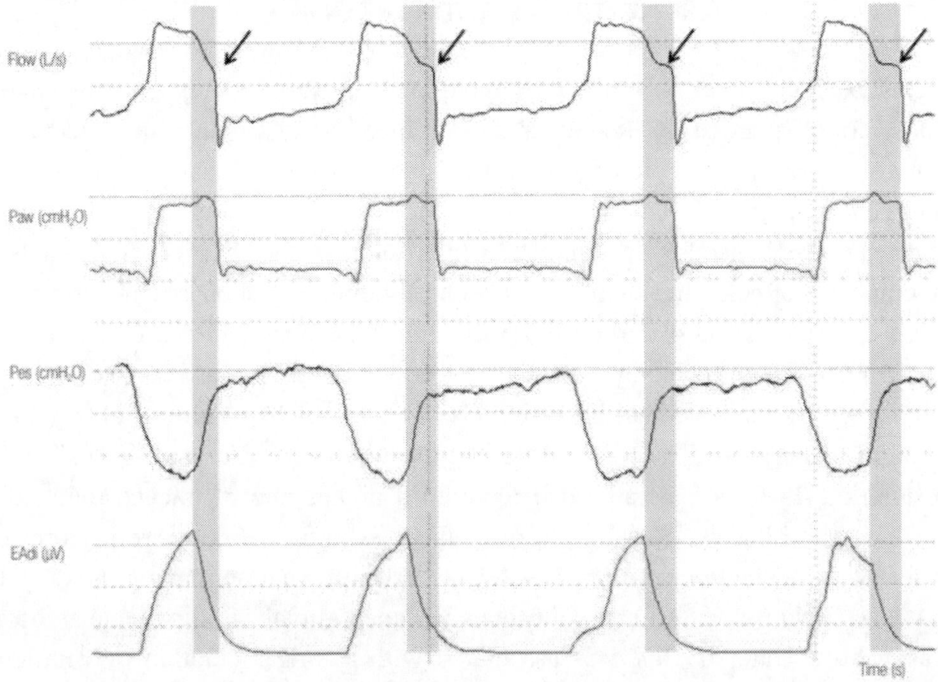

Figure 6. High assist in a patient ventilated with pressure support ventilation.

The Management of Patient-Ventilator Asynchrony

What to do?

- Proceed the mode patient-triggered
- Adjust trigger sensitivity to combine patient efforts and exclude cardiac auto-triggering
- Improve flow rate if it is unequal
- Manage the auto-PEEP
- Increase flow cycle-off to a higher value, terminating a breath early if the patient wants shorter breaths
- Reduce the flow cycle-off to a lower value if the patient requires longer breaths
- Clear the airway of sputum and secretions, and ensure its patency
- Increasethe sedation
- Use neuromuscular blockade

ASYNCHRONY AND OUTCOME

The existence and severity of asynchrony are associated with lengthened mechanical ventilation, more extended ICU stay, and mortality. Yet, we do not understand if asynchrony only serves as a pointer of the severity of disease or if asynchrony effects in prolonged continuation of ventilation. Corporations find it engaging to say that if asynchrony can be enhanced by new methods, the results can be changed. But, synchrony has no therapeutic effects, and increasing synchrony does not support better outcomes. Chao et al. described in 174 chronically ventilator-dependent patients that those with ineffective triggered breaths required a longer duration of mechanical ventilation (70 d vs 33 d) and a lower rate of eventual liberation (16% vs 57%) [16]. Thille et al. reaffirmed an association of prolonged mechanical ventilation with an asynchrony index [1] 10% (median duration 25 d vs 9 d) and also reported a higher rate of tracheostomy in the asynchrony group (33% vs 4%) [10]. Both of these essential works were performed in older critically ill medical populations (69–75 y old), with a quarter having the diagnosis of COPD. The study by de Wit and colleagues included a total of 60 patients and found that an asynchrony rate of 10% was associated with a longer duration of ventilation, reduced ventilator-free survival, and more prolonged ICU and hospital stay. The report by Robinson et al. in trauma patients does not demonstrate any variation in the duration of ventilation, ICU stays, or mortality in those patients with an asynchrony index 10% [17]. These findings likely represent the difference in indications for mechanical ventilation and type of respiratory dysfunction.

CONCLUSION

Assisted MV offers essential benefits over-controlled MV, but consideration should be paid on the presence of patient-ventilator asynchrony. Patient-ventilator asynchrony is universal; it may occur at any period of the respiratory cycle and can be due to time miscalculations or ventilator assist/respiratory demand discrepancies between the patient and the ventilator. It is associated with diverse unwanted effects and, may unfavourably affect the outcome. The gold standard for their acceptance is the documentation of patient effort. However, in several cases, careful examination of the ventilator screen, along with the clinical picture of the patient is adequate for the physician to recognize patient-ventilator dyssynchronies. Modern ventilators offer several modifiable settings to better patient-ventilator synergy. New comparable modes of ventilation are also significant in promoting.

REFERENCES

[1] Petrof BJ, Jaber S, Matecki S. Ventilator-induced diaphragmatic dysfunction. *Curr Opin Crit Care* 2010;16:19-25.

[2] Levine S, Nguyen T, Taylor N, Friscia ME, Budak MT, Rothenberg P, et al. Rapid disuse atrophy of diaphragm fibers in mechanically ventilated humans. *N Engl J Med* 2008;358:1327-35.

[3] Putensen C, Zech S, Wrigge H, Zinserling J, Stüber F, Von Spiegel T, et al. Long-term effects of spontaneous breathing during ventilatory support in patients with acute lung injury. *Am J Respir Crit Care Med* 2001;164:43-9.

[4] Blanch L, Villagra A, Sales B, Montanya J, Lucangelo U, Luján M, et al. Asynchronies during mechanical ventilation are associated with mortality. *Intensive Care Med* 2015;41:633-41.

[5] Elvira-Markela Antonogiannaki, Dimitris Georgopoulos, Evangelia Akoumianaki. Patient-Ventilator Asynchrony. Korean. Published online: 30 November 2017. *J Crit Care Med* 2017; 32(4): 307-322.

[6] Prinianakis G, Kondili E, Georgopoulos D. Effects of the flow waveform method of triggering and cycling on patient-ventilator interaction during pressure support. *Intensive Care Med* 2003;29:1950-9.

[7] Kondili E, Xirouchaki N, Georgopoulos D. Modulation and treatment of patient-ventilator asynchrony. *Curr Opin Crit Care* 2007;13:84-9.

[8] Georgopoulos D, Prinianakis G, Kondili E. Bedside waveforms interpretation as a tool to identify patient-ventilator asynchronies. *Intensive Care Med* 2006;32:34-47.

[9] Chiumello D, Pelosi P, Calvi E, Bigatello LM, Gattinoni L. Different modes of assisted ventilation in patients with acute respiratory failure. *Eur Respir J* 2002;20:925-33.

[10] Thille AW, Rodriguez P, Cabello B, Lellouche F, Brochard L. Patient-ventilator asynchrony during assisted mechanical ventilation. *Intensive Care Med.* 2006; 32:1515–22.

[11] Vaporidi K, Babalis D, Chytas A, Lilitsis E, Kondili E, Amargianitakis V, et al. Clusters of ineffective efforts during mechanical ventilation: impact on outcome. *Intensive Care Med* 2017;43:184-91.

[12] Vitacca M, Bianchi L, Zanotti E, Vianello A, Barbano L, Porta R, et al. Assessment of physiologic variables and subjective comfort under different levels of pressure support ventilation. *Chest* 2004;126:851-9.

[13] Carteaux G, Lyazidi A, Cordoba-Izquierdo A, Vignaux L, Jolliet P, Thille AW, et al. Patient-ventilator asynchrony during noninvasive ventilation: a bench and clinical study. *Chest.* 2012; 142:367–76.

[14] Prinianakis G, Plataki M, Kondili E, Klimathianaki M, Vaporidi K, Georgopoulos D. Effects of relaxation of inspiratory muscles on ventilator pressure during pressure support. *Intensive Care Med.* 2008; 34:70–4.

[15] Akoumianaki E, Lyazidi A, Rey N, Matamis D, PerezMartinez N, Giraud R, et al. Mechanical ventilation induced reverse-triggered breaths: a frequently unrecognized form of neuromechanical coupling. *Chest* 2013;143:927-38.

[16] Chao DC, Scheinhorn DJ, Stearn-Hassenpflug M. Patient-ventilatortrigger asynchrony in prolonged mechanical ventilation. *Chest* 1997; 112(6):1592-1599.

[17] Robinson BRH, Blakeman TC, Toth P, Hanseman DJ, Mueller E, Branson RD. Patient ventilator asynchrony in a traumatically in- jured population. *Respir Care* 2013.

In: Non-Invasive Mechanical Ventilation Complications ISBN: 978-1-53619-515-6
Editor: Antonio M. Esquinas

Chapter 15

NON INVASIVE MECHANICAL VENTILATOR. TECHNOLOGY FOR SAFETY APPLICATIONS

Carmen Rosa Vargas Arévalo
Hospital Clinic de Barcelona, Emergency service, Hospital de Palamós, Pneumology and Non-Invasive Mechanical Ventilation service, Barcelona, Spain

ABSTRACT

Non-invasive Mechanical Ventilation has had an exponential advance in the last four decades, offering us great advantages for the treatment of ventilatory support in patients with both acute and chronic respiratory failure.

It avoids in many cases to arrive to invasive ventilation; and we can control and monitor with the different ventilatory parameters that it has.

In the recent years, many technological advances have been added with different NIV equipment that allows us to perform an optimal and narrow monitoring of the ventilatory parameters, up to the point where it is possible to carry out telemonitoring and to connect telematically with these equipment and to be able to assess the various ventilatory parameters, make the corresponding adjustments in a safe manner, as well as to assess compliance, adhesion, evolution, detect early and treat acute exacerbation, disease progression, minimize and treat adverse effects and avoid complications.

1. INTRODUCTION

Non-Invasive Mechanical Ventilation (NIMV) is a great tool that allows us to provide respiratory support without reaching to invasive techniques, and that improves the quality of life of patients.

Delaubier and Rideau's description of a patient with Duchenne disease, effectively ventilated through a nasal mask, marked the beginning of a new era in the history of non-invasive mechanical ventilation.

In these last four decades, we are witnessing an important technological advance in NIMV [1].

2. Advantages of NIMV and the Path to New Technologies

NIMV has several advantages: the patient can stay awake, sedation is not usually required, the patient can speak or communicate, cough and expectorate, it facilitates an early weaning, avoids muscular atrophy and especially avoids large bronchial and parenchymal injuries resulting from high pressures and excessive volumes that could cause invasive ventilation.

In addition, decreases the morbidity and mortality rate, shortens the hospital stay and allows its continuity in an extra-hospital environment.

It is essential to monitor what happens between the patient and the ventilator using basic and advanced methods [2], monitoring and adjusting the entire system, from pressure management, interfaces, hours of use, etc.

Both, the decision to provide non-invasive ventilatory support according to the pathology to be treated, as well as the choice of ventilatory modes and their monitoring with dynamic adjustment of pressures and volumes, will depend on the success or failure of this treatment [3].

3. Use of Modern Technologies for NIMV Monitoring

We will discuss below all the technological tools that allow us to provide a NIMV more safely and avoid side effects and/or complications.

3.1. Patient Monitoring Patient

Follow-up is essential to assess compliance with the NIMV objectives.

With an appropriate follow-up program, we will be able to monitor treatment, detect early and treat acute exacerbation, as well as disease progression, minimize and treat adverse effects, avoid complications related to hospitalization and encourage lifestyle changes related to exercise, dieting and smoking cessation. In the treatment of acute and chronic pathologies, monitoring should be close, taking into account the following:

- Adequate frequency in case of unstable patients, and taking into account their dependence on the ventilator. In patients with total dependence as in neurodegenerative pathology a thorough surveillance is required.
- Hours of use of NIMV, since many of the ventilators have a time meter, a low time adherence can be observed, therefore, the patient should be assessed for the reason, correcting the causes that lead to this.
- Pulmonary function and monitoring of arterial gases; spirometric control with abrupt changes can determine acute complications such as possible over-added infections, atelectasis, pneumothorax, secretions, pleural effusion, etc.
- Interface surveillance; masks, tubes, harness, etc., are fundamental pieces, that although simple as it may seem, they are important pieces and that of the state in which they are will also be mandatory of the good or bad response that we object; For example, a harness larger in size than the patient needs will not allow a good sealing of the mask; tubing with the presence of liquids, or in the worst case with a hole will not allow a good flow, or condition large leaks respectively.

3.2. Adherence to Treatment

Adherence to treatment of patients with NIMV is essential to achieve therapeutic objectives.

The adaptation to the ventilation device is a process that requires some effort and if the equipment is not comfortable, makes noise or does not collect well the data, the patient will tend to abandon the treatment, a common situation in 30% of patients.

It is important for the treatment of acute and chronic pathology, to count with programs or adaptation steps, and interactive control of each patient, progressively adapting each parameter to the patient's tolerance, monitoring itself the progress, improvement and stability.

3.3. Platform Technology

The technology of the platform connected remotely with the medical team provides professionals and patients with information on the compliance of the therapy, control of hours of treatment and adaptation to it. Different devices have technology that allow the patient to monitor himself, taking into account the hours of use for example, so he can preselect objectives to put all his effort to achieve.

With these functionalities, the patient is involved in his treatment and the specialist has a daily and remote control of all his patients, with whom he can interact and work for the success of the therapy in a personalized way.

4. Monitoring Systems

We have different NIMV monitoring systems.

4.1. Alarm Systems

Provide the ability to control the patient, circuit and equipment. They must be precise, simple to program and interpret, audible and visual, and report when pre-established limits are reached.

There are certain parameters that are not programmable such as electric charge, exhalation valve failure, open safety valve.

The programmable parameters are: High and low airway pressure, high frequency, high and low exhaled minute volume, high and low exhaled current volume. It is advisable to program them at 10 or 20% above and below the established parameters [4]. In some cases, they are directly adjusted by the respirator.

4.2. Calibration

Prior to the use of a ventilator it is important to check that its operation is correct, for this purpose it is proceeded to its calibration. Like most computers, the same apparatus adjusts its initial systems, in this case it will calibrate the sensors of flow, volume, pressure, oxygen concentration and internal leaks. It is our responsibility to ensure that this process is carried out always and correctly.

4.3. Assembly According to Manual

With the advance and increasingly sophisticated programs of the ventilation equipment, they must be assembled according to their own manual.

It is recommended before any use of a ventilator, to do a preliminary test of 10 minutes to check the proper functioning of it.

4.4. Electronic Auto-Test

As all equipment that has a computer software, tests are carried out, which according to the model and brand may be automatic or can require to follow instructions programmed in the system or guided by the user's manual. Performing a quick auto test we will be able to check if there are leaks, measure the compliance of the circuits, so every time we make a change in the tubes we must do it.

5. Monitoring the NIMV. Doctor-Patient Relationship

It is essential to keep track of what happens between the patient and the ventilator using basic and advanced monitoring methods, in which we take into account from the vital functions, as well as the monitoring of positive and adverse effects on different patients and systems.

The technological advances also allow us to perfect the monitoring of the interaction of the patient and the mechanical ventilator which will facilitate us to optimize the ventilatory support that we provide to our patients.

It is important to monitor the respiratory parameters that we have programmed and their interaction with the patient, recognizing the physiological situation of the patient and how it evolves with the support of mechanical ventilation, with special emphasis on the safe levels of all pressures, the inspiration-expiration relationship, sensitivity, dead space, humidity, controlled leakage.

6. Telemonitoring

As previously mentioned, non-invasive mechanical ventilation has great advantages, it is important to add that, among the greatest advantages of this type of respiratory support, allows us to carry out Telemonitoring [5].

This allows us to have a wide range of possibilities: diagnosis, monitoring, work and management [6].

Subjects requiring NIMV are often complex and it should be noted that during nocturnal NIMV leaks, asynchronous events, central events, glotic closure, changes in resistance in the upper airway or secretions may occur.

All this can cause desaturations, awakenings, alterations in the architecture of sleep and poor night adherence.

The main success factors include: individualizing the subjects, determining the diseases and what stage they are in.

Not all clinical processes require telemonitoring (TM). Its implementation should be based on concrete, well-established situations and progressively to be implemented in a solid manner.

Its full application and transfer to the healthcare system on a large scale is not yet possible, although modern forms of cost-effective data processing using Big Data are currently being worked on.

6.1. Types of Telemonitoring [7]

There are two forms of Telemonitoring: synchronous and asynchronous.

6.1.1. Synchronous Telemonitoring

Synchronous telemonitoring, is done in real time, by videoconferencing or telephone coaching in verbal relation with the patient.

Video and phone contacts provide benefits for patients, such as the cost and time associated with travel or loss of hours at work [8].

6.1.2. Asynchronous Telemonitoring

Asynchronous telemonitoring, where we objective the data that is downloaded from the equipment.

With new technological advances, NIMV equipment also allows you to download usage data such as leaks, pressures, current volume and residual events. In addition, after downloading the device information in the corresponding software, the flow, pressure, current volume or leakage curves can be evaluated in detail, as well as estimating patient-ventilator asynchrony [8].

Telemonitoring needs to be simple and cost-effective. For this reason, manufacturers have been incorporating different forms of remote connectivity in their computers, either via wifi, 3G, Bluetooth, or a web platform in the «cloud». The ventilators automatically transmit the data at a certain frequency of time when the equipment is not in use and then the clinician accesses them using a secure code.

7. Safety of New Technological Systems

It is important that all the information provided by the different NIMV systems is at all times under data protection according to the regulations in the different health systems.

Therefore, from the legal point of view it is important that these types of treatment are governed under:

1) The regulation of medical devices involved in their treatment.
2) The involvement of the patient in the process (informed consent).

3) The collection and transmission of patient data through the most modern TM systems.

REFERENCES

[1] Modern Non-Invasive Mechanical Ventilation Turns 25. *Archivos de Bronconeumología* (English Edition), Volume 49, Issue 11, November 2013, Pages 475 - 479. [*Bronconeumology Archives*]

[2] Jubran, A. Advanced in Respiratory monitoring in Mechanical Ventilation. *Chest,* 1999; 116; 1416 - 1425.

[3] Telemedicine: science or fiction? *A Sist. Sanit. Navar*., (2005), pag. 309 - 323.

[4] Slutsky, A. et al. Mechanical Ventilation. ACCP Consensus Conference. *Chest,* 1993, 104:1833 - 59.

[5] Positioning of the Spanish Society of Pulmonology and Thoracic Surgery in the use of telemedicine in respiratory sleep disorders and mechanical ventilation. *Archives of Bronchopneumology*.

[6] A Health Telematics Policy in Support of the WHO Health for All Strategy for the Development of Global Health: *Report of the WHO Group Consultation on Health Telematics,* 11-16 December, Geneva, 1997. Geneva: World Health Organization; 1998.

[7] Information and telecommunications technologies: Telemedicine. *Rev. Clin. Med. Fam.,* (2011), p. 42 - 48.

[8] Non-invasive ventilation monitoring using integrated binivel home fan software: A bench study. *Chest,* 141 (2012), pp. 469 - 476.

In: Non-Invasive Mechanical Ventilation Complications
Editor: Antonio M. Esquinas
ISBN: 978-1-53619-515-6

Chapter 16

Complications during Non-Invasive Mechanical Ventilation. Acute and Chronic-Cardio - Hemodynamic Complications

Alejandro Úbeda[1,*], MD, PhD, Alonso Peinado[2], MD and Irene Fernández[1], MD

[1]Intensive Care Unit, Hospital Punta de Europa, Algeciras, Spain
[2]Department of Intermediate Care, Virgen del Mar-Vithas Hospital, Almería, Spain

Abstract

In general, NIMV is well tolerated hemodynamically, presumably due to the lower levels of insufflation pressures used, compared with invasive ventilation. The use of NIMV for a short period of time, not in the long term, has effects on heart rate, systolic blood pressure and systemic vascular resistance, depending on the type of patient and the clinical situation.

When initiating non-invasive mechanical ventilation (NIMV), many changes occur which end up affecting the patient haemodynamically. These hemodynamic effects are the result of positive airway pressure being transmitted to the surrounding structures of the thorax. The extent to which this occurs varies according to chest wall and lung compliance. Systolic volume can be compromised during NIMV because of the alteration that preload suffers due to thoracic pressure augmentation. It decreases venous return due to a pressure increased nearby RA. Additionally, LV's distensibility. This decreased preload compromises cardiac output as it affects RV. However, the use of NIMV can trigger significant hypotension and decreased cardiac output in patients with a previously altered haemodynamic state, especially with hypovolemia or with underlying heart disease without adequate drug therapy.

[*] Corresponding Author's E-mail: alubeda@gmail.com.

Keywords: non-invasive ventilation, cardiac output, hypotension, complications

INTRODUCTION

Spontaneous breathing is initiated by a muscular action which increased thorax volumen, generating a negative intrapleural pressure which allows to increase lung volumen and flow to the alveolar space. Simultaneously, that negative pressure makes easy blood entrance form thorax to the heart.

When initiating non-invasive mechanical ventilation (NIMV), many changes occur which end up affecting the patient haemodynamically. These hemodynamic effects are the result of positive airway pressure being transmitted to the surrounding structures of the thorax. The extent to which this occurs varies according to chest wall and lung compliance [1].

The Frank-Starling relationship is based on the link between the initial length of myocardial fibers and the force generated by contraction. There is a predictable relationship between the length between sarcomeres and the tension of the muscle fibers. The greater the ventricular diastolic volume, the more the myocardial fibers are stretched during diastole. Within a normal physiologic range, the more the myocardial fibers are stretched, the greater the tension in the muscle fibers, and the greater force of contraction of the ventricle when stimulated. The Frank-Starling relationship is the observation that ventricular output increases as preload (end-diastolic pressure) increase.

The left ventricular (LV) performance curves relate preload, measured as left ventricular end-diastolic volume or pressure, to cardiac performance, measured as ventricular stroke volume or cardiac output.

During states of increased LV contractility, for example, due to norepinephrine infusion, there is greater cardiac performance for a given preload. This is represented graphically as an upward shift of the normal curve. Conversely, during states of decreased LV contractility associated with systolic heart failure, there is less cardiac performance for a given preload as compared to the normal curve [2].

ACUTE COMPLICATIONS

Reduced Left and Right Ventricular Output

Alveolar inflation during positive pressure ventilation compresses the pulmonary vascular bed. This increases pulmonary vascular resistance, thereby reducing right ventricular (RV) output. Increased pulmonary vascular resistance can shift the interventricular septum to the left, impair diastolic filling of the LV, and reduce LV output.

When inspiration occurs during spontaneous breathing, right atrial pressure decreases, rising pressure gradient between both cavas and the right atrium (RA), which increases venous return. On the other hand, when breathing with positive pressure, pleural pressure increases, which also increases pressure inside the RA. It causes a decreased venous return which leads to a diminished RV filling.

EPAP reduces inspiratory deflections during systole diminishing transmural pressure (TP), venous return and preload of both ventricles. During diastole, EPAP increases intrathoracic and pericardial pressure which leads to a decreased TP and afterload. The effect on preload is the same in patients with systolic or diastolic dysfunction.

Systolic volume can be compromised during NIMV because of the alteration that preload suffers due to thoracic pressure augmentation. It decreases venous return due to a pressure increased nearby RA. Additionally, LV's distensibility. This decreased preload compromises cardiac output as it affects RV [2].

Decreased Cardiac Output

During NIMV, because of changes on the lung volumen it modifies alveolar capillaries causing that, at the beginning of the inspiration, as the volumen of blood increases inside those capillaries, that blood is forced to flow ahead if the pressure is too high.

That compression on the capillaries increases flow resistance, which has 2 consequences:

1. Higher RA pressure.
2. Higher blood flow resistance decreases left atrium blood flow, which also decreases LV blood flow.

Depending on how much volume is inside the RV, septum can be moved to the left which decreases even more LV flow causing even a lower cardiac output.

After initiating NIMV, LV preload is affected by a decreased venous return and a lower RV systolic volumen which can also cause a decreased cardiac output [2].

Since the resistance of venous return is very low, the normal small pressure gradient is adequate to drive 100% of the cardiac output back to the heart each minute. Thus, small increases in PEEP can causes relatively large decreases in preload and overall cardiac output [3]. Katira et al. [4], in an animal model, demonstrated the effect of large tidal volumes on decreases in RA pressures, RV end-diastolic volume and it since also created an increased RV ejection pressure developed progressive cor pulmonale. By adding 10cmH_2O PEEP and lowering tidal volumes, these detrimental effects were minimized.

During NIMV, changes in intrathoracic pressure (ITP) are the main determinants of changes in LV afterload. Particularly when high PEEP or large tidal volumes are employed, inspiration increases pleural pressure, decrease LV transmural pressure and decreases LV afterload, aiding in LV ejection. However, change in lung volume associated with ventilation can alter pulmonary vascular resistance and elastance as well as pulmonary arterial pressure [3]. The combination of ITP increase, decrease pressure gradient for venous return plus increased lung volume-induced increase in pulmonary vascular resistance may create a critically low output state [3].

In NIMV, inspiration-associated overinflation of lung volume will increase pulmonary vascular resistance increasing RV afterload. So, RV ejection can be impaired during inspiration if large tidal volumes are used [3].

Hypotension

The amount of venous return is determined by the pressure gradient from the extrathoracic systemic veins to the RA. Intrathoracic and RA pressure increase during positive pressure ventilation, thereby reducing the gradient for venous return. This effect is accentuated by auto-PEEP, applied PEEP, or intravascular hypovolemia [2].

CHRONIC COMPLICATIONS

As it has been previously detailed in this chapter, hemodynamic alterations belong to the group of major complications of non-invasive respiratory therapy. In order to avoid them, it is necessary to have a broad knowledge of the pathophysiology of the diseases that cause respiratory failure so that the optimal parameters can be applied to the ventilator without inducing an injury that could compromise the patient's life in the short and long term. Having always found the possibility of a protective ventilatory strategy.

NIMV, as a mode of positive pressure ventilation, affects the ventricular filling pressure mainly right, although secondarily and by biventricular interrelationship will affect the LV.

In insufficient ventricles and with high preloads the hemodynamic effects of NIMV may be beneficial because it decreases preload, increases contractility and decreases post-load, increasing LVEF and cardiac output. However, in patients with decreased LVEF and low preloads, it may produce deleterious effects, involving increased intrathoracic pressure, hypotension, pre- and post- load alterations and decreased cardiac output, as explained above.

With the use of NIMV a beneficial hemodynamic effect is produced as a consequence of the increase in intrathoracic pressure which is reflected in a decrease in the LV systolic ejection volume, filling pressure and tele-diastolic volume. As a final consequence, a decrease in cardiac output is observed which becomes more evident in patients with low left or RV ejection fraction, making it necessary to associate vasoactive pharmacies or vary the levels of pressures or ventilatory mode.

The decrease in afterload of the LV leads to an improvement in both mitral and aortic regurgitation as well as cardiac output and peripheral perfusion, however an increase makes it worse in the short or long term.

These pathophysiological mechanisms will not only lead to failure of the heart pump, but also to alterations in different target organs, producing serious short and long-term complications. It is also necessary to know that all critically ill patients have a higher demand for oxygen at the tissue level secondary to the stress caused by the disease and the misuse of respiratory therapy, which produces a prolonged admission and increases the probability of death in hospital due to cardiovascular disease or associated comorbidities (high blood pressure, low blood pressure, tachycardia, anemia, mechanical ventilation).

Hemodynamic effects. Artificial ventilation can have deleterious haemodynamic effects secondary to increased intrathoracic pressure, leading to a reduction in venous return and ventricular filling [5].

In general, NIMV is well tolerated hemodynamically, presumably due to the lower levels of insufflation pressures used, compared with invasive ventilation. The use of NIMV for a short period of time, not in the long term, has effects on heart rate, systolic blood pressure and systemic vascular resistance, depending on the type of patient and the clinical situation. In many cases, the application of positive intrathoracic pressure can improve the ventricular ejection fraction and cardiac output, especially in the patient with acute heart failure [6]. However, the use of NIMV can trigger significant hypotension and decreased cardiac output in patients with a previously altered haemodynamic state, especially with hypovolemia or with underlying heart disease without adequate drug therapy [7]. For years, the use of ventilation with double pressure level in cardiac patients with acute respiratory failure secondary to acute lung edema has been discussed, hypothesizing a relationship between the use of NIMV and the development of acute myocardial infarction, due to the hemodynamic deterioration produced by this mode of ventilation. This association has been ruled out, as no relationship has been demonstrated between the ventilatory mode and the development of acute myocardial infarction.

Cardiac dysfunction leads to a state of low cardiac output and systemic hypoperfusion to a greater or lesser degree. It is usually associated with a decrease in systolic blood pressure (< 90mmHg) and mean (< 65mmHg). Perfusion that is inadequate to meet tissue metabolic demands results in hypoxia and inadequate aerobic metabolism, and ultimately in cell injury, cell death, tissue injury, and organ failure. Patients with low output syndrome have more chronic or subacute manifestations of poor perfusion:

Heart

Venous or systemic congestion increases preload, leading to increased stress on the ventricular wall, valve regurgitation, myocardial stretching, remodeling, necrosis of ventricular myocytes, and a progressive decline in heart function [8]. Natriuretic peptides are released from the atria or ventricles under conditions of cardiac stress [9]. The contribution of O_2 to the myocardium is affected by three reasons: a) low diastolic blood pressure and high diastolic pressure in LV, which conditions a decrease in coronary perfusion; b) tachycardia which decreases the diastolic period and therefore the time of coronary perfusion; and c) concomitant presence of lesions in coronary arteries.

Lung

Increases in left atrial hydrostatic pressure and mitral regurgitation are transmitted retrogrades as increased pressure in the pulmonary capillaries. These changes increase the rate of fluid leak into the interstitium, causing lung stiffness and, in some patients, dyspnea. The lymphatic system regularly drains the interstitial fluid, but when the interstitial pressure exceeds the pleural pressure and exceeds the drainage capacity, fluid is displaced into the pleural and intra-alveolar spaces, causing pleural effusion and alveolar oedema. Increased permeability of the pulmonary vasculature caused by inflammation may play a role in patients who develop pulmonary oedema, despite relatively low hydrostatic pressures. Severe or repeated decompensations can result in cardiopulmonary remodelling, leading to deterioration of gas exchange, pulmonary vasoconstriction and eventually pulmonary hypertension [10].

Kidney

Cardiorenal syndrome has been defined as the simultaneous dysfunction of the heart and the kidneys, regardless of which of these two organs has suffered the initial injury. The cardiorenal syndrome is not a single entity, with different subtypes, being the most important type I cardiorenal syndrome, where rapid worsening of heart function leads to acute renal injury. Elevated central venous pressure can worsen renal function through a variety of mechanisms, including reduced renal blood flow induced by increased venous pressure, renal hypoxia, increased interstitial pressure and interstitial fibrosis.

Other contributors to acute kidney injury or worsening kidney function include inflammatory mediators (mediated by infection or tissue damage), transient renal function in conjunction with clinical improvement in heart failure. This pseudo-worsening of renal function is the result of a modification of hemodynamics, but only in a few patients with a response to treatment and improvement of heart function will renal tubular excision occur, and they will experience an irreversible decrease in glomerular filtration [11].

Liver

Dysfunction is present in 20-30% of patients with heart failure regardless of its origin, and elevated liver enzymes correlate with a worse prognosis [11]. Liver dysfunction is also closely related to renal dysfunction, and may have prognostic synergism. Venous congestion may cause cholestasis, with elevated alkaline phosphatase, bilirubin and γ-glutamyltransferase. Cholestasis is a more common finding, resulting from hypoperfusion in the context of hypoxic hepatitis [10].

Bowel

Altered intestinal permeability and an increased bacterial bio-layer may contribute to the process of chronic inflammation and malnutrition. Venous and systemic congestion, sympathetic vasoconstriction and low cardiac output all contribute to decreased flow in the splenic microcirculation and increased risk of intestinal ischemia. Ischemia causes epithelial cell dysfunction and loss of gut barrier function, which allows the passage of endotoxins produced by Gram-negative bacteria in the gut into the blood. These effects trigger systemic inflammation and cytokine generation, leading to various abnormalities of function and energy generation by cardiomyocytes [9, 10].

Brain

The neurological alteration that can be observed includes the presence of depression, cognitive dysfunction and delirium. The presence of brain dysfunction is associated with increased mortality in patients undergoing mechanical ventilation [10]. In the pathophysiology of cognitive impairment in the patient with low cardiac output, not only is hypoxemia implicated, but other factors, inflammation, stress and neurohormonal dysregulation are also involved.

For all that is developed throughout this chapter in relation to hemodynamic complications in the use of non-invasive ventilation, some authors have launched a call for caution on the use of NIMV in the patient with diastolic heart failure. In these cases, the decrease in preload and the decrease in volume at the end of the LV diastole that this entails and, therefore, in cardiac output, may produce a deterioration in cardiac function that leads to hypotension and organ dysfunction. It has also been postulated that pulmonary hyperinflation secondary to the use of NIMV may be harmful by activation of the parasympathetic nervous system resulting in a decrease in heart rate [10, 11]. The presence of severe dyspnea, anxiety and discomfort due to inadequate NIMV can lead to stress- related catecholamine release, with a consequent increase in oxygen demands on the myocardium and the possibility of cardiac ischemia or arrhythmias. In addition, coronary oxygen supply may be compromised by inadequate gas exchange due to alveolar occupation by oedema, accompanied by a decrease in mixed venous oxygen pressure secondary to increased oxygen consumption by the respiratory muscles.

Knowing well the pathophysiology of the disease we are facing, knowing how to adapt the ventilator parameters to the physiological needs of the patient, we will be prepared to act with caution and know when the technique is failing and we need to establish another type of therapy in advance.

Indicators of cardiovascular failure secondary to NIMV with non-protective parameters:

- Hemodynamic deterioration that does not respond to vasoactive drugs or malignant ventricular arrhythmias that are not controlled with the usual measures.
- Acute Coronary Syndrome-Acute Myocardial Infarction.
- Arrhythmia as a trigger for low cardiac output.

Knowledge of the factors related to the outcome of NIMV is essential to delimit the correct use of the ventilatory technique, by adequately selecting those patients in whom NIMV support treatment is most likely to fail. This would allow us to more safely determine which patients could benefit from the technique and which should be intubated directly, or after a short period of NIMV, and not expose them to a delay in invasive ventilation, which could be dangerous for the patient [12]. Finally, a delay in endotracheal intubation in patients who fail NIMV is associated with increased hospital mortality.

KEY MESSAGES

1. NIMV hemodynamic effects are the result of positive airway pressure being transmitted to the surrounding structures of the thorax.
2. During inspiration, NIMV increases pulmonary vascular resistance, thereby reducing RV output. Increased pulmonary vascular resistance can shift the interventricular septum to the left and reduce LV output.
3. NIMV-related hypotension is accentuated by auto-PEEP, applied PEEP or intravascular hypovolemia.
4. Extensive knowledge of the pathophysiology and application of respiratory parameters is necessary to avoid causing iatrogenesis in patients.
5. It is highly recommended to be realistic with the knowledge that each one has and thus be able to choose the best therapy that can be offered to a patient.

REFERENCES

[1] Rodríguez, I. J., Echeverry, J. C., Abello, M., Cruz, L. E. Changes in the hemodynamic profile when establishing mechanical ventilation in patients with ischemic heart disease and coronary disease: Measurement with thoracic bioreactance. *Rev. Colomb. Anestesiol.,* 2014; 42:76 - 82.

[2] Delicce, A., Makaryus, A. *Physiology,* Frank Starling Law. StatPearls. Jan. 2020.

[3] Mahmood, S. S., Pinsky, M. R. Heart-lung interactions during mechanical ventilation: the basics. *Ann. Transl. Med.,* 2018; 6:349.

[4] Katira, B. H., Giesinger, R. E., Engelberts, D., Zabini, D., Kornecki, A., Otulakowski, G. et al. Adverse heart-lung interactions in ventilator-induced lung injury. *Am. J. Respir. Crit. Care Med.,* 2017; 196: 1411 - 21.

[5] Baratz, D. M., Westbrook, P. R., Shah, P. K., Mohsenifar, Z. Effect of nasal continuous positive airway pressure on cardiac output and oxygen delivery in patients with congestive heart failure. *Chest,* 1992; 102: 1397 - 1401.

[6] Mehta, S., Hill, N. S. Noninvasive ventilation. *Am. J. Respir. Crit. Care Med.,* 2001; 163: 540 - 577.

[7] Díaz, O., Iglesia, R., Ferrer, M., Zavala, E., Santos, C., Wagner, P. D., Roca, J., Rodriguez – Roisin, R. Effects of noninvasive ventilation on pulmonary gas exchange and hemodynamics during acute hypercapnic exacerbations of chronic obstructive pulmonary disease. *Am. J. Respir. Crit. Care Med.,* 1997; 156: 1840 - 1845.

[8] Parrinello, G., Greene, S. J., Torres, D., Alderman, M., Bonventre, J. V., Di, P. P., Gargani, L., Nohria, A., Fonarow, G. C., Vaduganathan, M., Butler, J., Paterna, S.,

Stevenson, L. W., Gheorghiade, M. Water and sodium in heart failure: A spotlight on congestion. *Heart Fail Rev.,* 2015; 20:13 - 24.

[9] Ware, L. B., Matthay, M. A. Clinical practice. Acute pulmonary edema. *N Engl. J. Med.,* 2005; 353:2788 - 2796.

[10] MacIntyre, N. Physiologic effects of noninvasive ventilation. *Respir. Care*, 2019; 64:617 - 628.

[11] Núñez, J., Miñana, G., Santas, E., Bertomeu-González, V. Síndrome cardiorrenal en la insuficiencia cardiaca aguda: revisando paradigmas. *Rev. Esp. Cardiol.,* 2015; 68:426 - 435.

[12] Carrillo, A., Gonzalez-Diaz, G., Ferrer, M., Martinez-Quintana, M. E., Lopez-Martinez, A., Llamas, N., Alcazar, M., Torres, A. Non-invasive ventilation in community-acquired pneumonia and severe acute respiratory failure. *Intensive Care Med.,* 2012; 38:458 - 466.

In: Non-Invasive Mechanical Ventilation Complications ISBN: 978-1-53619-515-6
Editor: Antonio M. Esquinas

Chapter 17

Complications During Non-Invasive Mechanical Ventilation: Comorbidities Influence

M. Sevilla-Martínez**, MD, L. Olivencia-Peña, MD and A. Fernández-Carmona, MD

Intensive Care Unit, Hospital Universitario Virgen de las Nieves, Granada, Spain

Abstract

Compared with invasive mechanical ventilation, noninvasive ventilation (NIV) achieves the same physiological benefits of reduced work of breathing and improved gas exchange. Furthermore, it avoids complications of intubation and increased risks of ventilator-associated pneumonia especially in patients with comorbidities.

Use of NIV has spread in recent years, due in part to the change in patient profile: over time, the number of patients with baseline pathologies increases, due to the increasing age of the population and the possibility of applying NIV in patients to patients who previously required invasive measures.

Keywords: noninvasive ventilation; atelectasis, apnea, hypercapnia

Introduction

Non-invasive mechanical ventilation (NIV) is a method of ventilatory assistance with increasing relevance in management of respiratory failure in patients with different pathologies. Different frequent scenarios in clinical practice are mentioned.

* Corresponding Author's Email: sevillamartinezmaria@gmail.com.

NIV IN OBESE PATIENT

Morbid obesity is a major cause of chronic respiratory failure and an independent worse prognostic factor per se. Obesity is also associated with metabolic syndrome and facilitates the development of type 2 diabetes, hypertension, cardiac disease, obstructive sleep apnea (OSA), as well as cerebrovascular, liver, and kidney disease. Obesity therefore is a systemic illness involving many organ systems with complicated interactions [1].

From a purely respiratory point of view obesity produces [1-3]:

- Restriction of the rib cage and the diaphragm.
- Decreased lung compliance due to increased pulmonary blood volume and alveolar collapse as a consequence of closure of the small airway.
- Decreased oral pressure in case of massive obesity.
- Alteration of the resistance of respiratory muscles in massive obesity.

As a consequence ventilatory work is increased, so that in patients with body mass index (BMI) > 40 oxygen consumption at rest can reach up to 16% of the total, while it rarely exceeds 3% in the non-obese subject.

The most frequent functional anomaly in the obese is the decrease in the expiratory reserve volume with conservation of the residual volume, which produces a decrease in the functional residual capacity. While vital capacity is conserved, forced expiratory volume in the first second may be slightly reduced in patients with severe obesity.

Arterial blood gases are frequently altered proportionally to BMI due to: perfusion ventilation imbalance, responsible for isolated hypoxemia and alveolar hypoventilation, responsible for the hypoventilation obesity syndrome.

Based on the pathophysiology, the fundamental role of respiratory support therapies in these patients is understandable. This will aim to correct respiratory disorders during sleep, diurnal hypercapnia and residual hypoxemia that usually persists after correction of alveolar hypoventilation. The initial therapeutic management of these patients will depend on the clinical situation.

In the case of acute respiratory failure and outside of immediate life-threatening situations (shock, severe encephalopathy, multi-organ failure), NIV should be considered as first-line treatment in the management of ventilatory failure in these patients [4]. Currently the support pressure plus positive end-expiratory pressure (PEEP) mode, or Bilevel positive airway pressure (BiPAP) is the most widely used mode, to which supplemental oxygen can be added. Improvement in hypercapnia in obese patients may require higher PEEP levels and longer times than that of non-obese patients during acute hypercapnic respiratory failure (8-10cmH_20). Prolonging NIV in non-responders may dangerously delay EI and thus increase the risk of death, therefore the decision to EI and the time of non-invasive ventilation should be individualized. NIV failure in obese patients remain high in patients with pneumonia, on the other hand the mortality of obese intubated patients with systemic involvement is close to 30% according to series [5-6].

In case of the hypercapnic patient without acidosis, the choice of the initial ventilatory mode will depend on the coexistence of sleep apnea hypopnea syndrome (SAHS) and the severity of the hypercapnia [7].

- If $PaCO_2$ is < 50mmHg, and SAHS, it is advisable to start with a continuous positive airway pressure (CPAP) treatment. In addition to correcting apneas, this therapy can restore daytime normocapnia. However, in a significant number of patients, hypercapnia persists despite adequate treatment with CPAP. In this case, it must be assumed that hypercapnia responds to a different mechanism from SAHS, that is, obesity per se, which perpetuates hypoventilation. These patients require a change to non-invasive ventilation.
- If pCO_2 > 50mmHg, NIV is started, although once eucapnia is reached, go to CPAP if SAHS exists, since it has been shown that more than 30% of patients initially treated for NIV can be transferred to CPAP with good control in the patient. long-term.

NIV IN DIAPHRAGMATIC PARALYSIS

Diaphragm paresis or paralysis can be caused by diseases associated with motor neuron defects, metabolic or inflammatory myopathies, autoimmune polyneuropathies as well as surgery, trauma, mediastinal tumors or pleural infections. It can be uni or bilateral, producing very different clinical manifestations. Bilateral paralysis is frequently symptomatic, especially during supine and sleep [8].

Functionally it is a restrictive ventilatory defect with reduction of vital capacity> 20% in the supine position. The gas exchange is preserved and the monoxide diffusion is corrected to the alveolar volume. It is possible to find a reduction in the arterial pressure of oxygen related to alterations in the ventilation/perfusion ratio by microatelectasis [9].

Treatment and prognosis are determined by the underlying disease. In case of resorting to ventilatory support, NIV during the night is a well-established treatment for the management of this disease that facilitates the rest of the respiratory muscles, the relief of dyspnea, the treatment to respiratory failure with hypercapnia and correction of respiratory disturbances during sleep. In Khan's study of 66 patients with diaphragmatic dysfunction, control of sleep-disordered breathing with CPAP was possible in only 37.9% of patients and the rest required BiPAP. Patients with bilateral diaphragmatic dysfunction were 6.8 times more likely to fail with CPAP than those with unilateral diaphragmatic dysfunction [10].

NIV IN OBSTETRIC PATIENT

Acute respiratory failure (ARF) in the obstetric patient is the main cause of admission of pregnant women to Critical Care Units. It is mainly due to respiratory infection, asthmatic decompensation, acute lung edema and pulmonary thromboembolism.

NIV is indicated in pregnant women with ARF with adequate tolerance to the device, correct level of consciousness, hemodynamic stability and expectoration capacity. CPAP improves oxygenation and reduces afterload, and BIPAP also has the potential to increase tidal volume and reduce preload, so it could be more useful in pregnant women with asthma attacks and in severe cases.

The objective of using NIV is to optimize your clinical situation to improve gas exchange, maintaining adequate fetal oxygenation, obviating the need for endotracheal intubation (EI) (potentially difficult and at risk of aspiration).

It is important to know that the blood gas values that could be considered acceptable outside of pregnancy are lower than the minimum to ensure fetal well-being ($PaO_2 \geq 70$ mmHg, $PaCO_2 < 45$ mmHg).

NIV successful use for maternal ARF has been verified, allowing delayed fetal extraction. It has also been used during vaginal delivery and during cesarean delivery under neuroaxial anesthesia [11].

NIV IN PATIENTS WITH NEUROMUSCULAR DISEASE

Currently, NIV can be applied to all neuromuscular diseases that have in common, the compromise of the ventilatory function that will be determined by the behavior of the inspiratory, expiratory muscles or both, and of upper airways muscle groups.

Neuromuscular diseases are: Amyotrophic Lateral Sclerosis, Spinal Muscular Atrophy, Poliomyelitis and Post Poliomyelitis Syndrome, Congenital Infantile Hypotonia, Guillain Barré syndrome, Botulism, Steinert Muscular Dystrophy, Duchene, Myasthenia gravis.

Progressive muscle weakness will cause the inspiratory muscles to compromise chest movements, leading to decreased vital capacity and tidal volume. The respiratory pattern will be more superficial and the respiratory rate will increase, in order to maintain normal ventilation, but this compensation will be insufficient as the disease progresses. In situations with increased oxygen consumption such as infection or effort, alveolar hypoventilation with hypercapnia and hypoxemia manifested. Apnea-hypoapenea of central origin occurs, which during sleep can be accentuated since the obstruction of the upper airway is added (due to involvement of the lingual and retropharyngeal muscles.

Treatment is complex and depends on the disease. If it is hypercapnic, niv, negative pressure ventilation, oxygen therapy, and tracheostomy with mechanical ventilation are proposed.

An effective treatment is the use of CPAP devices. Its use, in addition to improving the work of the inspiratory muscles, increases intrathoracic pressure, decreasing cardiac post-load and increasing the left ventricular ejection fraction; it also reduces sympathetic tone and causes vasodilation by non-adrenergic mechanisms; Likewise, it moves the blood volume towards the extrathoracic compartment and, in the case of hypervolemia, increases the cardiac output. Despite these and other important immediate benefits (attenuation of central sleep apnea, improvement in nighttime oxygenation, decreased adrenaline levels, and increased exercise tolerance), treatment with CPAP does not appear to affect survival time in neuromuscular patients. In case of hypercapnia, the mechanical treatment of choice BiPAP device [12].

NIV IN POSTOPERATIVE PERIOD

Hypoxemia is frequent in the context of postoperative pulmonary atelectasis. Clinically, they are manifested by high respiratory rate and low tidal volumes, in the early postoperative period up to 7 days after surgery, being called post-surgical pulmonary restrictive syndromes.

The use of NIV in the postoperative period is widely described, since it reduce respiratory work, improve alveolar ventilation and reduce atelectasis, increasing functional residual capacity and thus improving gas exchange. These benefits, reducing need for invasive ventilation, are achieved with more evidence when NIV is started immediately and continuously after surgery in patients at risk, since it application hours after surgery or discontinued is should be individualized to the patient's situation.

Most of clinical practice guide guidelines of noninvasive ventilation for acute respiratory failure recommends NIV for patients with post-operative ARF. (Conditional recommendation, moderate certainty of evidence) [13].

NIV in Postoperative Period of Abdominal/Pelvic Surgery

Hypoxemia is found in up to 50% of postoperative abdominal surgery, with appearance of atelectasis in up to 90% of anesthetized patients.

It is produced by the reduction of diaphragmatic activity, direct manipulation or by injury to the phrenic nerve, increase in extravascular pulmonary water due to volume overload, as well as hypoventilation both due to pain and secondary to anesthetics (which also causes greater difficulty in eliminating secretions) leading to a decrease in functional residual capacity with consequent atelectasis. These mechanisms when added facilitate the appearance of respiratory failure and favors the development of respiratory infections.

NIV has beneficial effects on postoperative respiratory changes. Both the CPAP and PSV modes increase alveolar pressure favoring the re-expansion of atelectasis and the increase in lung volume. It is beneficial both prophylactic and therapeutic in the face of the development of ARF after abdominal interventions, studies have shown its usefulness both for PSV and CPAP in prophylaxis.

Evidence suggests that NIV, as a prophylactic or curative treatment, has proven to be an effective strategy to reduce intubation rates, nosocomial infections, intensive care unit and hospital stays, morbidity and mortality in postoperative patients [13].

NIV in the Postoperative Period of Supra-Diaphragmatic Surgery

Atelectasis and the inability to eliminate secretions are the most important etiological factors in the development of ARF in the postoperative period of thoracotomies, aggravated by intense pain affecting deep breathing and coughing.

There are few published works that study the effect of NIV after lung resection surgery, both in its prophylactic and therapeutic use. Thus, the case of lung resection is a procedure with significant postoperative morbidity and mortality. Pulmonary complications remain the leading cause of death post-operatively, and acute respiratory failure after lung resection is fatal in up to 60% to 80% of cases. This high mortality rate is largely related to the complications of postoperative reintubation and mechanical ventilation, therefore the role of NIV in this setting is very important. In Auriant's RCT study concludes that NIV can reduce the need for EI, thereby improving survival. The group treated with NIV obtained a significant decrease in the need for EI (50% vs. 20.8%, $p = 0.035$), as well as mortality at 120 days (37.5% vs. 12.5%, $p = 0.045$) [13].

In patients with ARF after upper gastrointestinal surgery, there is no certain evidence to base clinical action regarding non-invasive ventilation. ARF in these patientes frecuently is associated with anastomotic breakdown needing EI and aggressive treatment. Currently, some scientific Societies classifies upper gastrointestinal anastomotic surgery as a contraindication to NIV due to increased risk of esophageal suture dehiscence induced by pressure and gastrointestinal perforation, however NIV could have a role in the treatment of these patients: improving oxygenation and avoiding EI, correcting hypoxemia and ischemia (a frequent reason for suture breakdown). In 2015 a Cochrane systematic review concludes that CPAP or bilevel NPPV is an effective and safe intervention for the treatment of adults with acute respiratory failure after upper abdominal surgery (quality of the evidence low or very low). A more recent meta-analysis conducted by Charlesworth concludes that there is no evidence to definitively conclude that noninvasive positive pressure ventilation is either safe or dangerous following oesophagectomy [14-15].

KEY MESSAGES

- NIV provides a reduction in breathing work and an improvement in gas exchange. In addition, it avoids the complications of intubation and the increased risks of ventilator-associated pneumonia.
- Its benefits make it play an important role in patients with comorbidities.
- Its use has been studied in patients with neuromuscular disease and diagragmatic paralysis, improving their quality of life.
- It is especially useful in the postoperative period when patients frequently have hypoxemia due to atelectasis.

REFERENCES

[1] Marik P E, Desai H. Characteristics of Patients With the "Malignant Obesity Hypoventilation Syndrome" Admitted to an ICU. *J. Intensive Care Med.* 2013;28(2):124-30. doi: 10.1177/0885066612444261.

[2] Rabec, Claudio, Pilar de Lucas Ramos, and Daniel Veale. 2011. "Respiratory Complications of Obesity." *Archivos de Bronconeumologia* 47 (5): 252–61. https://doi.org/10.1016/j.arbres.2011.01.012. [*Bronconeumology Archives*]

[3] Lee, Mei-Yu, Ching-Chi Lin, Sheng-Yeh Shen, Chung-Hsin Chiu, and Shwu-Fang Liaw. 2009. "Work of Breathing in Eucapnic and Hypercapnic Sleep Apnea Syndrome." *Respiration; International Review of Thoracic Diseases* 77 (2): 146–53. https://doi.org/10.1159/000140491.

[4] Malcolm Lemyze, Pauline Taufour, Alain Duhamel, Johanna Temime, Olivier Nigeon, Nicolas Vangrunderbeeck, Stéphanie Barrailler, Gaëlle Gasan, Florent Pepy, Didier Thevenin, and Jihad Mallat. "Determinants of Noninvasive Ventilation Success or Failure in Morbidly Obese Patients in Acute Respiratory Failure". *PLoS One* 2014; 9(5): e97563. doi: 10.1371/journal.pone.0097563.

[5] G Gursel, M Aydogdu, G Gulbas, S Ozkaya, S Tasyurek, F Yildirim. "The Influence of Severe Obesity on Non-Invasive Ventilation (NIV) Strategies and Responses in Patients With Acute Hypercapnic Respiratory Failure Attacks in the ICU". *Minerva Anestesiol.* 2011;77:17-25.

[6] Pérez de Llano, Luis A, Rafael Golpe, Montserrat Ortiz Piquer, Alejandro Veres Racamonde, Manuel Vázquez Caruncho, Olga Caballero Muinelos, and Cristina Alvarez Carro. 2005. "Short-Term and Long-Term Effects of Nasal Intermittent

Positive Pressure Ventilation in Patients with Obesity-Hypoventilation Syndrome." *Chest* 128 (2): 587–94. https://doi.org/10.1378/chest.128.2.587.

[7] Qureshi, Asher. 2009. "Diaphragm Paralysis." *Seminars in Respiratory and Critical Care Medicine* 30 (3): 315–20. https://doi.org/10.1055/s-0029-1222445.

[8] McCool, F Dennis, and George E Tzelepis. 2012. "Dysfunction of the Diaphragm." *The New England Journal of Medicine* 366 (10): 932–42. https://doi.org/10.1056/NEJMra1007236.

[9] Khan, Akram, Timothy I. Morgenthaler, and Kannan Ramar. 2014. "Sleep Disordered Breathing in Isolated Unilateral and Bilateral Diaphragmatic Dysfunction." *Journal of Clinical Sleep Medicine* 10 (5): 509–15. https://doi.org/10.5664/jcsm.3698.

[10] Hutter, Deborah A, Robert Berkowitz, S Edward 3rd Davis, and Hormoz Ashtyani. 2006. "Application of Continuous Positive Airway Pressure in Hypoxemic Acute Respiratory Failure Associated with Diastolic Dysfunction in Pregnancy." *Congestive Heart Failure (Greenwich, Conn.)* 12 (3): 174–75. https://doi.org/10.1111/j.1527-5299.2005.05316.x.

[11] Bradley, T Douglas, Alexander G Logan, R John Kimoff, Frédéric Sériès, Debra Morrison, Kathleen Ferguson, Israel Belenkie, et al., 2005. "Continuous Positive Airway Pressure for Central Sleep Apnea and Heart Failure." *The New England Journal of Medicine* 353 (19): 2025–33. https://doi.org/10.1056/NEJMoa051001.

[12] Rochwerg B, Brochard L, Elliott M W, et al., "Official ERS/ATS clinical practice guidelines: noninvasive ventilation for acute respiratory failure". 2017. *Eur. Respir. J.* 50. https://doi.org/10.1183/13993003.02426-2016.

[13] Auriant, I, A Jallot, P Hervé, J Cerrina, F Le Roy Ladurie, J L Fournier, B Lescot, and F Parquin. 2001. "Noninvasive Ventilation Reduces Mortality in Acute Respiratory Failure Following Lung Resection." *American Journal of Respiratory and Critical Care Medicine* 164 (7): 1231–35. https://doi.org/10.1164/ajrccm.164.7.2101089.

[14] Debora A S Faria 1, Edina M K da Silva, Álvaro N Atallah, Flávia M R Vital. "Noninvasive Positive Pressure Ventilation for Acute Respiratory Failure Following Upper Abdominal Surgery." 2015. *Review Cochrane Database Syst. Rev.* 5;(10):CD009134. doi: 10.1002/14651858.CD009134.pub2.

[15] Michael Charlesworth, Tom Lawton, Stephen Fletcher. "Noninvasive Positive Pressure Ventilation for Acute Respiratory Failure Following Oesophagectomy: Is It Safe? A Systematic Review of the Literature." 2015. *Review J. Intensive Care Soc.*;16(3):215-221. doi: 10.1177/1751143715571698.

In: Non-Invasive Mechanical Ventilation Complications
Editor: Antonio M. Esquinas
ISBN: 978-1-53619-515-6

Chapter 18

COMPLICATIONS DURING NON-INVASIVE MECHANICAL VENTILATION. HYPERCAPNIC FAILURE. PHYSIOPATHOLOGY, DIAGNOSIS, PREVENTION AND TREATMENT

Fotis Yerosimou[1,*], MD and Eirini Papageorgiou[2], MD
[1]Department of Anesthesiology,
Cancer Hospital "Theageneio," Thessaloniki, Greece
[2]Department of Intensive Care Unit,
Cancer Hospital "Theageneio," Thessaloniki, Greece

ABSTRACT

Hypercapnia is a term that refers to the elevation of the partial pressure of carbon dioxide (PaCO2) above the value of 45 mmHg. This will occur if the gas exchange process that takes place in the lungs is compromised. Hypercapnia will result in acid-base balance disturbances due to the relationship between CO2 and hydrogen carbonate (HCO3) known as the pH buffering system. Hypercapnic respiratory failure is more commonly determined by the reduction of alveolar ventilation than by the increase of the rate of CO2 production. There are many causes of hypercapnic that include among others pre-existing lung conditions, thoracic wall deformities and neuromuscular disorders. Clinical examination is important part of the diagnostic process together with a detailed personal history. Diagnostic imaging tests, as well as laboratory tests, may be useful in discovering the etiology of hypercapnia. Treatment will depend on the cause of hypercapnic failure and instructions must be followed as given for the best possible outcome. Various prevention strategies exist in order to avoid more serious complications.

Keywords: hypercapnic failure, respiratory acidosis, non-invasive ventilation, response

---

* Corresponding Author's E-mail: yerosimoufotis@yahoo.com.

INTRODUCTION

The lungs are the primary organs of the respiratory system necessary for breathing through the gas exchange process. This process involves the extraction of oxygen from the atmosphere and transferring that oxygen through the bloodstream to all the organs and tissues, and the removal of carbon dioxide from the body. Respiratory failure will occur when this gas exchange process is compromised and the exchange between the oxygen and carbon dioxide is insufficient.

There are two main types of respiratory failure:

1. Hypoxemic respiratory failure (type I), which is characterized by an arterial oxygen tension (PaO2) lower than 60 mmHg with a normal or low arterial carbon dioxide tension (PaCO2) [1]. Main causes of hypoxemia include low ambient oxygen (e.g., high altitude), ventilation-perfusion (V/Q) mismatch, alveolar hypoventilation (due to decreased respiratory muscle activity), diffusion problems (e.g., ARDS and pneumonia) and shunt.
2. Hypercapnic respiratory failure (type II) which is characterized by a PaCO2 higher than 45 mmHg due to the body's inability to eliminate it. The main underlying causes include increased airway resistance (e.g., asthma, chronic obstructive pulmonary disease), decreased lung area for gas exchange (e.g., chronic bronchitis), decreased effort of breathing (drug effects, obesity), neuromuscular disorders (e.g., Guillain-Barré syndrome), and deformed, rigid or flail chest.

The classification of respiratory failure also includes two more types:

3. Perioperative respiratory failure (type III) which typically occurs in the perioperative period when factors that reduce functional residual capacity (FRC) combine with causes of increased closing volume to produce atelectasis [2]. This can be the result of obesity, ascites, excessive airway secretions and inadequate post-operative analgesia.
4. The last type of respiratory failure includes Shock (type IV) and it usually involves patients that are intubated and ventilated while in resuscitation for shock. This type of respiratory failure will result from the hypoperfusion of the respiratory muscles in the effort to reduce work of breathing of the patient.

Respiratory failure can also be distinguished into acute and chronic. Acute respiratory failure involves disturbances in the arterial blood gases (ABGs) and the acid-base balance status that can be life-threatening, while chronic respiratory failure develops over the course of few weeks or later and the disturbances are subtler and not so evident.

It is difficult to distinguish between acute and chronic hypoxemic respiratory failure using only ABGs. However, when there is an acute hypercapnic respiratory failure, the ABGs will reveal a drop on pH making it acidic. On the other hand, in the presence of chronic hypercapnic failure, there will be compensation by the renal system by increasing the bicarbonate concentration and as a consequence, the pH will only drop slightly. It should be noted that besides acute and chronic, there can be another category that includes acute exacerbation of existing chronic respiratory disturbances.

In this chapter we are going to discuss the type II respiratory failure, the hypercapnic failure and the basic physiopathology behind it, how to recognize and establish the diagnosis of hypercapnic failure, the possible measures for the prevention of hypercapnic failure, as well as treatment and management options available.

PHYSIOPATHOLOGY

Carbon dioxide (CO2) is a metabolic product of the many cellular processes within the body to process lipids, carbohydrates, and proteins [3]. Hypercapnia is a term that refers to the elevation of the partial pressure of carbon dioxide (PaCO2) above the value of 45 mmHg. There are many physiological mechanisms responsible for the regulations of CO2. These mechanisms include the pH buffering system, which occurs between CO2 and hydrogen carbonate (HCO3). Hypercapnia will result in acid-base balance disturbances due to this relationship.

As already mentioned, the respiratory system eliminates CO2 through the process of gas exchange. Retention of CO2 will occur when there are disturbances in this exchange process. Carbon dioxide is then hydrated with the formation of carbonic acid that subsequently dissociates with release of hydrogen ions (H+) in the body fluids [4]. As an outcome, this H+ concentration increase will cause the development of respiratory acidosis.

The normal level of carbon dioxide (CO2) tension in the arterial blood (PaCO2) results from the relationship between the rate of CO2 production and the portion of CO2 eliminated by the lung with alveolar ventilation [5]. Hypercapnic respiratory failure is more commonly determined by the reduction of alveolar ventilation (pump respiratory failure), than by the increase of the rate of CO2 production, even in high-risk patients with poor pulmonary reserve [6]. This is usually due to a decrease in minute ventilation relative to demand or an increase in the dead space.

Table 1. Causes of respiratory failure by type

Type I	Type II	Type III	Type IV
- Pneumonia - Cardiogenic pulmonary edema - Non-cardiogenic pulmonary edema - Pulmonary embolism - Atelectasis - Pulmonary Fibrosis.	- Asthma - COPD - Central hypoventilation - Neuromuscular and chest wall disorders - Obesity hypoventilation syndrome (OHS).	- Inadequate post - operative analgesia - Obesity - Ascites - Excessive airway secretions - Pre-operative tobacco smoking.	- Cardiogenic shock - Septic shock - Hypovolemic shock.

In order to minimize any changes that will occur in pH, the body's homeostatic mechanisms are activated. Due to the compensatory mechanisms, there will be an increase in bicarbonate levels. In the ABGs analysis we will observe a pH below the normal range, increased pCO2 value, and also increased bicarbonate concentration that results from the compensatory mechanism.

The etiology of hypercapnic respiratory failure can be categorized in 4 main causes; Pulmonary causes, Central Nervous System (CNS) disturbances, thoracic wall anomalies and neuromuscular disorders. Pulmonary causes include acute severe asthma, upper airways obstruction, COPD, bronchiectasis and obstructive sleep apnoea. Causes that involve the CNS may include among others increased intracranial pressure, head trauma, coma and drug usage. The main thoracic wall anomalies are flail chest, diaphragm rupture, scoliosis/kyphosis and other chest traumas such as fractured ribs if not given enough analgesia. Morbid obesity and distension of the abdomen can also result in hypercapnia. In the neuromuscular disorders we can include cervical cord lesions, poliomyelitis, Guillain-Barré syndrome, diphtheria, myasthenia gravis, organophosphorus poisoning and muscular dystrophy. In Table 1 we can see the causes of respiratory failure categorized by type.

DIAGNOSIS

Hypercapnia is diagnosed with the use of ABGs, usually by radial artery puncture. A detailed history together with physical findings is needed. Upon clinical suspicion of hypercapnia, an evaluation of hypercapnia is necessary as the list of differential diagnosis may be long. Laboratory tests will help establish the diagnosis and the cause of hypercapnia.

Depending on the cause of hypercapnia there will be different symptoms so history taking is important. Pneumonia is suggested by cough, sputum production, chest pain while pulmonary embolism may be presented with sudden onset of shortness of breath and chest pain. Sepsis is suggested by fever and chills. COPD exacerbation includes a history of heavy smoking, cough and sputum production. Exposure to chemicals, dust and other substances may help in diagnosing asthma, aspiration and inhalation injuries. Cardiogenic pulmonary oedema can be presented with chest pain, paroxysmal nocturnal dyspnoea and orthopnoea while non-cardiogenic pulmonary oedema can be evaluated with the presence of risk factors such as sepsis, aspiration, traumas and blood transfusions. The use of narcotic substances or exposure to toxins can be a cause for respiratory failure. As we have seen, a detailed history is essential and very helpful when trying to identify the cause of hypercapnia.

Clinical examination is another important part of the diagnostic process as it can offer valuable signs of the patient. Presence of wheezing indicates airway obstruction such as bronchospasm, secretions and airway pathology. Stridor also is a sign that indicates narrowed or obstructed upper airway in the larynx or trachea. Hypotension combined with poor perfusion signs may suggest sepsis or pulmonary embolism while hypertension combined with poor perfusion signs can be indicative of cardiogenic pulmonary oedema. In case of pulmonary hypertension, the right ventricle may be affected and there will be an elevated jugular venous pressure (JVP). Jugular venous distension is the visualization of the elevated JVP. If there is tachycardia and arrhythmias present, it may be due to cardiogenic pulmonary oedema.

Furthermore, laboratory work is needed to confirm the suspicion of hypercapnia and its cause. As already mentioned, ABGs will be the diagnostic tool that will help us establish the diagnosis of hypercapnia. Hypercapnia will present with a value of PaCO2 higher than 45 mmHg and a reduced pH below 7.35. ABGs analysis and evaluation help to establish a diagnosis and to the guide course of action according to these parameters and their changes during the treatment of the patient. A complete blood count may reveal findings that can help establish the cause of hypercapnia. Anemia can be the cause of cardiogenic pulmonary oedema, polycythemia may suggest chronic hypoxemia, while disturbances in white blood cells such as leukocytosis and leukopenia can indicate an infection. Respiratory, blood, urine and other body fluid cultures may be taken if deemed necessary.

Finally, diagnostic investigations such as chest x-ray, electrocardiogram, echocardiography, pulmonary function tests and bronchoscopy may be performed in order to facilitate the definite diagnosis.

PREVENTION

Prevention is important, especially for people with increased risks of hypercapnia, such as people with COPD, asthma, OHS, heavy smokers, people working with lung irritants and drug users. It is important to treat any existing lung condition, make lifestyle changes and follow correctly instructions given by the physician.

Firstly, cessation of smoking is one of the most important changes people should aim for in order to decrease the risks of ending up in a hypercapnic state. Stopping smoking can be a real challenge for many people, so people should consider asking help from their physician about existing programs that help with smoking cessation. It is especially of the essence with people suffering with respiratory problems to avoid worsening of their existing issues and minimize further irritation of the airways that could lead to exacerbation of their condition.

Additionally, maintaining a balanced diet, with healthy food while avoiding junk food is important. The excess of adipose tissue in the abdomen and surrounding chest wall reduces lung volume, namely functional residual capacity with a significant decrease in the expiratory reserve volume [7]. Losing excess weight is a must for obese people and people with sleep apnoea disorder as it can have a huge effect on the symptoms.

Furthermore, getting annual flu shots may reduce the risk of respiratory complications from infections such as influenza virus. Infections may be also avoided by frequently washing hands and avoiding crowds during flu season. Also, the use of antibiotics should be avoided if not prescribed by the physician since it can lead to antibiotic-resistant infections and increase the severity of complications.

It is crucial when are symptoms present, to visit a doctor as soon as possible to receive proper treatment. There is better prognosis if treatment starts at early stages. It is also crucial to take the medications as prescribed by the physician on time and not to miss any doses. Medical advices should be only received by specialized medical personnel. Self-treatment will not suffice and will only lead to worsening of the symptoms. Some diseases cannot be prevented but with the proper and early management we can prevent the most severe complications such as hypercapnia and hypercapnic coma.

TREATMENT

If left untreated, hypercapnia may lead to respiratory failure and hypercapnic coma. There is not a standard treatment plan or protocol for hypercapnia. The treatment regimen of hypercapnia will be depended on the severity of the status of the patient as well as the underlying cause.

If the symptoms are severe, then mechanical ventilation may be needed. Non-invasive ventilation (NIV) is often used in preference to invasive mechanical ventilation [8]. In case Non-Invasive mechanical ventilation cannot be used at the medical center, either due to unresponsiveness and low level of consciousness of the patient, or it is not available at that moment, or there is a lack of knowledge and experience of the treating physician, then endotracheal intubation may be deemed necessary. This will help to improve respiration and oxygenation of the patient while reducing the work of breathing of the patient. The duration of mechanical ventilation will depend on the underlying cause and the effectiveness of the treatment but should not be prolonged if not necessary. Delayed weaning can lead to complications such as ventilator induced lung injury (VILI), ventilator associated pneumonia (VAP), and ventilator induced diaphragmatic dysfunction [9]. The progress and effectiveness of the treatment can be monitored mainly with the use of ABGs analysis through which the parameters of the ventilator can be adjusted accordingly. In case hypercapnia is not too severe, the patient may benefit by oxygen therapy at home using CPAP (Continuous Positive Airway Pressure) or BiPAP (Bilevel Positive Airway Pressure) device. This is especially helpful in people suffering from obstructive sleep apnea syndrome to keep the airways open. Very severe respiratory failure, in which hypercapnia may also be present, is often treated with extracorporeal membrane oxygenation (ECMO), in which oxygen is added to and carbon dioxide removed directly from the blood [10].

It is never too late to make some lifestyle changes, even after the patient presents with hypercapnia. As already mentioned in the prevention segment, cessation of smoking is crucial, especially after symptoms and respiratory complications arise. Losing excess weight is essential, even more in case of morbidly obese patients and a strict diet regimen must be followed. All of the above should be combined with exercise if possible and incorporate physical activity into daily routine. In case of exacerbation due to exposure, patients should avoid contact with chemicals, fumes, dust and other irritants.

Certain medications may be prescribed by the physician and can very helpful and assist breathing. Antibiotics will help fight and treat pneumonia and other existing infections. Also, bronchodilators can decrease airway resistance and increase airflow to the lungs by dilating bronchi and bronchioles. Short-acting bronchodilators can provide relief during exacerbation episodes and acute onset of symptoms, while long-acting bronchodilators will help in the prevention and management of the symptoms. Furthermore, corticosteroids can be administered if necessary to reduce any inflammation of the airways.

Lastly, surgical treatment may be required in some patients. In cases where the tissue is affected and the damaged area can be removed, the patient will undergo lung resection and volume reduction surgery. More severe case may require lung transplant surgery and replace damaged lung from a healthy donor.

DISCUSSION

Hypercapnia is defined as an elevation in the arterial carbon dioxide tension. It is a very serious state and can lead to major complications. Hypercapnic respiratory failure may occur either acutely, insidiously or acutely upon chronic carbon dioxide retention. In all these conditions, pathophysiologically, the common denominator is reduced alveolar ventilation for a given carbon dioxide production [11].

There are many causes of hypercapnic failure. Symptomatology may vary and clinical examination together with personal history taking may not be sufficient, therefore further diagnostic tests may be required. Diagnostic imaging tests as well as laboratory tests may be useful in discovering the etiology of hypercapnia. It is necessary to establish the cause in order to follow the correct treatment.

It is crucial to seek proper medical treatment as soon as symptoms are present, in order to prevent complications that may increase risks and endanger the patient's life. Following the physician's recommendations and instructions regarding any ongoing treatment regimen is of great importance to improve existing respiratory conditions and avoid further problems. Patients must seek further medical advice if their current treatment is not bringing proper results. Also, proper treatment should be received for any other co-morbidities that may aggravate the situation. Lifestyle changes, especially smoking cessation and weight loss is a must especially in case of chronic lung conditions. Maintaining a healthy weight and a regular physical activity is also important in these situations.

Finally, Hypercapnic failure is a common phenomenon especially in people with pre-existing lung conditions. Time is of essence and as soon as symptoms present, people should seek medical attention immediately. Hypercapnia is serious and any delays in treatment will worsen the prognosis of the patient. Correct treatment and following instructions as given will improve the symptomatology and quality of life for the patients.

KEY MESSAGES

- Hypercapnic failure requires immediate medical attention;
- There are many causes of hypercapnic failure and must be identified for each patient;
- Correct treatment should be administered as soon as possible;
- Prolonging mechanical ventilation will worsen the prognosis;
- Prevention strategies can avert serious complications from arising.

REFERENCES

[1] Kaynar M. A., Sharma S. [Updated 2019 Jul 25] Respiratory Failure. *Medscape*.

[2] Respiratory Failure. (2019, December 12). *Physiopedia* https://www.physiopedia.com/index.php?title=Respiratory_Failure&oldid=227004.

[3] Rawat D., Sharma S. Hypercapnea. [Updated 2019 Jun 4]. In: *StatPearls* [Internet]. Treasure Island (FL): StatPearls Publishing; 2020 Jan-. Available from: https://www.ncbi.nlm.nih.gov/books/NBK500012/.

[4] Bruno C. M., and Valenti, M. (2012). Acid-base disorders in patients with chronic obstructive pulmonary disease: a pathophysiological review. *BioMed Research International*, 2012.

[5] Tobin M. J., Laghi F., Jubran A. Ventilatory failure, ventilator support and ventilator weaning. In: Dempsey J., editor. *Handbook of physiology: the respiratory system. Bethesda*, MD: American Physiological Society; 2012.

[6] Pisani L., Corcione, N., and Nava, S. (2016). Management of acute hypercapnic respiratory failure. *Current Opinion in Critical Care*, 22(1), 45-52. doi: https://10.1097/mcc.0000000000000269.

[7] Hodgson L. E., Murphy P. B., Hart N. Respiratory management of the obese patient undergoing surgery. *J Thorac Dis* 2015; 7: 943-952.

[8] Davidson A. C., Banham, S., Elliott, M., Kennedy, D., Gelder, C., Glossop, A., Church, Alistair C., Creagh-Brown, B., Dodd, J. W., Felton, T., Foëx, B., Mansfield, L., McDonnell, L., Parker, R., Patterson, C. M., Sovani, M., Thomas, Lynn (14 March 2016). "BTS/ICS guideline for the ventilatory management of acute hypercapnic respiratory failure in adults." *Thorax.* 71 (Suppl 2): ii1-ii35. doi: https://10.1136/thoraxjnl-2015-208209.

[9] Zein H., Baratloo, A., Negida, A., and Safari, S. (2016). Ventilator Weaning and Spontaneous Breathing Trials; an Educational Review. *Emergency* (Tehran, Iran), 4(2), 65-71.

[10] *Pisani L., Polastri, M., Pacilli, A. M. G., Nava, S. (2018). "Extracorporeal Lung Support for Hypercapnic Ventilatory Failure." Respiratory Care. 63 (9): 1174-1179.* doi: https://10.4187/respcare.06277.

[11] Roussos C., Koutsoukou A. *European Respiratory Journal* 2003 22: 3s-14s; doi: https://10.1183/09031936.03.00038503.

In: Non-Invasive Mechanical Ventilation Complications ISBN: 978-1-53619-515-6
Editor: Antonio M. Esquinas

Chapter 19

Complications during Non-Invasive Mechanical Ventilation. Chronic Obstructive Pulmonary Disease

Ana Isabel Santos*[*], MD, PhD
Pneumology Unit, Coimbra Hospital and University Centre, Coimbra, Portugal
Serviço de Pneumologia, Centro Hospitalar e Universitário de Coimbra, Coimbra, Portugal

Abstract

Chronic obstructive pulmonary disease (COPD) is one of the main causes of morbidity and mortality worldwide. Non-invasive ventilation (NIV) has been applied in the last decades for the treatment of exacerbations and end-stage COPD with remarkable results in the improvement of quality of life, lung function and survival. However, the use of NIV, and particularly high intensity-NIV, may result in some complications. The most frequent complications associated to NIV treatment in COPD patients include hemodynamic effects, the *deventilation syndrome*, pulmonary barotrauma, auto-positive end-expiratory pressure (auto-PEEP) and ventilator-associated pneumonia, which are addressed in this chapter. Although complementary studies are needed to clarify the reported complications, and in some cases the data is still sparce, clinicians should be aware of the risks associated with NIV in this particular subset of patients. Yet, current guidelines strongly recommend the use of NIV in patients with acute exacerbations of COPD.

[*] Corresponding Author's E-mail: anisa.rsantos@gmail.com.

1. INTRODUCTION

Chronic obstructive pulmonary disease (COPD) is a chronic lung disease with high morbidity and mortality worldwide [1], being the fourth leading cause of dead [2]. COPD exacerbations are a major cause of hospital admissions and they comprise high costs for national health care systems. In the past few decades, non-invasive ventilation (NIV) has been applied for the treatment of exacerbations and end-stage COPD in patients that frequently develop chronic hypercapnic respiratory failure (CHRF). The role of long-term nocturnal NIV in restrictive and neuromuscular diseases is well documented [3, 4]. Recent studies also demonstrated the benefits of long-term use of NIV, particularly high-intensity NIV (HI-NIV), in patients with COPD [5-7], however further investigation is required. Currently it is known that NIV improves pH, decreases the respiratory rate and $PaCO_2$, and consequently, reduces the intubation rate and mortality [8]. HI-NIV consists in using higher inspiratory pressures and respiratory frequencies to improve gas exchange, contributing to clinically relevant improvements in health-related quality of life, lung function, and survival as observed in patients with COPD, without undue loss of patient comfort [9]. Due to these advantages, the use of NIV in patients with acute exacerbation of COPD has been continuously increasing in the recent years [10, 11]. In fact, current guidelines strongly recommend the use of NIV in patients with acute exacerbations of COPD [2].

In this chapter, we aim to focus and describe the main complications of NIV in the treatment for patients with COPD.

2. HEMODYNAMIC EFFECTS

In physiological conditions, the respiratory system works as a negative pressure system. Thus, the excursion of the diaphragm down during normal inspiration generates a negative pressure in the pleural cavity and in the airways that pulls air into the lungs. This negative intrathoracic pressure also affects cardiac physiology, by decreasing the right atrial pressure and creating a sucking effect in the inferior vena cava which, in turn increases venous return [12].

Nevertheless, mechanical ventilation influences the main determinants of cardiac performance, including atrial filling, ventricular emptying, and myocardial contractility, thus affecting preload, afterload and heart rate, respectively. Actually, NIV, particularly the application of extrinsic positive end-expiratory pressure (PEEP), works by providing positive pressure to the upper airways until the alveoli, which is then transmitted to the alveolar space and thoracic cavity, creating a positive (or less negative) pressure. Therefore, the main acute effects of NIV on the heart result from the increase in pleural pressure and increase in lung volume [13]:

1. The rise in intrapleural pressure, leads to an increase in right atrial and mean systemic pressures, causing impairment in the heart filling as a result of the decrease in venous return and right atrium preload;
2. NIV reduces hypoxemia and hypercapnia, decreases pulmonary vasoconstriction, and also reduces right ventricle afterload. However, when the lung is hyperinflated, above functional residual capacity, alveolar vessels become compressed, as a result of alveolar distension;
3. The increase in lung volume and consequent compression of alveolar vessels increases left atrium preload temporarily, but it decreases once the right heart provides the pulmonary circuit, thus lefting the left heart with insufficient amounts of blood;
4. The positive pressure of NIV decreases transmural pressure ($P_{transmural} = P_{intravascular} - P_{pleural}$), and thus reduces left ventricle afterload.

Still, some long-term compensatory mechanisms may influence the long-term net effect on cardiac performance. Moreover, some groups have studied the acute effects of NIV [14-17] in patients with stable CHRF, however, long-term effects [18-22] are less clear and require further studies. A possible mechanism to explain the positive long-term effect of NIV was proposed by Budweiser *et al.* that observed a decrease in the prohormone of brain natriuretic peptide (NTproBNP) in patients with CHRF, both obstructive and restrictive, without significant differences between groups [18]. Therefore, NIV might reduce right and left heart stretching through mechanical compression of the heart and, on the other hand, the effects of NIV on right and left ventricle afterloads influence natriuretic peptide levels. A reduction in cardiac output can also decrease left ventricle stress. A decrease in natriuretic peptides leads to less diuresis, increased blood volume and restoration of right atrium pressure resulting in an increase in mean systemic pressure at long-term [13].

The relevance of these effects in the management of COPD patients treated with NIV is because a substantial proportion of COPD patients have cardiac comorbidities, including concomitant heart failure [23]. Potentially negative effects of NIV, particularly HI-NIV, on the heart should be considered. Actually, most trials investigating NIV in patients with stable hypercapnic COPD have excluded patients with heart failure, demonstrating the urgent need of further studies in COPD patients with cardiac comorbidities.

Moreover, the reported effects of mechanical ventilation in cardiac performance could be beneficial in some special circumstances such as in patients with cardiogenic pulmonary edema. In these patients there is a decrease in venous return meaning less blood pumped by the right ventricle and less pulmonary edema being generated [24].

In addition, it is important to consider the effects of extrinsic PEEP on cardiac output and in blood pressure in patients whom a cerebral perfusion pressure has to be maintained in straight levels, such as, after a stroke or a subarachnoid hemorrhage, when a drop in mean arterial pressure could disturb the cardiovascular autoregulation and cause adverse effects [25].

In conclusion, although largely unknown, we should be aware for the possible long-term effects of NIV in patients with CHRF and concomitant heart failure. NIV, and even HI-NIV with high PEEP, are commonly applied in patients with COPD, notwithstanding that the consequences of the acute effect on cardiac output reduction remain unknown.

3. Deventilation Syndrome

In patients with COPD treated with NIV, the removal of the ventilation mask in the morning, after nocturnal ventilation, may result in shortness of breath, commonly designated as *deventilation syndrome* [26]. Possible causes for the *deventilation syndrome* are the dynamic hyperinflation due to high-PEEP NIV [27] and patient-ventilator asynchrony [28]. *Deventilation syndrome* is described in nearly one third of patients with COPD under treatment with NIV [28], but also in many patients with obstructive sleep apnea syndrome and in the postoperative period [29].

A wide variety of ventilator modes are available for use in the treatment of patients with COPD, but until recently, no significant superiority had been demonstrated for any specific ventilation mode. However, in a recent study, Junger *et al.* demonstrated short-term improvements in exercise tolerance, in forced vital capacity, in quality of life and in morning dyspnea in patients with *deventilation syndrome* with their daily nocturnal HI-NIV, when ventilation mode was switched to pursed lips breathing ventilation (PLBV). This is a bilevel positive airway pressure (BiPAP) mode that mimics the pressure curve of spontaneous pursed lips breathing during the expiration phase. A possible mechanism for this may be that PBLV enables deeper and longer expiration, thus leading to a lower volume of end-expiratory intrathoracic gas, improved diaphragmatic relaxation, and, consequently, larger tidal volumes. PLBV may also improve the distribution pattern of ventilated air. In fact, contrarily to HI-NIV that leads to heterogeneous auto-PEEP and local areas of high-PEEP associated with inadequate ventilation, PLBV is remarkable to avoid auto-PEEP, minimizing these heterogeneous ventilated areas [27].

Even though many cases remain undiagnosed, the attending physician must be aware of this clinic entity that may compromise quality of life and adherence to the treatment. Screening of the *deventilation syndrome* must be assessed in each appointment with a patient treated with home ventilation. Even though diagnosis and monitoring of *deventilation syndrome* are complex, monitoring the parameters related to ventilation, patient lung function, severity of the disease and basal hypercapnia levels should be included [26]. Polysonography may help the diagnosis. Adjustment of the ventilator settings should be done in order to decrease ineffective inspiratory efforts, and to improve patient comfort during and after NIV [28]. Further studies in this field are needed to better clarify this entity and to find the best strategy to treat it.

4. Pulmonary Barotrauma

Pulmonary barotrauma is damage to lung tissue secondary to differences of pressure in the respiratory system, resulting in the presence of extra-alveolar air in locations where it is not present under normal circumstances. The most common origin of pulmonary barotrauma is due to alveolar rupture, which may result in other complications such as pneumothorax, pneumomediastinum and subcutaneous emphysema [30].

Barotrauma is a well-described complication of mechanical ventilation and is a cause of increased morbidity and mortality [31-33]. Breathing depends on negative intrathoracic pressures, however, mechanically ventilated patients are under mechanically applied non-physiological positive pressure. This increase in trans-alveolar pressure may result in alveolar rupture and consequent leakage of air into the extra-alveolar tissue [34]. Even though all modalities of mechanical ventilation can lead to barotrauma, the incidence of NIV-induced barotrauma is much lower when compared to patients receiving invasive mechanical ventilation. Furthermore, although virtually every patient on positive ventilation is at risk of developing barotrauma, patients with some respiratory conditions, including COPD, asthma, interstitial lung disease, *pneumocystis jiroveci* pneumonia, cystic fibrosis, neuromuscular disorders and acute respiratory stress syndrome, are more susceptible [30, 35-40]. In the particular case of COPD, there is an increased risk of dynamic hyperinflation and poor lung compliance, with a prolonged expiratory phase and difficulty in exhaling the full volume before the ventilator delivers the next breath, resulting in an increase in PEEP – auto-PEEP [41].

The relationship between PEEP and the development of barotrauma is controversial. Even though some groups report no association of high levels of PEEP and existence of barotrauma [41-45], others show that it is possible to minimize the occurrence of barotrauma by adjusting the ventilator settings [30, 35, 46-49]:

1. Pressure-controlled ventilation, particularly in patients with low compliance;
2. Maintain plateau and peak inspiratory pressures as low as possible: plateau pressures higher than 35 cmH_2O have been associated with increased risk for barotrauma;
3. Optimize inspiratory and expiratory times;
4. PEEP value should not exceed auto-PEEP – if higher PEEP is required for optimization of oxygenation, it should be titrated up slowly with close monitoring of the peak inspiratory and plateau pressures;

5. Avoid patient-ventilator asynchrony, by appropriate patient selection, choosing the adequate interface and size, optimization of ventilatory support, and checking for factors of desynchrony such as air leaks, noise and water in circuit.

Nowadays, increased awareness of clinicians for the dangers of excessive tidal volumes and airway pressures, has led to a decrease in the incidence of barotrauma and respective morbidity and mortality [41].

5. Intrinsic PEEP or Auto-PEEP

In a healthy person, a normal passive exhalation should allow the complete emptying of the air contained in the lungs until lung pressure is equalized with atmospheric pressure. However, in some conditions, the lungs may not empty effectively, and a certain amount of air may remain trapped at the end of exhalation, thus generating a positive pressure, the so-called intrinsic or auto-PEEP [12]. When repeated, cycle after cycle, the amount of air trapped increases, and there is an increase in intrathoracic pressure, leading to the hemodynamic effects described above, including a decrease in blood pressure, as well as an increase in plateau pressure and, consequently, barotrauma. In lung obstructive conditions, mainly COPD, there is an increase in air trapping that hampers ventilation mechanics. There is an increase in the consumption of oxygen and in CO_2 production, thus rising respiratory rate and worsening auto-PEEP in a vicious cycle. In COPD, there is a dynamic obstruction of airflow caused by airway inflammation and mucus plugs, increasing the expiratory effort and pressure around the airway. Thus, the airway becomes narrower and there is trapping of air in the alveoli that are dependent of that airway. Furthermore, the increased lung compliance that occurs in COPD, leads to airway collapse and air trapping. Other factors that can contribute to auto-PEEP, such as high tidal volume ventilation, high respiratory rate and slow inspiratory flow with a high inspiratory-to-expiratory time ratio.

In COPD patients dynamic hyperinflation with extrinsic obstruction of expiratory flow is the most common cause of auto-PEEP. Therefore, administration of low-level extrinsic PEEP can contribute to decrease auto-PEEP in these patients, by maintaining airways open, and leading to the easier release of air from the alveoli [12].

Quantification of auto-PEEP is complex since auto-PEEP can vary among individual lung units. It depends on the obstruction grade of each unit, consequently having a heterogeneous distribution throughout the lung and, changing proportionally to the airway resistance present at a particular lung unit. Several methods can be used to estimate auto-PEEP in a mechanically ventilated patient. For instance, auto-PEEP can be calculated by subtracting the external PEEP from the total PEEP, following a 2-second pause after de end of expiration in patients without spontaneous breathing [50].

Clinicians should rise suspicion of auto-PEEP when [12, 51]:

1. Exhalation is still ongoing when the next respiratory cycle starts;
2. Increasing plateau pressures;
3. Active exhalation with the use of accessory muscles;
4. Decrease in blood pressure;
5. Long expiratory times;
6. Respiratory distress.

The basic goal in the management of external PEEP in mechanically ventilated patients with auto-PEEP is to allow more time for exhalation so that all the air in the lung can be expelled. This can be accomplished by reducing the respiratory rate or inspiratory-expiratory ratio to 1:3 to 1:5, in order to allow more time to exhalation and reduce air trapping. However, the reduction in respiratory rate may cause hypercapnia, hypoxia or acidosis, thus increasing the resistance of pulmonary vasculature and worsening hemodynamic instability. Instead, a higher inspiratory flow rate with high peak pressures can be used, as it will assure fast delivery of air during inspiration and leading more time for expiration. However it should be used with caution as it increases the risk of barotrauma in these patients [51]. Possible strategies in these patients can be the use of a square waveform for ventilation delivery that can also speed up the inspiration process and, by decreasing the tidal volume that reduces the work of breathing [12]. Moreover, it is fundamental to control other factors that can increase respiratory demand, such as, fever, pain, anxiety and comorbidities. Also, before starting NIV in a COPD patient, pharmacological therapeutic should be optimized, by treating bronchoconstriction with bronchodilators, inflammation with corticosteroids and, when applicable, suction of mucus plugs. When used, in order to prevent auto-PEEP in patients with dynamic hyperinflation and, consequently, to avoid worsening of hyperinflation or circulatory compromise, external PEEP should be kept below 75 to 85% of auto-PEEP [52, 53].

Finally, NIV support can be a lifesaving procedure in patients with COPD exacerbations, by causing an improvement of gas exchange, resting of fatigued muscles, and relieve of respiratory distress. However, if not used properly, NIV can cause a considerable increase in morbidity and mortality, particularly in these patients due to the COPD pathophysiology and to the pattern of flow obstruction. Ventilation must be adapted to each patient needs and tolerance, and physicians must be aware of the potential drawbacks of this treatment.

6. Pneumonia

Mechanical ventilation is a risk factor for the development of nosocomial pneumonia. The risk of pneumonia is 3 to 5 times higher in invasive ventilation when compared to NIV, mainly in immunosuppressed patients and patients with comorbidities [35].

COPD patients are in higher risk of developing pneumonia, mainly those who are under treatment with steroids. Pneumonia may be the cause of exacerbation. However, patients with exacerbations of COPD appear to largely benefit from NIV, and even NIV was proven to be superior to standard medical therapy in preventing pneumonia, as shown by several studies [54-58]. Contrarily, a recent study from Chen *et al.* described the occurrence of nosocomial pneumonia as a cause for NIV late failure in patients with COPD and associated with higher mortality. However, this was a small study, including only 9 patients of a respiratory intensive care unit, a fact that limits extrapolation to other realities [59].

In the light of the existing evidence, we cannot point out nosocomial pneumonia as a complication of NIV in the particular subset of patients with COPD, as there are no clear studies demonstrating the higher frequency of pneumonia cases in COPD patients under NIV treatment. However, the risk of NIV-induced pneumonia can be minimized by excluding patients with compromised function of the upper airways or with difficulty in clearing secretions, as well as by avoiding or reducing sedatives, and positioning the patient in a sitting or semi-sitting position during NIV [35, 54, 56]. Also, current guidelines strongly recommend vaccination against *Streptococcus pneumoniae* as a strategy to avoid pneumonia by this agent [2].

Conclusion

In this chapter we addressed the most reported major complications of NIV that, due to the pathophysiology and progression of COPD, occur exclusively or have higher incidence in this particular subgroup of patients. However, studies concerning these complications in COPD patients are sparse. More studies are needed, including studies with larger number of patients, to clarify the relevance of these complications for initiating or suspending NIV treatment. In fact, each COPD patient is unique, and should be addressed based on his comorbidities, symptoms, and stage of the disease. Treatment and management of complications should be individualized. Moreover, besides the complications described in this chapter, many other factors can contribute to NIV failure. As any other patient, COPD patients are also susceptible to develop other minor complications of NIV. These include interface-related complications, such as arm edema and deep venous thrombosis, carbon dioxide rebreathing, claustrophobia, discomfort, facial skin lesions, noise disturbance, or patient-ventilator desynchrony. Air pressure and flow-related complications, such as air leaks, nasal or oral dryness, nasal congestion, airway dryness, and gastric insufflation are also commonly found. General complications of NIV are reviewed elsewhere [35].

In conclusion, communication with the patient is essential for the appropriate assessment and management of complications and therefore for NIV success. Further studies will help to improve management of COPD patients.

REFERENCES

[1] Mannino DM. Epidemiology and global impact of chronic obstructive pulmonary disease. *Semin Respir Crit Care Med*. 2005;26(2):204-10.

[2] 2020 Global Strategy for the Diagnosis, Management, and Prevention of COPD. *Global Initiative for Chronic Obstructive Lung Disease*. 2020.

[3] Simonds AK, Elliott MW. Outcome of domiciliary nasal intermittent positive pressure ventilation in restrictive and obstructive disorders. *Thorax*. 1995;50(6):604-9.

[4] Leger P, Bedicam JM, Cornette A, Reybet-Degat O, Langevin B, Polu JM, et al. Nasal intermittent positive pressure ventilation. Long-term follow-up in patients with severe chronic respiratory insufficiency. *Chest*. 1994;105(1):100-5.

[5] Duiverman ML, Wempe JB, Bladder G, Jansen DF, Kerstjens HA, Zijlstra JG, et al. Nocturnal non-invasive ventilation in addition to rehabilitation in hypercapnic patients with COPD. *Thorax*. 2008;63(12):1052-7.

[6] Duiverman ML, Wempe JB, Bladder G, Vonk JM, Zijlstra JG, Kerstjens HA, et al. Two-year home-based nocturnal noninvasive ventilation added to rehabilitation in chronic obstructive pulmonary disease patients: a randomized controlled trial. *Respir Res*. 2011;12:112.

[7] Köhnlein T, Windisch W, Köhler D, Drabik A, Geiseler J, Hartl S, et al. Non-invasive positive pressure ventilation for the treatment of severe stable chronic obstructive pulmonary disease: a prospective, multicentre, randomised, controlled clinical trial. *The Lancet Respiratory Medicine*. 2014;2(9):698-705.

[8] Lightowler JV, Wedzicha JA, Elliott MW, Ram FS. Non-invasive positive pressure ventilation to treat respiratory failure resulting from exacerbations of chronic obstructive pulmonary disease: Cochrane systematic review and meta-analysis. *BMJ*. 2003;326(7382):185.

[9] Dreher M, Ekkernkamp E, Walterspacher S, Walker D, Schmoor C, Storre JH, et al. Noninvasive ventilation in COPD: impact of inspiratory pressure levels on sleep quality. *Chest*. 2011;140(4):939-45.

[10] Chandra D, Stamm JA, Taylor B, Ramos RM, Satterwhite L, Krishnan JA, et al. Outcomes of noninvasive ventilation for acute exacerbations of chronic obstructive

pulmonary disease in the United States, 1998-2008. *Am J Respir Crit Care Med.* 2012;185(2):152-9.

[11] Stefan MS, Shieh M-S, Pekow PS, Hill N, Rothberg MB, Lindenauer PK. Trends in Mechanical Ventilation Among Patients Hospitalized With Acute Exacerbations of COPD in the United States, 2001 to 2011. *Chest*. 2015;147(4):959-68.

[12] Mora Carpio AL, Mora JI. Positive End-Expiratory Pressure. StatPearls. *Treasure Island* (FL)2020.

[13] Duiverman ML, Arellano-Maric MP, Windisch W. Long-term noninvasive ventilation in patients with chronic hypercapnic respiratory failure: assisting the diaphragm, but threatening the heart? *Curr Opin Pulm Med*. 2016;22(2):130-7.

[14] Ambrosino N, Nava S, Torbicki A, Riccardi G, Fracchia C, Opasich C, et al. Haemodynamic effects of pressure support and PEEP ventilation by nasal route in patients with stable chronic obstructive pulmonary disease. *Thorax.* 1993;48(5):523-8.

[15] Borghi-Silva A, Reis MS, Mendes RG, Pantoni CB, Simoes RP, Martins LE, et al. Noninvasive ventilation acutely modifies heart rate variability in chronic obstructive pulmonary disease patients. *Respir Med*. 2008;102(8):1117-23.

[16] Lukacsovits J, Carlucci A, Hill N, Ceriana P, Pisani L, Schreiber A, et al. Physiological changes during low- and high-intensity noninvasive ventilation. *Eur Respir J*. 2012;39(4):869-75.

[17] Marangoni S, Vitacca M, Quadri A, Schena M, Clini E. Non-invasive haemodynamic effects of two nasal positive pressure ventilation modalities in stable chronic obstructive lung disease patients. *Respiration*. 1997;64(2):138-44.

[18] Budweiser S, Luchner A, Jorres RA, Heinemann F, Hitzl AP, Schmidbauer K, et al. NT-proBNP in chronic hypercapnic respiratory failure: a marker of disease severity, treatment effect and prognosis. *Respir Med*. 2007;101(9):2003-10.

[19] Castro-Anon O, Golpe R, Perez-de-Llano LA, Lopez Gonzalez MJ, Escalona Velasquez EJ, Perez Fernandez R, et al. Haemodynamic effects of non-invasive ventilation in patients with obesity-hypoventilation syndrome. *Respirology*. 2012;17(8):1269-74.

[20] Dreher M, Schulte L, Muller T, Ekkernkamp E, Zirlik A. Influence of effective noninvasive positive pressure ventilation on inflammatory and cardiovascular biomarkers in stable hypercapnic COPD patients. *Respir Med.* 2015;109(10): 1300-4.

[21] Schonhofer B, Barchfeld T, Wenzel M, Kohler D. Long term effects of non-invasive mechanical ventilation on pulmonary haemodynamics in patients with chronic respiratory failure. *Thorax*. 2001;56(7):524-8.

[22] Sin DD, Wong E, Mayers I, Lien DC, Feeny D, Cheung H, et al. Effects of nocturnal noninvasive mechanical ventilation on heart rate variability of patients with advanced COPD. *Chest*. 2007;131(1):156-63.

[23] Chen W, Thomas J, Sadatsafavi M, FitzGerald JM. Risk of cardiovascular comorbidity in patients with chronic obstructive pulmonary disease: a systematic review and meta-analysis. *Lancet Respir Med*. 2015;3(8):631-9.

[24] Fellahi JL, Valtier B, Beauchet A, Bourdarias JP, Jardin F. Does positive end-expiratory pressure ventilation improve left ventricular function? A comparative study by transesophageal echocardiography in cardiac and noncardiac patients. *Chest*. 1998;114(2):556-62.

[25] Muench E, Bauhuf C, Roth H, Horn P, Phillips M, Marquetant N, et al. Effects of positive end-expiratory pressure on regional cerebral blood flow, intracranial pressure, and brain tissue oxygenation. *Crit Care Med*. 2005;33(10):2367-72.

[26] Esquinas AM, Ucar ZZ, Kirakli C. Deventilation syndrome in severe COPD patients during long-term noninvasive mechanical ventilation: poor sleep pattern, hyperinflation, or silent chronic muscular fatigue? *Sleep Breath*. 2014;18(2):225-6.

[27] Jünger C, Reimann M, Krabbe L, Gaede KI, Lange C, Herzmann C, et al. Non-invasive ventilation with pursed lips breathing mode for patients with COPD and hypercapnic respiratory failure: A retrospective analysis. *PLOS ONE*. 2020;15(9):e0238619.

[28] Adler D, Perrig S, Takahashi H, Espa F, Rodenstein D, Pépin JL, et al. Polysomnography in stable COPD under non-invasive ventilation to reduce patient–ventilator asynchrony and morning breathlessness. *Sleep and Breathing*. 2012;16(4):1081-90.

[29] Beyoglu CA, Koksal GM. Perioperative management of a patient with deventilation syndrome. *Obesity Research & Clinical Practice*. 2020;14(1):103-5.

[30] Diaz R, Heller D. Barotrauma And Mechanical Ventilation. StatPearls. *Treasure Island (FL)*2020.

[31] Gammon RB, Shin MS, Buchalter SE. Pulmonary barotrauma in mechanical ventilation. Patterns and risk factors. *Chest*. 1992;102(2):568-72.

[32] Gattinoni L, Bombino M, Pelosi P, Lissoni A, Pesenti A, Fumagalli R, et al. Lung structure and function in different stages of severe adult respiratory distress syndrome. *JAMA*. 1994;271(22):1772-9.

[33] Schnapp LM, Chin DP, Szaflarski N, Matthay MA. Frequency and importance of barotrauma in 100 patients with acute lung injury. *Crit Care* Med. 1995;23(2): 272-8.

[34] Boussarsar M, Thierry G, Jaber S, Roudot-Thoraval F, Lemaire F, Brochard L. Relationship between ventilatory settings and barotrauma in the acute respiratory distress syndrome. *Intensive Care Med*. 2002;28(4):406-13.

[35] Carron M, Freo U, BaHammam AS, Dellweg D, Guarracino F, Cosentini R, et al. Complications of non-invasive ventilation techniques: a comprehensive qualitative review of randomized trials. *Br J Anaesth*. 2013;110(6):896-914.

[36] Carron M, Gagliardi G, Michielan F, Freo U, Ori C. Occurrence of pneumothorax during noninvasive positive pressure ventilation through a helmet. *J Clin Anesth.* 2007;19(8):632-5.

[37] Gupta D, Nath A, Agarwal R, Behera D. A prospective randomized controlled trial on the efficacy of noninvasive ventilation in severe acute asthma. *Respir Care.* 2010;55(5):536-43.

[38] Diaz O, Iglesia R, Ferrer M, Zavala E, Santos C, Wagner PD, et al. Effects of noninvasive ventilation on pulmonary gas exchange and hemodynamics during acute hypercapnic exacerbations of chronic obstructive pulmonary disease. *Am J Respir Crit Care Med.* 1997;156(6):1840-5.

[39] Gammon RB, Shin MS, Groves RH, Jr., Hardin JM, Hsu C, Buchalter SE. Clinical risk factors for pulmonary barotrauma: a multivariate analysis. *Am J Respir Crit Care Med.* 1995;152(4 Pt 1):1235-40.

[40] de Latorre FJ, Tomasa A, Klamburg J, Leon C, Soler M, Rius J. Incidence of pneumothorax and pneumomediastinum in patients with aspiration pneumonia requiring ventilatory support. *Chest.* 1977;72(2):141-4.

[41] Anzueto A, Frutos-Vivar F, Esteban A, Alia I, Brochard L, Stewart T, et al. Incidence, risk factors and outcome of barotrauma in mechanically ventilated patients. *Intensive Care Med.* 2004;30(4):612-9.

[42] Weg JG, Anzueto A, Balk RA, Wiedemann HP, Pattishall EN, Schork MA, et al. The relation of pneumothorax and other air leaks to mortality in the acute respiratory distress syndrome. *N Engl J Med.* 1998;338(6):341-6.

[43] Stewart TE, Meade MO, Cook DJ, Granton JT, Hodder RV, Lapinsky SE, et al. Evaluation of a ventilation strategy to prevent barotrauma in patients at high risk for acute respiratory distress syndrome. Pressure- and Volume-Limited Ventilation Strategy Group. *N Engl J Med.* 1998;338(6):355-61.

[44] Brochard L, Roudot-Thoraval F, Roupie E, Delclaux C, Chastre J, Fernandez-Mondejar E, et al. Tidal volume reduction for prevention of ventilator-induced lung injury in acute respiratory distress syndrome. The Multicenter Trail Group on Tidal Volume reduction in ARDS. *Am J Respir Crit Care Med.* 1998;158(6):1831-8.

[45] Ventilation with Lower Tidal Volumes as Compared with Traditional Tidal Volumes for Acute Lung Injury and the Acute Respiratory Distress Syndrome. *New England Journal of Medicine.* 2000;342(18):1301-8.

[46] Eisner MD, Thompson BT, Schoenfeld D, Anzueto A, Matthay MA, Acute Respiratory Distress Syndrome N. Airway pressures and early barotrauma in patients with acute lung injury and acute respiratory distress syndrome. *Am J Respir Crit Care Med.* 2002;165(7):978-82.

[47] Argiras EP, Blakeley CR, Dunnill MS, Otremski S, Sykes MK. High PEEP decreases hyaline membrane formation in surfactant deficient lungs. *Br J Anaesth.* 1987;59(10):1278-85.

[48] Woodring JH. Pulmonary interstitial emphysema in the adult respiratory distress syndrome. *Crit Care Med*. 1985;13(10):786-91.

[49] Zimmerman JE, Dunbar BS, Klingenmaier CH. Management of subcutaneous emphysema, pneumomediastinum, and pneumothorax during respirator therapy. *Crit Care Med*. 1975;3(2):69-73.

[50] Reddy RM, Guntupalli KK. Review of ventilatory techniques to optimize mechanical ventilation in acute exacerbation of chronic obstructive pulmonary disease. *Int J Chron Obstruct Pulmon Dis*. 2007;2(4):441-52.

[51] Mowery NT. Ventilator Strategies for Chronic Obstructive Pulmonary Disease and Acute Respiratory Distress Syndrome. *Surg Clin North Am*. 2017;97(6):1381-97.

[52] Ranieri VM, Giuliani R, Cinnella G, Pesce C, Brienza N, Ippolito EL, et al. Physiologic effects of positive end-expiratory pressure in patients with chronic obstructive pulmonary disease during acute ventilatory failure and controlled mechanical ventilation. *Am Rev Respir Dis*. 1993;147(1):5-13.

[53] Petrof BJ, Legare M, Goldberg P, Milic-Emili J, Gottfried SB. Continuous positive airway pressure reduces work of breathing and dyspnea during weaning from mechanical ventilation in severe chronic obstructive pulmonary disease. *Am Rev Respir Dis*. 1990;141(2):281-9.

[54] Hess DR. Noninvasive Positive-Pressure Ventilation and Ventilator-Associated Pneumonia. *Respiratory Care*. 2005;50(7):924-31.

[55] Kohlenberg A, Schwab F, Behnke M, Geffers C, Gastmeier P. Pneumonia associated with invasive and noninvasive ventilation: an analysis of the German nosocomial infection surveillance system database. *Intensive Care Med*. 2010;36(6):971-8.

[56] Gay PC. Complications of Noninvasive Ventilation in Acute Care. *Respiratory Care*. 2009;54(2):246-58.

[57] Echevarria C, Steer J, Hartley T, Lane N, Bourke SC. Predictors of NIV Treatment in Patients with COPD Exacerbation Complicated by Respiratory Acidaemia. *Copd*. 2020;17(5):492-8.

[58] Gungor S, Mocin OY, Tuncay E, Aksoy E, Goksenoglu NC, Ocakli B, et al. Risk factors of unfavorable outcomes in chronic obstructive pulmonary disease patients treated with noninvasive ventilation for acute hypercapnic respiratory failure. *The Clinical Respiratory Journal*. 2020;14(11):1083-9.

[59] Chen T, Bai L, Hu W, Han X, Duan J. Risk Factors Associated with Late Failure of Noninvasive Ventilation in Patients with Chronic Obstructive Pulmonary Disease. *Can Respir J*. 2020;2020:8885464.

In: Non-Invasive Mechanical Ventilation Complications ISBN: 978-1-53619-515-6
Editor: Antonio M. Esquinas

Chapter 20

NEUROMUSCULAR DISORDERS. MOTOR AND INTELLECTUAL DISABILITIES. RARE NEUROLOGICAL DISEASES

S. Fernández Huerga
Médico Adjunto, Servicio Neumología,
Complejo Hospitalario Universitario de León, Adjunto al Servicio de Neumología

ABSTRACT

The impact of these neuromuscular disorders on the respiratory muscles and the upper airway results in swallowing and breathing problems, as well as the appearance of ineffective cough, all of which leads to a higher risk of recurrent respiratory infections. Most patients need to exceed hours of continuous use of NIV, with pressure ulcers, irreversible malformations, dryness in the nasopharyngeal mucosa, sleep disorders, and many other complications. Special equipment is also needed in order to adapt ventilation for day, night or social activities, besides a backup one in case of failure. Finally, an early diagnosis of the pathology and its complications are essential in order to avoid failure of NIV.

INTRODUCTION

Non-invasive mechanical ventilation (NIV) has been used for many years in a number of diseases, being the group of patients with neuromuscular disorders where there is the longest experience, starting with its use in the 1930s poliomyelitis epidemic and how it then reduced the mortality rate.

Randomised studies on the use of NIV in patients with neuromuscular diseases are not possible due to ethical reasons, but it has indeed been possible to demonstrate an enhancement of life quality and survival.

Since patients require this treatment chronically, for long hours and even continuously, NIV might cause complications, which have been greatly reduced nowadays with the implementation of new methods and materials.

Physiopathology of Neuromuscular Diseases

The common feature of this group of patients is respiratory muscles involvement, although not all of them are necessarily affected, neither in the same extent nor in their evolution across time.

Compromising the upper airway results in swallowing impairment, risk of bronchoaspiration and ineffective cough, all of which leading to a higher risk of recurrent respiratory infections. Inspiratory and expiratory muscles involvement contributes to daytime hypercapnia, which along with ineffective cough deteriorates the reaction to acute episodes and eventually increases mortality.

Mechanism of Action of NIV

NIV main function in patients with neuromuscular diseases is to reach muscular rest, improve the sensitivity of the respiratory centre and pulmonary mechanics, and correct the recurring sleep disorders of these patients, along with the consequent correction of daytime hypercapnia and dyspnoea. The main indications for NIV are listed in Table 1 and the contraindications in Table 2.

Table 1. NIV indications

- Clinical:
  - Daytime hypersomnolence
  - Dyspnoea
  - Cognitive changes
- Physiological:
  - Hypercapnia
  - 5 min nocturnal continuous desaturation or intermittent nocturnal desaturation over 10% of the register
  - Vital capacity inferior to 50%

Table 2. NIV contraindications (relative)

• Facial trauma or burns
• Vomiting
• Confusion or agitation
• Upper airway obstruction
• Recent facial, upper airway or upper gastrointestinal tract surgery
• Life threatening hypoxaemia
• Inability to protect upper airway
• Decreased level of consciousness
• Fixed upper airway obstruction
• Bowel obstruction
• Respiratory secretions in excess

The use of NIV on patients with neuromuscular diseases may be performed as chronic home ventilation, or acute hospital ventilation in infectious exacerbations or significant stress generated situations (i.e., invasive procedures).

MAIN NEUROMUSCULAR DISEASES REQUIRING NIV

Multiple neuromuscular diseases require NIV, such as motor neuron diseases (namely Amyotrophic Lateral Sclerosis -ALS-) and muscular dystrophies (i. e., Duchenne's dystrophy) besides other conditions with a lower incidence.

Genetic diseases:

- Mitochondrial myopathy
- Muscular dystrophies
- Congenital neuropathies
- Congenital myotonic dystrophies
- Endocrinopathies
- Spinal muscular atrophies

Acquired diseases:

- Polymyositis
- Secondary spinal injuries
- Myasthenia gravis
- Cerebral palsy
- Poliomyelitis
- Secondary polyneuropathies

Complications of NIV in Patients with Neuromuscular Diseases

The use of NIV should not generally exceed 8-10 hours of continuous use, although in some cases, especially in palliative care, it can significantly surpass that time.

The most frequent complication, as in other pathologies requiring NIV, is pressure sores. Early monitoring of their emergence is essential in order to avoid irreversible malformations or poor tolerance towards NIV caused by pain in the pressure area. Patches or fabrics with hydrocolloids prevent the appearance of these lesions. Once present it is advisable to alternate different interfaces or their material. It should be also considered the possibility to use a pipette in certain patients with equipment prepared and programmed for that mode. Moreover, wrong adaptation of interfaces could generate air leakage towards the eyes, facilitating possible outbreaks of conjunctivitis, and exert an excessive and continuous pressure over the dental arch, which could constrain movement or even inflict the loss of dental pieces.

Another frequent complication resulting from continuous use of NIV is the appearance of dryness in the nasopharyngeal mucosa when the ventilator is not equipped with a humidifier.

One of the characteristics of patients with neuromuscular diseases is that the use of NIV tends to be increasingly prolonged, which means that potential equipment failures must be considered. Thus, for those patients with high dependency or those who exceed the 12 hours of use, it is highly recommended to have at least two programmed life-sustaining devices and spare batteries, which allow to change the equipment in the presence of any failure or to use batteries if there is any issue with the power source. If possible, use of alternative interfaces without nasal support must be considered. Equipment should also be adapted to be used outside home (in wheelchairs), allowing the patient to engage in social activities and the use of pipette if well tolerated.

The appearance of asynchronies may be principally related to problems occurring at the interface due to leaks, or to alterations in the evolution of the disease with dependence on the equipment for longer than 12 hours, which would involve a change of mode from ventilatory to controlled or from pressure to volumetric. The appearance of paradoxical glottic closure is common in patients with bulbar ALS, resulting in obstructive events. Therefore, an early diagnosis should be made in order to ponder whether performing a tracheostomy and/or pressure adjustment.

It is also advisable to conduct conventional polysomnography to find out sleep disorders and correct them by using different ventilation equipment and programmes according to sleep and daytime.

The appearance of atelectasis can be corrected by altering the PEEP, whereas the barotraumas and pneumothorax, although rare, require the adjustment and decrease of pressures or volumes. Abdominal distension caused by aerophagy due to very high pressures or volumes must also be corrected by adjusting the parameters of the ventilator.

Conclusion

Patients with neuromuscular diseases require the use of NIV, which helps both to improve quality of life and to reduce mortality. The prolonged use of NIV equipment as the disease evolves is related to the appearance of complications, the most frequent being the formation of pressure sores and air leaks. In addition, there are complications inherent to the pathology itself that must be examined and corrected early, either with new equipment programming or with several ventilators with different programmes depending on the patient's needs and ventilation periods.

References

[1] Lisboa C, Díaz O y Fadic R. Ventilación mecánica no invasiva en pacientes con enfermedades neuromusculares y en pacientes con alteraciones de la caja torácica. Serie Sobre Enfermedades Respiratorias, Músculos y Rehabilitacion. Serie 4: Los músculos respiratorios en las enfermedades neuromusculares y de la caja torácica. *Arch Bronconeumología* 2003;39(7):314-20. [Non-invasive mechanical ventilation in patients with neuromuscular diseases and in patients with alterations of the rib cage. Series On Respiratory Diseases, Muscles and Rehabilitation. Series 4: The respiratory muscles in neuromuscular and rib cage diseases. *Arch Bronconeumology*]

[2] Vega-Briceño L, Prado F, Bertrand P, Sánchez I. *Soporte ventilatorio no invasivo en enfermedades neuromusculares.* ISSN 07 I8-322I. [*Non-invasive ventilatory support in neuromuscular diseases*]

[3] Maquilón C, Castillo S, Montiel G, Ferrero G, Toledo A y Siroti C. Consenso Chileno De Ventilación No Invasiva. IV. Ventilación no invasiva en pacientes con enfermedades neuromusculares *Rev Chil Enf Respir* 2008; 24:192-198. [Chilean Consensus on Non-Invasive Ventilation. IV. Non-invasive ventilation in patients with neuromuscular diseases *Rev Chil Enf Respir*]

[4] Camargo Rubio, Rubén Darío. Bioética en la ventilación mecánica invasiva: enfermedades crónicas/terminales. *Acta Colombiana de Cuidados Intensivos*. 2020. [Bioethics in invasive mechanical ventilation: chronic / terminal diseases. *Colombian Act of Intensive Care*]

[5] Ferrero E et al. Normativa Separ: normativa sobre el manejo de las complicaciones respiratorias de los pacientes con enfermedad neuromuscular. *Archivos de Bronconeumología*. 2013;49(7):306-313. [Separ Regulations: regulations on the management of respiratory complications in patients with neuromuscular disease. *Archives of Bronconeumology*.]

In: Non-Invasive Mechanical Ventilation Complications
Editor: Antonio M. Esquinas
ISBN: 978-1-53619-515-6

Chapter 21

COMPLICATIONS DURING NON-INVASIVE MECHANICAL VENTILATION. SLEEP BREATHING DISORDERS

Vânia Caldeira*

Department of Pulmonology, Hospital S. Bernardo (Centro Hospitalar Setúbal), Lisboa, Portugal

ABSTRACT

Positive airway pressure is a well-known treatment for multiple sleep breathing disorders. In order to choose the best therapy for each patient it is important to recognize the different pathophysiology beside each clinical entity (sleep apnoea, obesity hypoventilation syndrome,), but also the more common adverse events of therapy to avoid and solve them. CPAP and APAP are the first line therapies in moderate to severe OSAS, servoventilation is an adequate therapy for CSA with Cheyne Stokes respiration and bilevel pressure or CPAP could be used in OHS. Although the differences between equipments and modalities for each pathology, the side effects are usual very similar. The majority of side effects are in relation with the interface or the pressure administered, and a careful follow-up is essential to identify and resolute the common problems with ventilation. Finally, is also important to know that some serious but rare adverse events have been reported as pneumothorax, pneumocephalon and massive epistaxis.

Keywords: PAP therapy, non-invasive ventilators, OSAS, CSA, OHS, PAP side effects

* Corresponding Author's E-mail: vania.medicina@gmail.com.

Introduction

Sleep related breathing disorders (SRBD) are conditions characterized by disordered respiration during sleep and include a range of different entities that share common features: sleep apnoea - which includes obstructive sleep apnoea syndrome (OSAS) and also central sleep apnoea (CSA) -, sleep-related hypoventilation syndromes - such as obesity-hypoventilation syndrome (OHS) and neuromuscular disorders (NMD) - and SRBD with hypoxaemia associated with chronic respiratory diseases as chronic obstructive pulmonary disease (COPD) [1].

This chapter will focus essentially on sleep apnoea (OSAS and CSA) and OHS as NMD, COPD and other respiratory chronic diseases will be discussed in other chapters.

Obstructive Sleep Apnoea Syndrome

OSAS is a common disorder characterized by increased collapsibility of the upper airway with repetitive apnoeas or reduced breathing during sleep and affects about 26% of the United States adult population [1-4]. Patients usually present with loud snoring, witnessed apnoeas and excessive daytime sleepiness [1]. Obesity is the major risk factor for OSAS and there is an increased cardiovascular risk in these patients [2]. Other risk factors are male gender, advanced age, post-menopausal women and craniofacial abnormalities. Besides that, it is associated with poor quality of life, disruption of sleep and increased accidents [4].

Positive airway pressure (PAP) therapy is the gold standard treatment in adults with moderate to severe OSAS and in all OSAS patients with sleepiness [3]. Oral devices that causes mandible protrusion and stabilization are a valid alternative in mild to moderate OSAS or as a second-line therapy in severe OSAS patients that are not compliant or not responsive to PAP therapy [5, 6]. Various surgical techniques are available for the treatment of OSAS: however, only maxillomandibular advancement surgery (MMA) showed to be as effective as PAP in severe OSAS. The other types of surgery (as the largely used uvulopalatopharyngoplasty - UPPP) are only valid alternatives in patients with mild OSAS and severe obstructive anatomy or as adjunct therapies when only PAP is not enough [6, 7].

The most widely used modality of PAP treatment is continuous positive airway pressure (CPAP), applying a constant pressure throughout the respiratory cycle to splint the airway open [4, 6]. In the last years, because of the low access to therapeutic polysomnography in order to titrate the optimal pressure of CPAP, auto-adjusting PAP (APAP) had become a valid alternative [2]. In fact, literature demonstrated no clinically significant difference in PAP adherence when comparing treatment using home APAP versus CPAP after in-laboratory titration. Besides that, APAP allows a faster therapy initiation with lower costs and a continuous regulation of pression to adjust to variations in patient weight, body position or alcohol ingestion. American Academy of Sleep Medicine (AASM) recommends the use of APAP only in patients without significant comorbidities and continues to indicate the use of titration polysomnography in patients with congestive heart failure, significant pulmonary disease, CSA or severe nocturnal desaturation [4].

In cases of failure because of coexisting central hypoventilation or uncompliant patients with high pressure CPAP/APAP and difficulty exhaling against a fixed pressure, bilevel positive airway pressure (BiPAP) or auto-adjusted BiPAP (autoBiPAP) must be tried [2, 3, 6].

Central Sleep Apnoea

CSA is characterized by a lack of respiratory effort during sleep and also presents with symptoms common to OSAS as witnessed apnoeas, sleepiness and gasping, but usually without significant snoring and frequently associated with cardiovascular or neurological diseases. CSA can be associated with hypercapnia where it is typically associated with chronic hypoventilation (in stroke or neurodegenerative diseases) or normocapnia, such as in Cheyne-Stokes breathing (CSB), primary CSA and high-altitude periodic breathing. CSB is associated with instability of the respiratory drive and is more common in male patients, older than 60 years old and with congestive heart failure (CHF), occurring in about ~25-40% [1, 8].

The indications to start CPAP therapy in CSA and data in outcomes are not as well established as in OSAS. CPAP may be an appropriate first-line therapy in moderate to severe CSA, particularly in patients with CHF, as it showed to attenuate CSA, improve nocturnal oxygenation and increase ejection fraction [1].

BiPAP-ST provides a higher inspiratory pressure (IPAP), a lower expiratory pressure (EPAP) and a respiratory backup rate and although the insufficient evidence available it is sometimes used in primary CSA and in CSB patients. Besides many patients do not tolerate the treatment, there are also concerns over excessive augmentation of tidal ventilation conducting to hypocapnia that exacerbates CSB [1].

A growing alternative in CSA with CSB pattern is adaptive servo-ventilation (ASV): the EPAP is settled to prevent obstructive events (as in CPAP modality) and there is administered a variable breath-by-breath IPAP (between settled limits) in response to the current pattern of patient breathing. Thus, this IPAP is adaptative and inversely proportional to the instantaneous tidal volume and there is a backup respiratory rate allowing to stabilize the respiratory pattern and prevent periodic breathing and central events. The support pressure (IPAP/EPAP difference) is minimal during normal breathing or hyperpneic periods and increases during central apnoeas [1, 9]. Some studies showed that ASV improved not only the SRBD but also cardiac function in CHF patients. In these patients ASV versus CPAP improves apnoea-hypopnea index (AHI), sleep quality, left ventricular ejection fraction and decrease the levels of plasma BNP [9].

However, because of the results of SERVE-HF showing an increase mortality in a group of patients, ASV is not recommended in CHF patients for the treatment of moderate to severe CSA-CSB if ejection fraction is below 45%. Further studies are needed to clarify the CHF patient that benefits with ASV without severe adverse events. In the light of current evidence ASV should be offered to all CHF patients with mild CSA-CSB and those with moderate to severe CSA-CSB with preserved ejection fraction [10]. Instead CHF patients with CSA-CSB seems to be more compliant with ASV than conventional PAP [9].

Beyond its major use in CHF patients with CSB, ASV could be a second-line therapy in patients non-responsive to CPAP and has been used in idiopathic CSA, complex sleep apnoea, opioid-associated CSA and CSA after stroke [1].

Obesity Hypoventilation Syndrome

Obesity Hypoventilation Syndrome (OHS) is defined by the combination of obesity, sleep-disordered breathing and daytime hypercapnia during wakefulness, not secondary to other causes - neuromuscular, metabolic, lung or chest wall diseases [1, 11]. About 90% of patients with OHS have OSAS and 10% of patients with OSAS have OHS [4, 11]. The prevalence of OHS is estimated to be 0,3-0,4% but in the last years it is increasing with the burden of severe obesity. Like OSAS, there is an association with cardiovascular morbidity but that seems to be worse than in OSAS patients [11]. Untreated OHS patients have an 18-month mortality of 23%, which falls to 3% in NIV-treated patients [1]. OHS patients are in great risk of hospitalization with acute-on-chronic hypercapnic respiratory failure and consequent death [11].

Although extensive use of nocturnal NIV in OHS patients, the evidence of efficacy is limited. While CPAP is not theoretical a hypoventilation treatment, just preventing obstructive events, in the last years some studies have focused on CPAP treatment as an effective alternative to BiPAP. The Pickwick study was a large RCT that compared three alternative treatments for OHS - lifestyle modification (control group), CPAP and NIV (bilevel pressure with assured volume modality). It showed that patients with OHS and OSAS (with higher AHI) can achieve reductions in daytime PaCO2 with CPAP treatment and that nocturnal oxygenation and sleep quality improved significantly with both CPAP and NIV [11].

The American Thoracic Society guidelines recommend the use of PAP during sleep in all stable ambulatory patients diagnosed with OHS. In patients with concomitant severe OSA it is recommended CPAP as first-line therapy, rather than NIV [12].

NIV COMPLICATIONS

Although PAP therapy has consistent evidence on improved survival in severe OSAS, the benefit depend substantially on the daily PAP use and adherence is still a major clinical challenge. The current literature emphasizes that the pattern of adherence is established early [13]. Patient education, management of expectations and problem resolution in the first weeks are essential to adherence [3, 13]. Long-term follow-up in PAP-treated patients by trained health care providers and sleep specialists is recommended [3].

The potential benefits of CPAP in OSAS are reduction in AHI severity, improvement in symptoms as sleepiness, sleep disruption, car accidents and reduction in blood pressure. Potential cardiovascular and mortality benefits cannot be ruled out [4]. CPAP and BiPAP therapy are safe and adverse events are mainly minor and reversible [3]. The side effects may be annoying but usually do not pose major health problems [1]. Potential benefits of PAP therapy outweighed the harms in most patients with moderate to severe OSAS. However, side effects with PAP therapy can result in poor sleep quality having impact on long-term adherence to therapy and making it so important [4, 13].

One interesting real-life study about PAP treatment showed discontinuation in a large group of OSAS patients [13], with only 63% definitely users. In the nonusers group (37,4%), the majority discontinued the therapy within the first 3 months. In this study, side effects were the most common reported reason for discontinuation of PAP therapy. Most patients complained about side effects of the interface (24,1%) - leakage, skin dermatitis -, discomfort with the PAP device (13,3%), claustrophobia (12,1%), rhinitis (6%), insomnia (4,8%). The attention to side effects during long-term follow-up enables to troubleshoot PAP interfaces, machine or usage problems [3].

Regarding complications, one study reported that 43,4% of patients with OHS under PAP therapy in the ICU during an episode of acute-on-chronic hypercapnic respiratory failure experienced an adverse event. The most common were skin lesion (36%), eye irritation (13%), claustrophobia (9%), gastric distention (4%). On the other hand, in the ambulatory scenario the most common side effects were rhinitis (13%) and oral dryness (7-9%) [14].

Although rare and usually minor, there are a wide variety of possible side effects. Most of the side effects are in relation with the interface, as mask leak, skin abrasion or ulceration, mask allergy, facial dermatitis, conjunctivitis or sore eyes or claustrophobia [4, 9]. There is a small group of patients for whom the idea of wearing a mask is psychological unacceptable because of anxiety, apprehension or claustrophobia. In these patients a slow approach by the NIV team and the use of adjunctive options as hypnosis or cognitive behavioral therapy seems important. Mask leak can cause xerophthalmia, conjunctive irritation and xerostomia. If not well fitted to the patient face the mask can cause pain impairing quality of sleep or skin lesions [15]. A variety of masks available continues to evolve, with new designs focusing in improving comfort with better fitting to each patient and reducing leaks. Various types of interfaces are available as nasal masks, nasal pillows, oral masks and full-face masks. However, side effects have been reported with all kind of interfaces. In general, nasal masks are better tolerated and have less side effects (leakage, sore eyes, claustrophobia, oronasal dryness) versus oronasal masks [1, 4, 9].

Other important and common side effects are pressure-related as rhinitis/rhinorrhea, sneezing, desiccation, sinusitis, headache, epistaxis, otitis, aspiration, belching, mouth or mask leak (dry mouth), pressure intolerance, sense of difficulty exhaling, tinnitus and aerophagia [4]. Nasal and oral dryness is a common side effect, and this may be approached with passive or heated humidifiers. Literature demonstrated clinically significant reduction in nasal discharge, nasal and oral dryness and epistaxis with the current use of humidifiers. The most common side effects of humidified PAP are condensation of water into the PAP circuit and accumulation of humidity in face, nose or mouth. However, literature favors routine use of these humidified systems to improve comfort and reduce side effects. The development of systems of modified pressure, that transiently lowers the pressure during expiration, have improved patient comfort, even with higher pressures. Gastric insufflation from NIV increases with the increase of pressure, being 20 cmH2O the safe limit. Moreover, the treatment of OSAS with PAP also could lead to the development of treatment-emergent central sleep apnea associated with PAP [4, 9].

There are equipment-related side effects, as noise, smell, tubing condensation, cumbersome equipment, spousal intolerance, ramp overuse and equipment maintenance and cleaning; the possibility of equipment-failure with recurrence of OSAS and other general side effects (anxiety, insomnia, headache, fatigue, chest discomfort, periodic limb movements) [4, 9].

Although major device and interface improvements in the last years, this seems to have only a little impact on adherence to therapy. Thereby, careful attention should be given to educational and behavioral interventions [4].

Finally, it is still important to highlight that serious adverse effects have been reported, as pneumothorax, pneumocephalon and massive epistaxis. Also, in home-ventilated children the development of mid-facial hypoplasia is a well-known complication [1]. Aspiration pneumonia has been reported in about 5% of ventilated patients, which decreased by excluding patients with compromised upper airway function or problems in secretions management. Barotrauma is a rare but well-recognized complication of NIV although the risk is lower than with invasive mechanical ventilation and it usually is associated with some pulmonary diseases as COPD and cystic fibrosis. Caution is also needed in patients with unstable hemodynamic status or severe cardiac disease without appropriate treatment because of the risk of significant hypotension and reduced cardiac output [9].

Regarding side effects, differences between CPAP and APAP are not clinically significant. Some patients experience less pressure discomfort, less nasal irritation or less machine noise with APAP, while others refer more discomfort with pressure variation of APAP. Individual patterns justify a trial with the alternate modality in intolerant patients. Also, there was no significative difference in side effects between BiPAP and CPAP treatment [4]. Side effects with BiPAP are in general the same as with CPAP, although more difficult in tolerating the higher pressures is common [1]. Finally, adverse effects with ASV are similar to CPAP but usually, in patients with CHF, treatment compliance is better [1, 9].

In conclusion, the adequate comprehension of SRBD differences and the underlying pathophysiology allows the clinician to choose the best therapy and the most appropriate PAP modality for each patient, minimizing discomfort, thus representing a nuclear first step toward patient adherence and efficacy of treatment. In addition, a wide knowledge of the PAP equipment, different interfaces and side effects of therapy with a careful follow up of the patients enables the fast identification of adverse effects and its resolution.

REFERENCES

[1] Bassetti C., Dogas Z. and Peigneux P. 2014. *Sleep Medicine Textbook*, 95-110; 215-220; 259-273. European Sleep Research Society.

[2] Slouka D et al. 2018. "Risk factors for failure of continuous positive airway pressure treatment in patients with obstructive sleep apnoea." *Biomed. Pap. Med. Fac. Univ. Palacky Olomouc Czech Repub*. 162 (2): 134-138.

[3] Kushida C et al. 2006. "Practice parameters for the use of continuous and bilevel positive airway pressure devices to treat adult patients with sleep-related breathing disorders." *Sleep*. 29: 375-379.

[4] Patil S et al. 2019. "Treatment of adult obstructive sleep apnea with positive airway pressure: an American Academy of Sleep Medicine systematic review, meta-analysis and GRADE assessment." *Journal of Clinical Sleep Medicine*. 15(02):301-34.

[5] Ramar K et al. 2015. "Clinical practice guideline for the treatment of obstructive sleep apnea and snoring with oral appliance therapy: an update for 2015." *Journal of Clinical Sleep medicine*. 15;11(07):773-8.

[6] Epstein LJ et al. 2009. "Clinical guideline for the evaluation, management and long-term care of obstructive sleep apnea in adults." *Journal of Clinical Sleep Medicine*. 15;5(03):263-76.

[7] Aurora RN et al. 2010. "Practice parameters for the surgical modifications of the upper airway for obstructive sleep apnea in adults." *Sleep*. 1;33(10):1408-13.

[8] Darien IL et al. 2014. *International Classification of Sleep Disorders*. 3rd ed.: American Academy of Sleep Medicine.

[9] Aurora RN et al. 2016. "Updated adaptive servo-ventilation recommendations for the 2012 AASM guideline: the treatment of central sleep apnea syndromes in adults: practice parameters." *Journal of Clinical Sleep Medicine*. 15;12(05):757-61.

[10] Esquinas A. 2010. Noninvasive Mechanical Ventilation, 93-98; 107-117. Springer.

[11] Masa J et al. 2015. "Efficacy of different treatment alternatives for Obesity hypoventilation syndrome: Pickwick study." *American Journal of Respiratory and Critical Care Medicine*. 192(1): 86-94.

[12] Mokhlesi B et al. 2019. "Evaluation and management of Obesity hypoventilation syndrome: an official American Thoracic Society clinical practice guideline." *American Journal of Respiratory and Critical Care Medicine*. 200(3): 6-24.

[13] Galetke W et al. 2011. "Long-term therapy with continuous positive airway pressure in obstructive sleep apnea: adherence, side effects and predictors of withdrawal - a real life study." *Respiration*. 82: 155-161.

[14] Afshar M et al. 2019. "The role of positive airway pressure therapy in adults with obesity hypoventilation syndrome: a systematic review and meta-analysis." *Annals of American Thoracic Society*. In press.

[15] Simonds A. 2015. *Handbook Noninvasive Ventilation*, 234-245. European Respiratory Society.

In: Non-Invasive Mechanical Ventilation Complications
Editor: Antonio M. Esquinas
ISBN: 978-1-53619-515-6

Chapter 22

Complications During Non-Invasive Mechanical Ventilation: Oncology/ Hematology Clinical Conditions

Raffaele Scala*, MD, FCCP and Luca Guidelli, MD
Pulmonology and Respiratory Intensive Care Unit,
San Donato Hospital Arezzo, Italy

Abstract

Acute respiratory failure (ARF) is the most frequent and challenging complication in onco-hematologic patients. Early referral to ICU, multidisciplinary cooperation, new therapeutic, large application of NIV has contributed to improve the prognosis of malignancies complicated by ARF. Among all, non-invasive ventilation (NIV) has been considered crucial for the "turning point" in the mortality of critically ill patients with malignancies as it averts IMV-associated life-threatening complications The actual evidence suggests benefits from a trial of "prophylactic" CPAP or NIV in the early phase of ARF in onco-hematologic patients without multiple organ dysfunctions. However, delayed intubation after prolonged NIV failure is associated with poor hospital survival. Concerning the setting, starting early CPAP/NIV in the ward to reduce ICU admission is still controversial. Finally, NIV is feasible as "palliation" in selected terminally onco-hematologic patients.

Keywords: noninvasive ventilation, high flow nasal therapy, endotracheal intubation, intensive care unit, do not intubate status

* Corresponding Author's E-mail: raffaele_scala@hotmail.com.

Introduction

Acute respiratory failure (ARF) is the most frequent and challenging complication in cancer as it occurs in up to 40-50% of patients with solid tumors, hematological malignancies and bone marrow transplantation recipients. Mechanical ventilation was required in 44-69% of cancer patients admitted to intensive care unit (ICU) [1].

Among the variables recorded at ICU admission, the severity of patient's clinical condition and the institution of invasive mechanical ventilation (IMV) are the only two which are independently associated with hospital mortality [1].

The mortality of mechanically ventilated cancer patients remains high but it has significantly decreased over the past two decades from 80-90% in the 1980s to 65-75% in the 1990s and even less than 50% in specialized centres. The improved outcome in mechanically ventilated cancer patients could be attributed to: 1) a better and earlier referral to ICU with the exclusion of patients with poor functional status or those wishing no life-prolonging treatment; 2) a better management of septic complications; 3) a closer cooperation between onco-hematologist and intensivists [1]. Among all, non-invasive ventilation (NIV) has been considered crucial for the "turning point" in the mortality of critically ill patients with malignancies as it averts IMV-associated life-threatening complications [1].

This chapter will focus on the use of NIV as a means to treat ARF in adult onco-hematologic patients, with and without a status of "do not intubate" (DNI) choice, as well as the still controversial usefulness of NIV as "palliation" in terminal neoplastic patients.

Pathophysiology of NIV in Onco-Hematologic Patients

While a good outcome in ARF essentially requires reversal of the underlying mechanisms, correction of hypoxaemia and oxygen delivery as well as hypercapnic acidosis is pivotal to ensure patient survival in the meantime. The primary approach in hypoxaemic patients is to raise alveolar oxygen content by increasing the inspired fraction of oxygen (FiO2); more profound hypoxaemia can be reversed by pushing up alveolar oxygen pressure and inducing alveolar recruitment with continuous positive airway pressure (CPAP) [1]. Furthermore, CPAP is effective in cardiogenic pulmonary edema thanks to its favourable hemodynamic effects. Recently, high-flow nasal oxygen-therapy (HFNO) HFNO has been proposed as either preventive or alternative or integrative treatment of NIV in milder degrees of hypoxemia, included those occurring in cancer patients, due to its advantages over conventional oxygen-therapy (e. g., delivery of high FiO2, adequate humidification, patient comfort, provision of low PEEP values) [1].

Correcting hypercarbia on the other hand requires increasing alveolar ventilation and unloading of respiratory muscles by means of NIV that, differently from CPAP, delivers two different levels of pressures, being higher during the inspiration than during the expiration [1].

The likelihood of success of NIV depends on the patho-physiological pattern of ARF, being greater in hypercapnia (i.e., "pump failure") than in hypoxemia (i.e., "lung failure") [1]. ARF in malignancies could develop as a consequence of both, isolated or combined, patho-physiological dysfunctions in patients with or without pre-existent cardiopulmonary diseases. ARF may result from direct pulmonary involvement by the malignancy, opportunistic infection, therapy-induced pulmonary toxicity, pulmonary embolism, post-operative complications and diffuse alveolar haemorrhage [1]. In addition, ARF may be caused by exacerbations of comorbid illness as chronic obstructive pulmonary disease (COPD) or congestive cardiac failure [1].

While mechanical ventilation supports the failing respiratory system and reverses the physiopathological derangements, the aetiology of ARF should be aggressively investigated to guide therapy and estimate prognosis. Some aetiologies such as bacterial sepsis or cardiogenic pulmonary oedema carry a better prognosis than others, such as invasive fungal disease or direct airway invasion by the malignancy [1]. It has been shown that ARF directly caused by haematological malignancy can be reversed by aggressive chemotherapy; in contrast, pulmonary involvement by solid tumours still carries a grim prognosis [1]. Being able to identify the aetiology of ARF itself appears to be associated with a better outcome, as in patients without a clear diagnosis there is very high mortality [1].

Although NIV is a widely accepted treatment of ARF in cancer patients who desire life-support measures, in some advanced malignancies prolonging survival is not a desirable goal and, conversely, palliation of symptoms is the main target of the care [1]. The use of NIV for cancer patients with ARF could be classified into three categories: 1) NIV as "life support" without limitations of life-sustaining treatments; 2) NIV as "ceiling ventilation" for patients refusing ETI; 3) NIV as a "palliation" for patients wishing to receive only comfort measures (e.g., relief of dyspnea).

CLINICAL USE OF NIV IN ONCOHEMATOLOGIC PATIENTS

The evidence about the use of NIV in onco-hematologic patients consists of five interventional randomized controlled trials (RCTs), [2-5] as well as of a larger set of observational studies. We analysed separately the role of NIV in onco-hematologic patients without and with limitations of care (i.e., DNI status)

NIV in Patients Without Limitations of the Care

Nonpalliative use of NIV has been investigated in 4 RCTs [2-4] mainly focused on haematological malignancies, two of them showing favourable and two unfavourable findings.

In the first French RCT, Hilbert et al., [2] compared the effectiveness of intermittent NIV plus standard medical therapy with supplemental of oxygen versus no ventilator support in an heterogeneous population of 52 immunocompromised patients, 30 of whom had haematological malignancies, with pulmonary infiltrates, fever, and moderate acute respiratory distress syndrome (ARDS) ($PaO_2/FiO_2 < 200$). Rate of ETI (46% versus 77%; $p = 0.03$) and of serious complications (13% versus 21%; $p = 0.02$), as well as ICU (38% versus 69%; $p = 0.03$) and hospital mortality (50% versus 81%; $p = 0.02$) were significantly reduced in NIV as compared to control group. Subgroup analysis demonstrated a reduced mortality with NIV only in haematological malignancies patients.

In the subsequent Italian RTC, Squadrone et al., [3] compared the effects of early CPAP delivered with the helmet plus oxygen versus the only oxygen in 40 patients with leucopenia and mild ARDS (PaO_2/FiO_2 between 200 and 300) in absence of infectious causes. The study was performed in the ward under the supervision of an emergency ICU team. CPAP reduced the relative risk for developing more severe ARF needing ICU admission for invasive or noninvasive ventilatory support (i.e., primary outcome) to 0.25 (95% confidence interval: 0.10-0.62). As compared to control group, CPAP group showed lower incidence of pulmonary (25% versus 65%; $p = 0.025$) and systemic infections (10% versus 65%; $p = 0.001$), fewer ICU admissions (4 versus 16 patients; $p = 0.0002$), lower ETI (10% versus 70%; $p = 0.0001$) and mortality rate (25% versus 85%; $p = 0.0004$).

In a German mono-centric RCT, Wermke et al., [4] evaluated the impact of the adjunct of intermittent NIV to the oxygen-therapy in 86 patients undergoing an allogeneic hematopoietic stem cell transplantation (HSCT) at the initial phase of ARDS (i.e., $PaO_2/FiO_2 < 300$) in the hematological ward. Although early ARF treatment with NIV was associated with a non-significant decreased rate of failure to achieve sufficient oxygenation (24% versus 39%; $p = 0.17$), neither ICU admission rate nor need for intubation or survival parameters were significantly improved by NIV. Unfortunately, the study has several drawbacks (eg. use of NIV as "rescue" in 16 out 17 patients worsening with oxygen; low power for insufficient sample size; unreported values of baseline PaO_2/FiO_2 and respiratory rate) and, therefore, one should also consider that the life expectancy of patients undergoing HSCT is poor as this is the last-line of treatment after several disease relapses.

More recently, in a large multicenter French RCT Lemiale et al., [5] investigated whether early intermittent NIV in adjunct to only oxygen-therapy improved survival in

374 critically ill immunocompromised patients (317 in treatment for malignancies), who were admitted in ICU for moderate ARDS (median PaO2/FiO2: 130 in oxygen versus 156 in NIV group). Compared to oxygen, early NIV did not reduce the day-28 all-cause mortality (24.1% versus 27.3%). Furthermore, there were no differences on all the secondary outcomes (ICU-acquired infections, duration of mechanical ventilation, lengths of ICU and hospital stays). Unfortunately, the study has several limitations, such as limited power for a lower than expected mortality rate with oxygen-therapy, higher proportion of patients receiving HFNO in oxygen versus NIV group, undefined criteria for intubation.

Several observational studies have related outcome in cancer patients with ARF to the prognosis of invasively ventilated patients. NIV was provided to 4-59% of patients and intubation averted in a range varying from a third to more than 90%. In most but not in all studies, [1, 6-12]. NIV as compared with IMV was associated with better survival, but only few studies corrected this for differences in severity of illness between invasively and non-invasively ventilated patients. Results were equivocal, with some, studies finding a protective effect associated with the use of NIV, and others finding none [1, 6-12]. Some of these studies reported mortality rates above 90% in patients failing a trial of NIV; in other reports, both intubation following NIV and NIV failure after 24 h were independent predictors of mortality [1, 6-12]; At present it is not clear whether the excess mortality in patients failing NIV is due to irreversibility of the underlying disease process and they would have died if they were intubated earlier or to harm caused by inappropriate use of NIV which suggests that earlier intubation would have been associated with better outcome [1].

Weighting the Clinical Evidence of NIV

Several factors are to be kept in mind when analyzing the results of the different NIV studies in cancer patients.

First, interventional studies compared NIV to standard care with supplemental oxygen only, considering worsening of hypoxemia and/or intubation as the endpoint [1-12]. In contrast, most of the observational studies compared patients treated with NIV or IMV as initial mode of ventilatory support [1-12]. Patients who required immediate intubation, eg, because of septic shock, were excluded in the interventional trials. Inclusion of these sicker patients in the observational studies may have biased the results to the disadvantage of IMV patients. Moreover, in non-RCT studies criteria for ETI are usually not reported and, some patients where intubated for less than 48 hours, probably for not-ARF reasons (eg. interventional procedures) [1]. Due to these bias, outcome's data of non-RCT studies should be taken cautiously.

Second, in the interventional studies, patients were likely to receive NIV earlier in the course of their critical illness, as either "prophylactic" (prevention of ARF) or "curative" treatment (avoidance of ETI). In the observational studies, the time lag to ICU referral remains unknown and is probably variable. In a large observational study [11] involving 1302 subjects with hematological malignancies, in three quarter of cases NIV was started later in the course of ARF (i.e., PaO2/FiO2 < 200). A longer delay to the start of NIV has been shown to be an independent predictor of NIV failure which may explain the high failure rates in some non-interventional trials.

Third, the association between initial ventilatory support and outcome may have been confounded by case mix of the patient population, as the underlying cause of ARF has been shown to be a strong predictor of outcome. Higher chances of NIV success are expected in cancer patients with hypercapnic ARF due to decompensation of chronic cardiopulmonary disease (e.g., COPD exacerbation, cardiogenic pulmonary oedema) as compared to those experiencing de novo" hypoxemic ARF [1].

Finally, it is striking that several studies were single-centre trial and some dated back to the 1990s, which creates additional bias of variable expertise in ventilatory management of cancer patients [1].

Predicting the Success of NIV

Since intubation after NIV failure strongly predicts mortality in cancer patients and survival of IMV-patients has recently decreased, it's crucial to find accurate criteria that predict NIV success. Hence, in selected subjects at high-risk of NIV failure, IMV could be considered as a preferable first-line ventilatory support at an earlier stage of ARF [1, 13]. Failure of NIV was significantly associated with a delay in initiating NIV, severe hypoxemia at baseline (i.e., PaO2/FiO2< 200), and presence of extrapulmonary organ failure (i.e., need for vasopressors and for renal replacement therapy); in addition, increasing respiratory rate under NIV was an early predictor for failure [13]. Moreover, a NIV trial is likely to fail when the underlying cause of ARF is unknown or not rapidly reversible. Like for non-cancer patients, NIV should be avoided in presence of absolute contraindications (i.e., imminent respiratory arrest, haemodynamic instability, life-threatening arrhythmia, acute coronary syndromes, inability to protect the airway or vomiting). Conversely, excessive respiratory secretions, recent upper gastrointestinal or airway surgery, decreased consciousness or agitation related to hypercapnic encephaloptahy are considered relative contraindications [1, 13]. In fact, in expert hands, cautious use of sedatives may be helpful to control anxiety and discomfort, while copious secretions could be managed with bronchoscopy under NIV [1, 13].

Aside from patient characteristics, success of NIV may depend upon the appropriate choice of the type of ventilator, the mode of NIV and the patient-ventilator interface. In mildly hypoxemic cancer patients, CPAP, especially if delivered with helmet, could be a well tolerated and cheaper alternative to NIV [1]. A better tolerance of prolonged NIV delivered by helmet instead of face mask is reported by two centers. However, application of CPAP/NIV with helmet requires expertise and adequate monitoring of the patient for the risk of carbon dioxide re-breathing and rapid hypoxia in case of ventilatory flow disconnection [1].

Concerning the setting of treatment, the strategy based on the early application of NIV outside the ICU is still debated. In fact, starting NIV in the ward may be risky because of the lack of tight monitoring by ICU nurses and the unavailability 24-hours a day of an intensivist to make adequate and timely decisions [1]. Accordingly, the delayed admission in ICU of patients who do not improve with NIV may worsen their outcome. The favorable findings of the Italian RCT may be explained by a long experience in using a simple technology (i.e., CPAP) in the hematology ward under the strict supervision of a ICU team [1].

NIV in Patients with Limitations of the Care

An increasing amount of published data have described the use of NIV in ARF patients refusing intubation, or considered to be poor candidates for intubation because of severely impaired functional status or advanced malignancy [1]. Whereas the subgroup of DNI patients with advanced cancer experienced 85 per cent failure of NIV in one report, other studies described successful reversal of ARF and ICU survival in more than half of DNI cancer patients [1]. In a recent multicenter observational study performed on 780 patients (a quarter of them affected by cancer) admitted in ICU, Azoulay et al., [14] demonstrated that NIV used as “ceiling treatment” was not associated with increased anxiety, depression, or stress among both patients and relatives, compared to NIV used without treatment-limitation decisions. Of note, “ceiling NIV” should be withdrawn and palliative care has to be intensified if NIV fails and/or is not tolerated any longer [1].

In patients with terminal malignancy, who do not want any form of life-prolonging therapy as their quality of life is found unacceptable, “palliative” NIV could be considered only if it improves dyspnoea, provides time to come to terms with death, as well as allows to get their personal affairs in order [1]. The more controversial point is whether the benefit of NIV in palliate dyspnea may be outweighed by the discomfort and the limited communication induced by a tight-fitting face-mask. Few studies reported that NIV is feasible and reduced dyspnoea in advanced solid cancer patients with ARF [1, 15, 16].

In the first multicentre feasibility RCT on “palliative” NIV performed in 200 advanced solid cancer patients, Nava et al., [15] showed that, compared with only oxygen-therapy, the adjunct of NIV is more effective in reducing dyspnea and the amount of the needed doses of opiates and their side effects (e.g., depressed sensorium). This may mean a better capability of communication for the patient at the end-of-life, with a good control of symptoms.

Since the prognosis appears to be limited in these patients, it's questionable whether ICU is the best place for "palliative" NIV. In fact, failure of NIV requires rapid intensification of comfort measures which could be more adequately performed in other environments (i.e., Respiratory High-Depencency Units, wards, hospice). It must be underlined that in a setting where clinicians are unfamiliar with NIV the chance of benefit is low and the risk of increasing discomfort at the end-of-life is high [1, 16].

Key Messages

- ARF requiring MV is the most frequent reason for ICU admission in onco-hematologic patients,
- Early referral to ICU, multidisciplinary cooperation, new therapeutic strategies, large application of NIV has contributed to improve the prognosis of malignancies complicated by ARF.
- The actual evidence suggests benefits from a trial of "prophylactic" CPAP or NIV in the early phase of ARF (i.e., PaO2/FiO2> 200) in onco-hematologic patients without multiple organ dysfunctions.
- Delayed intubation after prolonged NIV failure is associated with poor hospital survival
- Starting early CPAP/NIV in the ward to reduce ICU admission is still controversial.
- NIV is feasible as "palliation" in selected terminally onco-hematologic patients.

References

[1] Scala R, Maccari U, Ciarleglio G, Granese V, Madioni C. NIV in cancer patients. In: Elliott MW, Nava S, Schönhofer B. *Principles and practice of non-invasive ventilation and weaning.* Second Edition. CRC Press. Taylor and Francis Group. New York (US) 2019; pp. 481-486.

[2] Hilbert G, Gruson D, Vargas D *et al.* Noninvasive ventilation in immunosuppressed patients with pulmonary infiltrates, fever, and acute respiratory failure. *N. Engl. J. Med.* 2001;344:481–7.

[3] Squadrone V, Massaia M, Bruno B, et al. Early CPAP prevents evolution of acute lung injury in patients with hematologic malignancy. *Intensive Care Med.* 2010;36:1666-74.

[4] Wermke M, Schiemanck S, Höffken G, et al. Respiratory failure in patients undergoing allogeneic hematopoietic SCT--a randomized trial on early non-invasive ventilation based on standard care hematology wards. *Bone Marrow Transplant*. 2012;47:574-80.

[5] Lemiale V, Mokart D, Resche-Rigon M, et al. Effect of Noninvasive Ventilation vs Oxygen Therapy on Mortality Among Immunocompromised Patients With Acute Respiratory Failure: A Randomized Clinical Trial. *JAMA*. 2015;314:1711-9.

[6] Hilbert G, Gruson D, Vargas D, et al. Noninvasive positive airway pressure in neutropenic patients with acute respiratory failure requiring intensive care unit admission. *Crit. Care Med.* 2000;28:3185–90.

[7] Varon J, Walsh GL, Fromm RE. Feasibility of noninvasive mechanical ventilation in the treatment of acute respiratory failure in postoperative cancer patients. *J. Crit. Care* 1998;13:55–7.

[8] Depuydt PO, Benoit DD, Roosens CD. The impact of the initial ventilatory strategy on survival in hematological patients with acute hypoxemic respiratory failure. *J. Crit. Care 2010;25:30-6.*

[9] Adda M, Coquet I, Darmon M et al. Predictors of noninvasive ventilation failure in patients with hematologic malignancy and acute respiratory failure. *Crit. Care Med.* 2008;36: 2766–72.

[10] Azevedo L C, Caruso P, Silva U V, et al. Outcomes for patients with cancer admitted to the ICU requiring ventilatory support: results from a prospective multicenter study. *Chest* 2014;146:257-66.

[11] Gristina G R, Antonelli M, Conti G, et al. Noninvasive versus invasive ventilation for acute respiratory failure in patients with hematologic malignancies: a 5-year multicenter observational survey. *Crit. Care Med.* 2011;39:2232-9.

[12] Ferreira JC, Medeiros P Jr, Rego FM, et al. Risk factors for noninvasive ventilation failure in cancer patients in the intensive care unit: A retrospective cohort study. *J. Crit. Care* 2015;30:1003-7.

[13] Ozyilmaz E, Ugurlu A O, Nava S. Timing of non-invasive ventilation failure: causes, risk factors, and potential remedies. *BMC Pulm. Med.* 2014;14:19.

[14] Azoulay E, Kouatchet A, Jaber S, et al. Noninvasive mechanical ventilation in patients having declined tracheal intubation. Intensive Care Med 2013;39:292-301.

[15] Nava S, Ferrer M, Esquinas A, et al. Palliative use of non-invasive ventilation in end-of-life patients with solid tumours: a randomised feasibility trial. *Lancet Oncol.* 2013;14:219-27.

[16] Scala R, Nava S. NIV and palliative care. *Eur. Respir. Mon.* 2008;41:287-306.

In: Non-Invasive Mechanical Ventilation Complications
Editor: Antonio M. Esquinas
ISBN: 978-1-53619-515-6

Chapter 23

Complications of Non-Invasive Ventilation in Chronic Respiratory Failure

Anoro Abenoza Laura[1,*], MD and Buisán Esporrín Cristina[2,†], MD

[1]Department of Pneumologia,
Hospital Clínico Universitario Lozano Blesa, Zaragoza, Spain
[2]Department of Cardiology, Hospital Clínico Universitario Lozano Blesa,
Zaragoza, Spain

Abstract

Noninvasive mechanical ventilation (NIMV) is a therapeutic procedure that aims to supplement or improve ventilatory function. In recent decades its benefit and multiple indications have been demonstrated in the treatment of patients with chronic heart failure (CHF) and acute complications [1].

However, the use of this therapy in patients with chronic heart failure, is not exempt from risks and complications, so it must be carefully individualized and requires close monitoring when ischemic heart disease and/or arterial hypotension also coexist.

Special mention requires the revision of the indication of servo ventilation in patients with severe chronic heart failure, due to its possible adverse effects.

Keywords: non invasive mechanical ventilation, chronic health failure, hypotension, ischemic heart disease, servo ventilation

* Corresponding Author's E-mail: lauraanoro@hotmail.com.
† Corresponding Author's E-mail: crisitnabuisanesporrin@gmail.com.

CHRONIC HEART FAILURE, ARTERIAL HYPOTENSION AND NIMV

The application of positive intrathoracic pressure through NIMV causes changes at different levels. It can increase ventilation in dead space areas and hyperventilate more perfused areas, due to differences in alveolar compliance. This involves alterations in the ventilation-perfusion ratio (V/Q), alveolar distension and atelectasis due to hypoventilation of the most perfused areas [2].

At cardiovascular level, it decreases venous return and therefore cardiac output, causing hypotension. In addition, it increases pulmonary vascular resistance, affecting right ventricular function (Figure 1).

These patients are usually polymedicated with various hypotensive drugs for chronic heart failure (betablockers, angiotensinal-converting enzyme inhibitors, diuretics...). The application of the NIMV must be careful avoided when high pressures, and it is necessary that this therapy is subjected of close monitoring due to the risk of a marked decrease in the blood pressure figures.

On the other hand, hydrosaline retention is generated by different mechanisms such as the reduction of glomerular filtration or the stimulation of baroreceptors. These changes are also proportional to the applied pressure [2].

Elevated positive intrathoracic pressure produced by NIMV, reduces venous return with the consequent decrease in cardiac output and renal hypoperfusion. This leads to the activation of the renin-angiotensin-aldosterone system, increasing sodium reabsorption to compensate arterial hypotension. Therefore, in patients presenting a reduced ejection fraction, decompensation of their chronic heart failure can be developed.

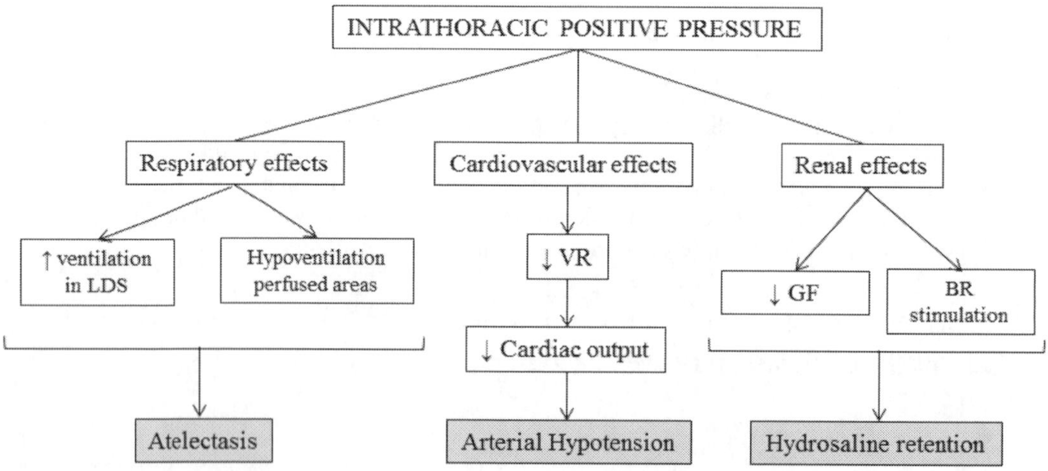

Figure 1. BR (baroreceptors), GF (glomerular filtration), LDS (lung dead space), VR (venous return).

CHRONIC HEART FAILURE, ISCHEMIC CARDIOMYOPATHIE AND NIMV

NIMV has demonstrated to be beneficial for the treatment of obstructive sleep apnea (OSA) and its cardiovascular complications, reducing the risk of acute myocardial ischemic, its recurrences, and cardiac arrhythmias in these patients [3].

Some studies describe an increase number of acute myocardial infarctions attributed to coronary vasoconstriction due to a rapid correction of blood oxygen levels, secondary to treatment with NIMV [4].

These studies are subject of series of biases such as sample size or the presence of confounding factors (intrinsic characteristics of patients that make them more susceptible), limiting the validity of these results [5]. Therefore, more conclusive scientific studies would be necessary to confirm or discard these findings.

CHRONIC HEART FAILURE AND ADAPTATIVE SERVO VENTILATION

Respiratory disorders related to sleep (RDS) are found in a high number of patients with heart failure, and can be manifested as obstructive, central (Cheyne-stokes respiration) or mixed events [6]. Cheyne-stokes respiration is characterized by episodes of apnea followed by an increase in respiratory rate and tidal volume, being detected mainly in patients with heart failure with depressed left ventricle ejection fraction (less than 45%) [7]. Although these respiratory events can be seen with some frequency in heart failure, are not exclusive to this disease, and can be seen, for example, in neuromuscular disorders [8].

However, the presence of RDS increases the severity of heart failure and cardiac dysfunction, being an independent risk marker of poor prognosis and mortality in these patients. This fact is a consequence of an increased sympathetic activity, facilitating diastolic dysfunction during apnea [9]. Taking all this into account, in obstructive sleep apnea with an apnea and hypopnea index equal to or greater than 30, it could be treated depending on carbon retention, and several factors such as patient adaptation, among others, with continuous positive airway pressure (CPAP), bilevel positive airway pressure (BIPAP) or adaptive servo ventilation with the goal of improving sleep quality, ejection fraction and functional grade.

Servo ventilation consists of a ventilatory mode that offers an expiratory positive airway pressure (EPAP) and an inspiratory positive airway pressure (IPAP) depending on the detection of central apneas. The IPAP is automatically adjusted according to the respiratory effort and the EPAP prevents the collapse of the airway, when patient does apnea (Figure 2) [6].

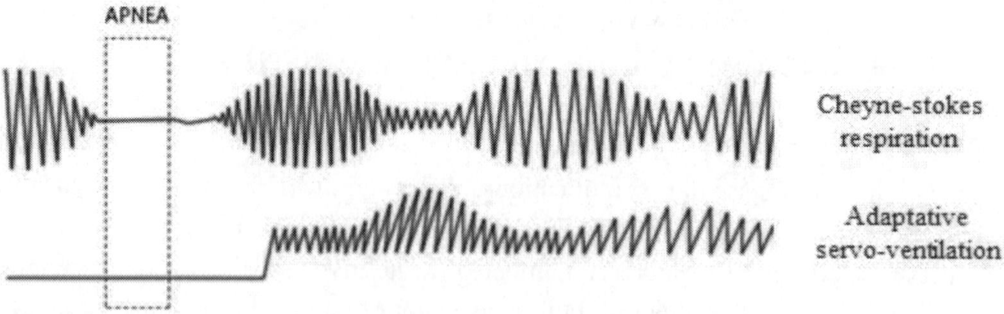

Figure 2. Adaptative servo ventilation recognises apneas and increases IPAP.

A study published in 2016 [9] shows an increase of mortality in those patients who received adaptive servo ventilation compared to the control group, and there was no benefit in terms of improvement in quality of life and symptoms.

The justification of these results is uncertain, although it seems that the cause involved would be the elimination of the compensatory mechanism (in this case Cheyne-stokes respiration) that arises in heart failure. In conclusion, authors do not recommend this ventilatory mode in patients with heart failure with a reduced ejection fraction. However, more studies are necessary to assess the validity of these results and to evaluate if there are more complications that have not been described so far.

Key Messages

1. NIMV is a proven therapy for chronic heart failure and its complications, but it is not without risks.
2. Due to its reducing effect on venous return and therefore on cardiac output, it can cause a drop-in blood pressure, especially in patients with hypotensive treatments.
3. More studies are needed to reliably confirm or rule out the risk of acute myocardial infarction and NIMV treatment.
4. Recent studies have warned of an increase in mortality in patients with depressed left ventricle ejection fraction who received treatment with adaptive servo ventilation.

References

[1] Uña Orejón R., Ureta Tolsada P., Uña Orejón S., Maseda Garrido E., Criado Jiménez A. Ventilación mecánica no invasiva. *Rev Esp Anestesiol Reanim.* 2005; 52(2):88-100.

[2] Gallardo Romero J. M., García T. G., Sancho Chust J. N., González Martínez M. Ventilación no invasiva. *Arch Bronconeumol.* 2010; 46(Suppl. 6):14-21.

[3] Facultad de medicina universidad autónoma de madrid. *Thesis Doctoral Carlos Javier Carpio Segura.* 2006. [Faculty of Medicine, Autonomous University of Madrid.]

[4] Peter J. V., Moran J. L., Phillips-Hughes J., Graham P., Bersten A. D. Effect of non-invasive positive pressure ventilation (NIPPV) on mortality in patients with acute cardiogenic pulmonary oedema: a meta-analysis. *Lancet.* 2006; 367(9517):1155-63.

[5] Ho K. M., Wong K. A comparison of continuous and bi-level positive airway pressure non-invasive ventilation in patients with acute cardiogenic pulmonary oedema: A meta-analysis. *Crit Care.* 2006; 10(2):1-8.

[6] Cowie M. R., Woehrle H., Wegscheider K., Angermann C., D'Ortho M. P., Erdmann E., et al., Adaptive servo-ventilation for central sleep apnea in systolic heart failure. *N Engl J Med.* 2015; 373(12):1095-105.

[7] Giannoni A., Raglianti V., Taddei C., Borrelli C., Chubuchny V., Vergaro G., et al., Cheyne-Stokes respiration related oscillations in cardiopulmonary hemodynamics in patients with heart failure. *Int J Cardiol* [Internet]. 2019; 289:76-82. Available from: https://doi.org/10.1016/j.ijcard.2019.03.033.

[8] Deak M. C., Kirsch D. B. Sleep-disordered breathing in neurologic conditions. *Clin Chest Med* [Internet]. 2014; 35(3):547-56. Available from: http://dx.doi.org/10.1016/j.ccm.2014.06.009.

[9] Yang H., Sawyer A. M. The effect of adaptive servo ventilation (ASV) on objective and subjective outcomes in Cheyne-Stokes respiration (CSR) with central sleep apnea (CSA) in heart failure (HF): A systematic review. *Hear Lung J Acute Crit Care.* 2016; 45(3):199-211. Available from: http://dx.doi.org/10.1016/j.hrtlng.2016.02.002.

In: Non-Invasive Mechanical Ventilation Complications
Editor: Antonio M. Esquinas
ISBN: 978-1-53619-515-6

Chapter 24

Complications of Non-Invasive Ventilation in Palliative Care

Jithin K. Sreedharan[1] and Gokul Krishna G.[2]
[1]Department of Respiratory Care,
Prince Sultan Military College of Health Sciences,
Dammam, Kingdom of Saudi Arabia
[2]Department of Respiratory Therapy,
Batterjee Medical College,
Jeddah, KSA

Abstract

Non-invasive ventilation (NIV) has to be used meticulously in patients with terminal illnesses. Evidence supporting the palliative role of NIV in end-stage lung diseases is still lacking.

In patients with respiratory failure and limited life-expectancy, NIV helps to reduce dyspnea and opiate requirements and has more acceptability than conventional oxygen therapy.

Facial skin breakdown, claustrophobia, aerophagia, aspiration, discomfort, dead space, dryness, and persistent leak are known complications of NIV, which pose more challenges to the intended purpose of palliative care. However, it helps the patient feel more comfortable and perhaps improve communication abilities. In the past decade, the use of palliative NIV has increased substantially.

Keywords: End of life care, palliative care, chronic respiratory disease, non-invasive ventilation

ABBREVIATIONS

COPD	Chronic Obstructive Pulmonary Disease
CO_2	Carbon dioxide
HRQOL	Health-related quality of life
ICU	Intensive Care Unit
NIV	Non-Invasive Ventilation
NMD	Neuromuscular diseases
RICU	Respiratory intensive care unit
V/Q	Ventilation/perfusion

INTRODUCTION

Palliative care is a concept in medical care which includes the supportive care modalities providing for patient comfort care in end-stage diseases or in terminally ill patients. The concept addresses numerous aspects in the trajectory of lung diseases such as chronic obstructive pulmonary disease (COPD), cardiogenic pulmonary edema, lung cancer, upper and lower respiratory tract infections, restrictive thoracic disorders, and neuromuscular diseases [1]. Acute on chronic respiratory failure is generally the end-stage pathological manifestation of these diseases. Palliative care patients can often experience many symptoms, along with the incidence of an acute exacerbation of such diseases leading to acute respiratory failure (ARF). Due to the disease or its impediments, patients with respiratory failure might travail from severe dyspnea, which is not preserved by conventional pharmacological therapy [2]. Sudden dyspnea necessitates the treatment of any reversible cause and necessitates supportive measures to curtail its sensation. Non-invasive ventilation (NIV) in palliative care can either be administered to offer a chance for endurance, as a strategy to resolve acute respiratory failure (ARF), or to relieve respiratory distress symptoms in terminal stage care. NIV may help to forego endotracheal intubation and avoid the need for mechanical ventilation in such patients [2].

In patients who require life support with pre-set limits, such as those with do-not-intubate (DNI) orders, NIV's goal is to alleviate respiratory distress symptoms and improve ventilation-oxygenation, evade intubation, and reduce mortality [3]. In the midst of such patients, it appears that those with reversible causes of dyspnea remarkably benefit from NIV when used as a life-support intervention, with no compromise in health-related quality of life (HRQOL) and no surge in apprehension, depression, or symptoms related to stress disorders after hospital discharge. Essentially the mechanism of symptom relief through NIV remains the same in all the aforementioned clinical conditions. NIV eases the work of breathing, improving alveolar ventilation, functional residual capacity, reviving collapsed alveoli, reducing shunts, and improving the ventilation/perfusion (V/Q) ratio. Taken together, NIV helps scale down the respiratory rate, carbon dioxide (CO_2) retention, and improves the overall of symptoms of respiratory distress in patients near the end of life. However, there is a paucity of evidence to state what type of patients and diseases are more inclined to benefit from palliative NIV or its impact on improvement in overall health care quality of life [15].

INDICATIONS

Indication for NIV in a palliative care setting consists of providing symptomatic relief of dyspnea as a means of allowing the patient time to make substantial decision-making regarding end-of-life care and to allow for time to achieve end-of-life goals. Moreover, NIV may be used as a transitory conduit to more definitive dyspnea relief [13].

Patients with obstructive lung disease have increased ventilator demand, hyperinflated lung, and generalized respiratory muscle weakness, leading them to live with severe breathlessness despite aggressive conventional treatment strategies. Exacerbations increase the ventilatory demand, and hyperinflation of the lung with restricted diaphragmatic movement will reduce the volume generation and increase the respiratory rate. Non-invasive ventilation meritoriously relieves the respiratory muscles, increases volume and decreases the respiratory rate, and decreases the diaphragmatic work of breathing. As a result of an improvement in oxygenation and hypercapnia reduction, an overall improvement in dyspnea is witnessed. Due to the rapid reversibility in COPD exacerbations, NIV is considered to be an essential adjunct to pharmacotherapy and other conventional treatment modalities. COPD patients have a high incidence of sleep-disordered breathing, together with nocturnal desaturation and hypoventilation. Nocturnal NIV might help lessen desaturation and hypoventilation occurrences during sleep; it improves sleep quality and diurnal respiratory failure [4]. The palliation of dyspnea may benefit beyond symptom relief and palliative NIV, contributing to symptom relief without adding to the care burden.

NIV successfully palliates distressing aspects of the chest wall and neuromuscular diseases (NMDs). It helps to assist the respiratory muscles to counterbalance the alveolar hypoventilation and achieve better gas exchange. NIV helps to slow down the forced vital capacity decay, thus improving the patient's quality of life, physical activity and hemodynamic normalization of blood gases. This provides a slight improvement in other physiological measures and a prolonged survival with marginal hospitalizations. Depending on neuromuscular disease development to respiratory distress or dyspnea, NIV may be introduced in the management of amyotrophic lateral sclerosis, Duchenne's muscular dystrophy, Steinert's muscular dystrophy, myasthenia gravis, and spinal muscular atrophy. In neuromuscular patient care, NIV should be considered early when the patient shows signs and symptoms of dyspnea, elevated carbon dioxide levels, reduced forced vital capacity, and various incidences of nocturnal hypoventilation [5].

The sensation of dyspnea has been shown to associate firmly with inspiratory load, and NIV may help mitigate the sense of breathlessness that is incredibly distinct in terminally ill patients with cancer and palliative care. Indeed, NIV conceivably disregards the requirement for intubation or tracheostomy and perpetuates normal swallowing, speech, and cough mechanisms in such patients. The need for oxygen supplementation, opioids and pain relievers can also be reduced inherently when NIV is established [6]. A vast majority of patients and their families are worried about comfort in the advanced phases of their disease. However, some might also want to safeguard cognition and the capability to communicate; from this perspective, NIV would be useful if it improves dyspnea and respiratory distress without having other undesirable consequences [7]. End-stage cancer patients are highly susceptible to having pleural effusion, fever, sepsis, or pulmonary embolism. In such cases, NIV support may temporarily assist the respiratory muscles, allowing the patients to recuperate the strength to breath without additional breathing aids [10].

Goals of NIV for Palliative Care

NIV is a well-established treatment strategy in an acute care setting, but its effective use in palliative care is still debatable. The use of NIV in palliative care has both positive and negative aspects as some believe it to be a measure to alleviate respiratory distress and control symptoms, whereas others consider it an unnecessary prolongation of the dying process. The goals of NIV in palliative care are similar to those in acute care, but the selection of these goals is based on physician and patient family preferences. Improving gas exchange, avoiding intubation, relieving/improving respiratory distress symptoms, maximizing patient comfort, avoiding hospitalization, and improving mobility are the most common goals for initiating NIV in palliative care [11].

The Society of Critical Care Task Force on "Palliation Use of NIV" suggested the classification of use of NIV into 3 categories [4]. The first category emphasizes NIV as life support with no pre-set limitations on life-sustaining treatments. NIV must be initiated if it improves gas exchange and if it is reasonably tolerated, provides efficient support, and buys time to treat the predisposing factor causing ARF. The second category acts as life support when patients and families have decided to forego endotracheal intubation. The third and last category involves critically ill patients, those who do not want any form of life-prolonging treatment. NIV is chosen to forego all life support, receiving "comfort measures only". In most setups, clinicians themselves may be unclear about the goals of NIV for end-of-life conditions, considering the adverse consequences, unmet patient/family expectations, indecorous use of medical recourses, unintended prolongation of dying process, and escalating patient/family anxiety and stress. Specific concerns have been raised about whether patients and their families have an adequate understanding of care goals when NIV is used in the end-of-life context with DNI/DNR and "comfort measures only" (CMO) [7].

When applied for palliative purposes compared with "conventional" use, the difference in goals of NIV must be stressed. In patients with no pre-set limitations on advanced life support, NIV must be considered only if there is a significant improvement in oxygenation and there is a subsequent reduction in symptoms. Even some extent of discomfort while using the NIV is acceptable for these patients if NIV helps to avoid endotracheal intubation and improves oxygenation and ventilation and thereby the survival rate. NIV should be provided in a controlled setup, where patients are monitored continuously by skilled and experienced clinical teams. Discontinuation of NIV will be considered in case of improvement in patient status and in case of poor tolerance or failure of NIV with the need for invasive ventilation. The goals and the appropriate time for discontinuation of NIV are similar for those patients who decline endotracheal intubation and invasive mechanical ventilation, with the difference that NIV will be withdrawn if not successful and/or tolerated any longer, and CMO will be intensified. From the ethical point of view, before applying NIV to DNI patients, it is crucial to have their informed consent. In patients who choose CMO to palliate their symptoms, NIV will be considered successful only if it comforts the patient without having any negative consequences and allows them to communicate with the family. The CMO patients can be transferred home to continue their end stage of life with palliative use of NIV. The Critical Care Medicine Task Force advises that the goals of the care should be continually reassessed because risks, benefits, and treatment preferences change over time and, therefore, the goals of the care and the category of NIV also change in the same patient [4].

THE LOCATION FOR THE PALLIATIVE USE OF NIV

The choice of where to start palliative NIV is based on the patient's need for monitoring, staff expertise, monitoring skills and time-response to NIV. The best location for treating patients with ARF is always in the ICU itself, where immediate response is available [12]. However, for patients with DNI or DNR orders, the palliative use of NIV can be considered in an outpatient or inpatient setup based on the patient's end of life choices. The initiation of NIV and titration can be started in the hospital setting. Respiratory Intensive Care ICU represents a balanced setting where there is proficiency in NIV, cost-effective application of its use, understanding of the history of chronic respiratory patients, and an awareness of end-of-life issues. The RICU should act as a "step-down unit" for stabilized patients transferred from the ICU and as a "step-up unit" for cases not resorting to medical therapy in emergency departments or wards and for those who transferred from home or palliative care facilities [12].

Privacy for the patient and easier family access to palliative care centers may contribute to the remedial process and facilitate discharge, especially for those patients requiring long-term oxygen therapy and/or palliative mechanical ventilation. Conversely, discharge from the palliative care centers to home care becomes possible for patients who have recovered from the initial phase of symptoms but still need special attention and monitoring. Compared to the direct and indirect resources required by traditional hospital care and palliative care facilities, the advantages for home care are linked to the lower nursing staff requirements and the improved quality of life and psychosocial comfort of the patient. The issue of where to start palliative NIV continues to be debated due to the divergence of settings capable of delivering NIV even within the same hospital. This is often dependent on the relevant team's experience, the availability of prompt ETI, and the existence/lack of well-defined step-down and/or step-up pathways.

Complications of NIV in Palliative Care Patients

The prompt identification of complications of NIV is of pivotal importance in palliative care as the undue deferment of alternative or advanced treatment strategies may be associated with increased mortality. Immediate complications are associated with improper understanding, patient agreement to the use of NIV, feeble cough reflex, excessive secretions, hypercapnic encephalopathy syndrome, intolerance, agitation, and patient-ventilator asynchrony. Early complications are expected from 1 to 48 hours due to agitation, leakage, eye irritation, patient-ventilator asynchrony, an inappropriately sized interface, poor gas exchange, the inability to promptly correct these mistakes, rapid onset of severe dyspnea, claustrophobia, and the persistence of a high frequency with respiratory muscle's distress. Late complications usually develop after 48 hours and may be related to sleep disturbance, severe comorbidities, pressure ulcers, gastro-distension, eye irritation, and pneumothorax. One of the major apprehensions with the use of NIV is the supposed low acceptance rate, exclusively when patients are severely dyspneic and anxious. However, it is recommended to explain the technique prudently; patients should undergo a brief trial period on NIV under expert monitoring before prescribed with palliative NIV. The assurance shall be given to the patients that the withdrawal from NIV is possible at any time; in such cases, NIV might be accepted and tolerated with better results [8].

Skin breakdown, from transient erythema to skin necrosis, is a frequent NIV complication which can limit interface tolerance and duration of NIV. Nasal lesions, frequently developed on the nose bridge, account largely for mask-related NIV complications after 48 hours. Progressive tightening of the harness along with high volume with solidity or low volume with wrinkles in the mask cushions are factors that contribute to this complication. Prolonged use of NIV in palliative patients causes nasal, oral, and airway dryness which then leads to the release of inflammatory mediators. This in turn results in alterations in lung dynamics and patient comfort. High pressure and volumes, flow, increased airway resistance, low compliance, and short inspiratory time all lead to aerophagia and gastric distension.

NIV should be used very cautiously in aspiration pneumonia as NIV itself can results in aspiration of gastric contents. Caution should be taken in patients with excessive gastric distension, ileus, nausea or vomiting, or in those who are deemed to be at high risk for gastric aspiration. The risk of aspiration pneumonia can be curtailed by excluding patients with a compromised upper airway function or trouble in clearing secretions, allowing at-risk patients nothing by the mouth until they are stabilized, and by placing the patient in the sitting or semi-sitting position during NIV. Lack of awareness about appropriate gastric decompression measures and NIV application immediately after consumption of a meal are potential threats for palliative NIV. NIV has more obvious hemodynamic effects in patients with severe disease who are hypotensive or have a low circulating blood volume and in patients with an underlying cardiac disease without adequate pharmacological therapy.

Due to poor lymphatic drainage, upper extremity edema is observed due to uncompensated fluid filtration from blood vessels to the tissue when helmet NIV is used. Improper brace fixation while stabilizing the helmet interface may cause prolonged compression to the armpit, leading to venolymphatic stasis and, consequently, edema. Carbon dioxide rebreathing related to the interface, circuitry, and NIV mode itself is common in palliative NIV, which conversely affects the outcome [17].

The intensity of breathlessness in patients receiving palliative care often gets worse the closer individual approaches the end of their life. Anxiety, depression, low quality of life, and cognitive deficits could play a detrimental role in their clinical conditions, and it may be worsened during the adaptation process to NIV.

Brief psychological support and counseling are appropriate for the acceptance and adherence to NIV in palliative care. The physician and clinical team should make sure and inform the patient and their family about all the possible complications of palliative ventilation and NIV.

The proper selection of the optimal device, patient and caregiver education, tolerable management of ventilatory support, availability of a skilled team, and accurate clinical and instrumental monitoring are crucial to minimizing the risk of complications during palliative NIV.

Complications in Pediatric Palliative Care

In certain instances, decisions regarding mechanical respiratory support determine the expected disease outcome. The level and modality of provided respiratory support can ultimately preclude the question of life or death. Palliative NIV is a special treatment aimed to alleviate breathing and thereby improve the quality of life. Clinicians consider NIV an essential tool in palliative care to provide comfort to patients, relieve suffering, and improve the quality of life of both children and their families. The use of NIV has proven an appropriate measure to relieve dyspnea due to acute respiratory failure in children with a do-not-intubate (DNI) order. Tolerability may be limited by mask discomfort, discomfort from the air pressure, claustrophobia, poorly managed initial setup, and child or parent anxiety. The use of NIV cannot be designed only to prolong the dying process with no improvement, with a possible detriment to the child's symptom burden and quality of life. Complications with NIV are seen in the most fragile patients, and they include gastric distention, aspiration, pneumothorax, and pressure ulcerations [14].

The most common cause of NIV failure in the pediatric population is the lack of patient-specific interfaces and therapy intolerance. Serious complications such as skin ulcerations and deep tissue injury are common among infants and children on NIV as palliative support. Skin ulcerations are also the most preventable complication in these populations with adequate preventative measures such as cushioned masks and intermittent breaks if tolerable. Aspiration is another concern; these patients require additional precautions related to the delivery interface, feeding, and monitoring to reduce aspiration risk. Continuously monitoring the pressures and alarm settings will avoid the chance of pneumothorax. Providing adequate humidification will improve tolerance and will help to hydrate secretions. In some cases, the child will be so uncooperative and/or non-compliant that attempting to apply NIV will produce more anxiety and possibly more hemodynamic instability. The use of NIV for pediatric patients is fraught with difficulties. Hence the paramedical and medical staff, family members, and caregivers should have proper training and adequate experience, which is sometimes difficult in a palliative care setup [16].

Withdrawal of NIV in Palliative Patients

Non-invasive ventilation (NIV) is a method of supporting breathing. It is administered by a cushioned mask and does not involve an artificial airway. The air is pressurized at different pressures throughout the breathing cycle to help the patient take breaths and keep the airway open. Most patients will only use NIV for parts of the day or night. However, some are dependent on NIV for all 24 hours of the day. For these patients, withdrawal of NIV may cause distressing symptoms, and death may occur soon after withdrawal. For these reasons, meticulous planning is required. A patient who is not 24-hours dependent on NIV can discontinue NIV at any point by merely not replacing their masks. It is also essential to involve the right people to plan and support this process; palliative care physicians, nurses who have taken care of the patient/s, and family members should all be a part of this process. What the patient will experience during and after withdrawal of NIV should be explained to non-medical personnel like family members and caregivers. The patient and family ought to deliberate which family member/s or friends should remain with the patient. A professional involved in the withdrawal will remove the mask. If the patient and family specifically ask for a family member to do this, it should be given scrupulous consideration, and discussion should occur with those involved. No family member should feel pressured to undertake this responsibility [9].

Consideration should be given for anything the patient wishes to attend to before withdrawal such as saying important things to family and friends and resolving related affairs. Principally, withdrawal should be planned to take place in regular working hours and when all necessary staff is available to support this. Although it can be particularly difficult at a home setup, the withdrawal process can occur at home or in the hospital setup. If at home, all the professionals involved will be present in the home for this process. At home, this will be by complete removal of the NIV after the patient's comfort has been ensured. In general, this is the preferred option in all settings [7]. However, in the hospital, some patients may undergo a gradual reduction of the ventilation pressure called weaning. At this time, a specific medication is used to ensure the patient is not aware of the NIV being withdrawn and does not become uncomfortable or distressed. Practices such as replacing the NIV mask with a simple oxygen therapy mask can be discussed, and a decision shall be made for each patient individually. If a patient requires NIV 24 hours a day, they will likely die soon after the NIV is withdrawn, possibly within minutes. However, in some cases, it can take hours or even days. Inform the patient and family that physical changes will occur, including that the patient may change color, and their breathing may change and become shallower and eventually stop [16].

When NIV Should Not Be Used in Palliative Care

Palliative NIV should not be used or recommended in specific clinical situations. NIV should not be compelled if proper consent of the patient is not obtained. NIV is also not recommended for patients who do not comfortably fit multiple interfaces. Similarly, if the patient is not relieved of dyspnea after several hours of titration, then NIV should not be used. Palliative NIV is also not advised for unconscious patients or those who cannot communicate properly since they do not feel the potential impact of NIV on their associated symptoms. Palliative NIV is not suitable for patients at the end-stage of a chronically progressive disease like COPD, neuromuscular disorders, CHF or those with fatal malignancy and those who do not want any form of life-prolonging therapy as their baseline quality of life cannot be achieved despite conventional therapies [10].

Ethical Considerations

Decisions about stopping the treatment at the end of life are emotionally distressing, and some may involve ethical dilemmas. The healthcare team or the patient's friends and family may find it difficult to contemplate the withdrawal of life-sustaining treatment. However, the withdrawal of medical treatment does not directly correlate with actively rushing a patient's death. The withdrawal of the treatment, even if at the request of a competent patient or subsequent to the consideration of best interests in a patient who lacks capacity, permits the underlying disease to take its natural progression which had been temporarily delayed by the NIV. These issues need to be explained to all involved before withdrawal [16].

NIV, when used for patients in palliative care, is often used in situations that are progressive and life-limiting. Patients may reach a stage when the benefits they get from NIV do not outweigh the burdens of continuing it. This may prompt a resolution to withdraw NIV. Patients with no plan for advanced care have to decide when to stop NIV. If the patient lacks the potential to make decisions on the withdrawal of life-sustaining treatment, the healthcare team should carefully assess their care. Discussions should include the palliative care clinicians and should take place with the patient, family, and caregivers to ensure that all understand the reasons for withdrawing NIV, to plan how it will come about, and to explain what will happen to the patient as a result of the withdrawal [9]. This is a big decision to make, and those involved should be given time to discuss these issues several times if needed. It is vital to involve the right people to plan and support this process. The need for mourning support should be addressed at the earliest opportunity. Staff support mechanisms, including debriefing sessions, need to be considered.

Conclusion

NIV is a crucial adjunct to medications for patients suffering from dyspnea during end-stage lung diseases, and it has been used sporadically as a potential treatment for acute respiratory failure in patients with a do-not-intubate order [9]. The prevalence of severe dyspnea in terminally ill patients is more than 65% with heart failure, 70% with lung cancer, and 90% with COPD. However, substantial disagreement exists as to whether NIV should be used to relieve dyspnea at the end of life; continuing NIV in a deteriorating medical condition could potentially prolong the dying process without any benefit. The success of NIV in palliative care relies on careful evaluation of patient goals and finding an appropriate time to initiate, withhold and withdraw NIV [13]. The patient and family must be aware of the risks associated with the use of NIV, and alternative measures in the event of NIV failure must be identified before beginning [10]. An integrated approach across illnesses is essential, and the goals of care should be reviewed periodically because the hazards, benefits, and treatment choices can change over time.

REFERENCES

[1] Saunders, C. The evolution of palliative care. *J. R. Soc. Med.,* 2001; 94(9):430 - 432.

[2] Azoulay, E., Demoule, A., Jaber, S., Kouatchet, A., Meert, A. P., Papazian, L., Brochard, L. Palliative noninvasive ventilation in patients with acute respiratory failure. *Intensive Care Med.,* 2011; 37(8):1250 - 1257.

[3] Tanvetyanon, T. Which patient with a do-not-intubate order is a candidate for noninvasive ventilation? (Editorial). *Crit. Care Med.,* 2004; 32(10):2148 - 2150.

[4] Curtis, J. R. (2008). Palliative and end-of-life care for patients with severe COPD. *The European Respiratory Journal,* 32(3), 796 - 803. https://doi.org/10.1183/09031936.00126107.

[5] Gifford, Alex H. *Noninvasive ventilation as a palliative measure.* Current Opinion in Supportive and Palliative Care: September 2014 - Volume 8 - Issue 3 – p. 218 - 224 doi: 10.1097/SPC.0000000000000068.

[6] Leblanc, T. W., Abernethy, A. P. Building the palliative care evidence base: Lessons from a randomized controlled trial of oxygen vs room air for refractory dyspnea. *J. Natl. Compr. Can. Netw.,* 2014; 12(7):989 - 992.

[7] Wilson, M. E., Majzoub, A. M., Dobler, C. C., Curtis, J. R., Nayfeh, T., Thorsteinsdottir, B. et al. Noninvasive ventilation in patients with do-not-intubate and comfort-measures-only orders: A systematic review and meta-analysis. *Crit. Care Med.,* 2018; 46(8):1209 - 1216.

[8] Gay, P. C. Complications of noninvasive ventilation in acute care. *Respir. Care,* 2009; 54:246 - 257.

[9] Kacmarek, R. M. Should noninvasive ventilation be used with the do-not-intubate patient? *Respir. Care*, 2009; 54:223 - 229.

[10] Nava, S., Ferrer, M., Esquinas, A. et al. Palliative use of noninvasive ventilation in end-of-life patients with solid tumours: a randomised feasibility trial. *Lancet Oncol.*, 2013; 14:219 - 227.

[11] Curtis, J. R., Cook, D. J., Sinuff, T. et al. Noninvasive positive pressure ventilation in critical and palliative care settings: Understanding the goals of therapy. *Crit. Care Med.*, 2007; 35:932 - 939.

[12] Azoulay, E., Soares, M., Darmon, M. et al. Intensive care of the cancer patient: Recent achievements and remaining challenges. *Ann. Intensive Care,* 2011; 1:5.

[13] Levi, B. H., Heverley, S. R., Green, M. J. Accuracy of a decision aid for advance care planning: Simulated end-of-life decision making. *J. Clin. Ethics,* 2011; 22:223 - 238.

[14] Mellies, U., Ragette, R., Dohna Schwake, C. et al. Long-term noninvasive ventilation in children and adolescents with neuromuscular disorders. *Eur. Res. J.,* 2003; 22:631 - 636.

[15] Windisch, W. Impact of home mechanical ventilation on health-related quality of life. *Eur. Respir. J.,* 2008; 32:1328 - 1336.

[16] Krivec, U., and Caggiano, S. (2020). Noninvasive Ventilation in Palliative Care and Ethical Dilemma. *Frontiers in pediatrics*, 8, 483. https://doi.org/10.3389/fped.2020.00483.

[17] Hess, D. R. Noninvasive ventilation in neuromuscular disease: Equipment and application. *Respir. Care,* 2006; 51:896 - 911.

In: Non-Invasive Mechanical Ventilation Complications ISBN: 978-1-53619-515-6
Editor: Antonio M. Esquinas

Chapter 25

COMPLICATIONS DURING NON-INVASIVE MECHANICAL VENTILATION - BRONCHOFIBEROSCOPY AND OTHER PROCEDURES

Sara Moura Cabral*
Pulmonology Department –
Coimbra Hospital and Universitary Centre (CHUC), Portugal

ABSTRACT

Non-invasive ventilation (NIV) during endoscopic procedures has been considered an extremely useful and safe approach for either diagnostic or therapeutic purpose [1]. Bronchofiberoscopy, carried out for difficult intubation and to perform bronchoalveolar lavage and biopsies, is one of the upper endoscopic exams in which NIV is used the most [2]. In clinical practice peri-procedural NIV improves oxygenation operating with masks that allow the insertion of endoscopic probes. [3]. The full face Janus mask is a device with an opening covered by a membrane and two separable halves with a midline port that allows the insertion of endoscopic probes into patients mouth or nose, without interrupting continuous positive airway pressure.

To reduce patients unpleasant sensations during the procedure, a mild degree of sedation is usually administered, which furthermore compared with general anesthesia, results in no need for hospitalization, reducing costs and complications. Despite these advantages, NIV support is not free of complications, especially because the unprotected airway may lead to a higher risk of aspiration and the occurrence of cough, when under sedation, might cause intraprocedural anatomic lesions [3]. Hypoventilation and desaturation may also be associated with the procedure, resulting in its no completion or leading to acute respiratory failure and intubation [4]. Bronchoalveolar lavage (BAL) is known to induce significant hypoxemia and therefore previous severe hypoxemia may represent a contraindication for this procedure. Additionally, the indications to perform endoscopic maneuvers in the cardiac and gastrointestinal settings are clearly expanding

* Corresponding Author's E-mail: saramouracabral@hotmail.com.

because they represent a considerable less invasive approach compared with surgical interventions [1].

Keywords: peri-procedural non-invasive ventilation, bronchofiberoscopy, full face Janus mask, bronchoalveolar lavage, hypoxemia, complications

In the recent years, peri-procedural NIV has been used during endoscopic maneuvers to improve oxygenation in high-risk patients [1]. Bronchofiberoscopy, carried out for difficult intubation and to perform bronchoalveolar lavage and biopsies, is one of the upper endoscopic exams in which NIV is used the most [2].

Peri-procedural NIV is been considered an extremely useful and safe approach in patients who undergo bronchofiberoscopy for either diagnostic or therapeutic purpose. Several studies suggested that peri-procedural NIV is superior to high-flow nasal cannula oxygen in avoiding hypoxia during bronchofiberoscopy [1].

In clinical practice, peri-procedural NIV improves oxygenation operating with masks that allow the insertion of endoscopic probes. To reduce unpleasant sensations, patients are usually under a mild degree of sedation, which furthermore compared with general anesthesia results in no need for hospitalization, reducing costs and complications. Despite these advantages, NIV support is not free of complications, especially because the unprotected airway may lead to a higher risk of aspiration and the occurrence of cough, when under sedation, might cause intraprocedural anatomic lesions [3].

Patient compliance is required to avoid possible complications, such as airway tract perforation, due to patient movements. Hypoventilation and desaturation may also be associated with the procedure, resulting in its no completion or leading to acute respiratory failure and intubation [4].

Standard NIV masks are not suitable for intra-procedural ventilation. Thus, to apply NIV to endoscopic procedures, the system should be sealed enough to provide an effective positive pressure and, at the same time, versatile to be opened allowing the insertion of an endoscopic probe during intra-procedural time [1].

The first known interface was the Patil-Syracuse mask. It had an additional opening, closed with a plastic cap, and a silicone membrane to take in endotracheal tubes or endoscopic devices. Maitre et al., developed a full facemask connected to a continuous positive airway pressure device with four funnel-shaped microchannels linked to an external oxygen source, and therefore delivering pressure by constant flow oxygen insufflation. As the gas was injected into the capillaries, the high-velocity jets created a constant positive pressure into the mask, dependent on the oxygen flow rate and on the capillaries diameter. This system also had a second opening to allow oxygen delivery without positive pressure when required. The great advantage of this device was the connection to the atmosphere, preventing excessive airway pressure and allowing endoscopy to be performed without disconnection or leaks [1].

In 2009, Heunks et al., presented positive results with a full facemask modified with a plastic cylinder, allowing the insertion of a bronchoscope through the mouth and equipped with a disposable cap from a swivel connector that could seal the cylinder and prevent air leakage during endoscopy.

The full face Janus mask (figure 1) is a more recent device, with an opening covered by a membrane and two separable halves, with a midline port that allows the insertion of endoscopic probes into patients mouth or nose, without interrupting continuous positive airway pressure. Therefore, it can be placed on or removed, even during the endoscopic examination. This is relevant, especially in cases of unexpected and sudden acute respiratory insufficiency, restoring patients oxygenation and the conclusion of the procedure, avoiding intubation [1].

In spontaneous breathing hypoxemic patients is known that NIV, during bronchofiberoscopy, ensures appropriate gas exchange, avoiding intubation. It can be used before the procedure, to pre-oxygenate the patient, increasing the respiratory reserve; during the procedure, to prevent hypoventilation and hypoxia or to treat these conditions in case of its occurrence; and after the procedure, to enhance patients recovery [4].

In critically ill patients, with acute hypoxemic respiratory failure ($PaO_2/FiO_2 < 300$) prior to decision to perform bronchoscopy and already under NIV, bronchofiberoscopy can be useful for diagnostic or therapeutic purpose. It is generally considered safe, but BAL is known to induce significant hypoxemia and therefore previous severe hypoxemia may represent a contraindication for this procedure. Particularly in hypoxemic patients, the benefits have to be weighed against possible risks, but it can generally be performed with an acceptable risk [4].

Since these patients *per se* have high odds for subsequent endotracheal intubation due to NIV failure, bronchoscopy should only be performed by experienced clinicians in bronchoscopy and endotracheal intubation, and performed in an environment with a high monitoring level [4].

Bronchoscopy can generally be completed in all patients without subsequent complications such as oxygen desaturation and endotracheal intubation during the first eight hours, and BAL can yield diagnostic information in about 60-80% of the patients [4].

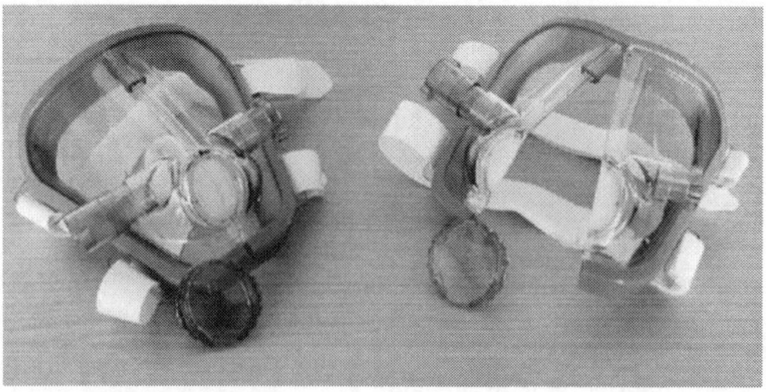

Figure 1. Full face Janus mask - adapted from "Noninvasive Ventilation during Endoscopic Procedures: Rationale, Clinical Use, and Devices."

Additionally, the indications to perform endoscopic maneuvers in the cardiac and gastrointestinal settings are clearly expanding because they represent a considerable less invasive approach compared with surgical interventions [1].

In regards to cardiovascular procedures, we can enhance transesophageal echocardiography (TEE), as it can provide superior information compared with the transthoracic approach, and transfemoral aortic valve replacement. This procedure is routinely performed with the patient under sedation and requires prolonged TEE periprocedure. In these cases, we can successfully administer ventilatory support through a full facemask, that allows the insertion of an endoscopic probe and ventilatory support in sedated patients [1].

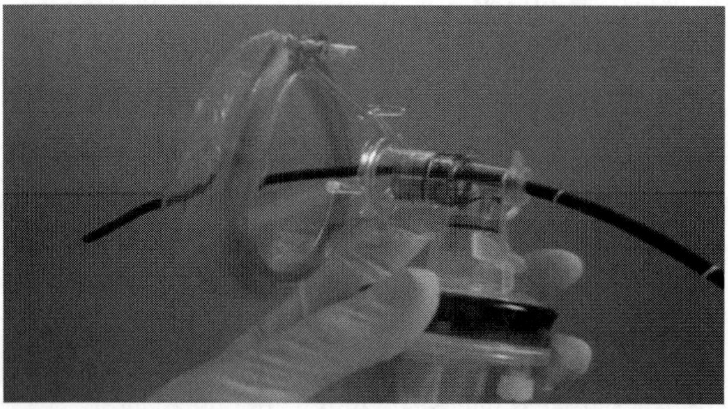

Figure 2. Bronchoscope inserted through swivel connector into the face mask - adapted from "Fiber optic bronchoscopy in patients with acute hypoxemic respiratory failure requiring noninvasive ventilation - a feasibility study."

Gastrointestinal procedures, such as esophagogastroduodenoscopy, endoscopic retrograde cholangiopancreatography and percutaneous gastrostomy, are also quite frequent nowadays. During these procedures, to prevent hypercapnia and respiratory acidosis, NIV has shown to be extremely useful in high-risk patients. The most common cause for procedure failure, requiring endotracheal intubation, is respiratory failure which can be manifested by agitation and delirium [1].

In conclusion, regarding upper endoscopic maneuvers, the possibility of granting adequate ventilation through NIV, avoiding general anesthesia and intubation is very promising. Advantages and disadvantages should be considered, and the most appropriate strategy performed according to clinical context for each patient.

REFERENCES

[1] Pieri, M., Landoni, G., Cabrini, L., Noninvasive ventilation during endoscopic procedures: rationale, clinical use, and devices. *Journal of Cardiothoracic and Vascular Anesthesia* - 2018 Apr; 32(2):928-934.

[2] Cabrini, L., Nobile, L., Cama, E., Borghi, G., Pieri, M., Bocchino, S., A Zangrillo Non-invasive ventilation during upper endoscopies in adult patients. A systematic review. *Minerva Anestesiol.* 2013 Jun; 79(6): 683-94.

[3] Cabrini, L. and Landoni, G. A novel non-invasive ventilation mask to prevent and manage respiratory failure during fiberoptic bronchoscopy, gastroscopy and transesophageal echocardiography. *Heart, Lung and Vessels.* 2015; 7(4): 297-303.

[4] Baumann, H. J., Klose, H., Simon, M., Ghadban, T., Braune, S. A., Hennigs, J. K. and Kluge, S. Fiber optic bronchoscopy in patients with acute hypoxemic respiratory failure requiring noninvasive ventilation - a feasibility study. *Critical Care - BioMed Central.* 2011 Jul; 15(4): R179.

In: Non-Invasive Mechanical Ventilation Complications
Editor: Antonio M. Esquinas ISBN: 978-1-53619-515-6

Chapter 26

COMPLICATIONS DURING NON-INVASIVE MECHANICAL VENTILATION. HYPOXIA. PREOXYGENATION, ENDOTRACHEAL INTUBATION

Oguzhan Kayhan and Yalim Dikmen*
Department of Anaesthesiology and Intensive Care, Istanbul University-Cerrahpasa, Cerrahpasa Medical Faculty, Istanbul, Turkey

ABSTRACT

Non-invasive respiratory support methods have been increasingly used in recent years for patients receiving treatment for acute respiratory failure. Avoiding invasive methods provides better results here, as in every field of medicine. However, patients with respiratory distress are not intubated at the right time and delayed intubation causes an increase in mortality.

Various preoxygenation methods are applied to avoid hypoxemia during the apnea period after anesthesia induction until intubation occurs in patients undergoing surgery. The apnea period, which is limited to only a few minutes in healthy lungs, is very short in lung diseases. Therefore, preoxygenation is of particular importance before the intubation of patients with respiratory failure.

Preoxygenation is the process of filling lung reserves with oxygen. Determining which method to use in which patient for preoxygenation is an issue that should be considered, as it can directly affect patient outcomes.

Keywords: hypoxia, preoxygenation, non-invasive ventilation, intensive care

* Corresponding Author's E-mail: yalim.dikmen@gmail.com.

Introduction

Today, conventional oxygen therapy (COT), nasal high flow oxygen (NHFO), non-invasive ventilation (NIV) or invasive mechanical ventilation (IMV) are applied alone or in combination in patients treated for acute respiratory failure (ARF), depending on the severity of the failure. While COT or NHFO are sufficient in mild and moderate respiratory insufficiency, NHFO and NIV are used in severe respiratory insufficiency and IMV is used in case these methods are ineffective. IMV requires intubation, a life-threatening procedure for intensive care patients.

The decision to intubate the patients with ARF is made as a result of failure of COT, NHFO and NIV, persistence or progression of respiratory failure symptoms. For intubation, patients are sedated, curarized, and a tube is inserted into the trachea by laryngoscopy. This process is not always as easy as described. Intubation of even the healthiest person brings some risks. The scenario takes place in a wide range from "easy intubation" to "can't ventilate, can't intubate," where the patient can not be intubated but can not be ventilated through a face mask either. Therefore, preoxygenation methods are used to delay desaturation in an event of unexpected prolonged apnea.

Preoxygenation can be summarized as giving the patient a high concentration of oxygen to replace nitrogen in the functional residual capacity of the patients who are planned to be intubated. All methods applied for preoxygenation perform the process of removing nitrogen from the alveoli and replacing it with oxygen, also known as denitrogenization. In this way, while the high concentration of oxygen in the alveoli meets the oxygen uptake during apnea for seconds or minutes, and this is vital in difficult intubation.

Preoxygenation was first defined in the 1960's and was primarily used for anesthesia induction with full stomach (Nolan, 1967). In the following years, it was started to be applied in all intubations in order to gain time in unexpected difficult intubations. Various methods have been used over the years. Mask oxygen, balloon-valve-mask (BVM) ventilation, NHFO, NIV are some of the methods used. With a mask sealed over the nose and mouth of the patient breathing with 100% oxygen that does not mix with the room air, and a fresh gas flow that meets the patient's inspiratory flow makes it easier to achieve preoxygenation targets. The more the preoxygenation method used cannot meet these conditions, the more difficult it is to reach sufficient preoxygenation.

It is important to determine whether the preoxygenation has been done adequately. In order to determine the effectiveness of preoxygenation, end-tidal O_2 (ETO_2) monitoring is recommended, and an $ETO_2 \geq 90$ is defined as adequate preoxygenation (Langeron et al., 2018; Tanoubi et al., 2009). End-tidal O_2 indicates the oxygen concentration at the alveolar level, that is how much of the FRC is consisted of oxygen. Since the oxygen concentration in the alveolar air increases with the decrease of nitrogen concentration, the increase of ETO_2 indicates that denitrogenization takes place.

Apneic oxygenation is the delivery of oxygen to the upper airways via the oropharynx or nasopharynx to prevent arterial oxygen desaturation. Even in the absence of respiration, oxygen passes through the alveoli into the bloodstream. In this way, a pressure difference occurs between the upper airways and the alveoli. Oxygen flows through the upper airways to the alveoli due to this pressure difference and a continuous oxygen flow occurs. Theoretically, arterial desaturation is delayed in this way.

In a healthy adult breathing normal room air, the oxygen reserve in the lung with normal FRC is up to 400 ml. During the apnea period, when the the oxygen reserve in the lung decreases to 250 ml, oxygen saturation begins to fall towards 90%. The time until this happens is less than a minute. After preoxygenation by breathing 100% oxygen, lung oxygen reserve increases by 2375 ml. In this case, the calculations show that the lung oxygen reserve can be increased ten times by preoxygenation with 100% oxygen under suitable conditions (Tanoubi et al., 2009).

The situation is slightly different in patients with acute respiratory failure. The most important complication that may occur during intubation is desaturation and related cardiac arrest. In intensive care patients cardiac arrest occurs at a rate of 2.7% during intubation (De Jong et al., 2018). In patients with normal lungs, intubation may be delayed depending on anatomical features and desaturation may develop accordingly. However, even if there is no delay in intubation, desaturation and related consequences may occur in acute respiratory failure. Desaturation develops rapidly when the patient is curarized for intubation due to failing lungs that already function well below their normal capacity due to reasons such as decrease in FRC, deterioration in gas exchange, ventilation and perfusion mismatch. In addition, increased oxygen consumption due to reasons like infection contributes to the acceleration of oxyhemoglobin desaturation. Complications due to low saturation are more common, since the duration of normal saturation, which may take 4 minutes with preoxygenation in healthy lungs, is very short in intensive care patients with lung pathology (Weitzner et al., 1959).

PREOXYGENATION METHODS

For preoxygenation, the patient must breathe 100% oxygen with a sealed mask. Various techniques have been described to increase the speed and efficiency of preoxygenation. These techniques include tidal breaths, deep breaths, and combinations of these (Nimmagadda et al., 2017). In addition, apneic oxygenation was recommended in addition to preoxygenation to delay oxyhemoglobin desaturation (Nimmagadda et al., 2017). These methods are also applied in intensive care patients with acute respiratory failure, although they are mostly based on studies conducted for preoxygenation applied during anesthesia induction for surgical procedures.

In order to breathe 100% oxygen without re-breathing with a sealed oxygen mask and without mixing the room air, first of all, the importance and benefits of the preoxygenation process should be explained. In this way, it can be easier to achieve the desired result by increasing the patient's compliance with the procedure.

The goal in preoxygenation should not be to reach 100% SpO_2 with pulse oximetry. Because this value does not indicate that the body's oxygen reserves are filled, but only the oxyhemoglobin saturation. To achieve 100% oxyhemoglobin saturation, it is sufficient to provide a slightly higher FiO_2 from the room air. The main target in preoxygenation should be to follow the functional residual capacity, which is the main oxygen store of the body, is filled with maximum oxygen and nitrogen is removed from this space. For this, ETO_2 and ETN_2 must be monitored. Anesthesia devices generally, and some intensive care ventilators show only ETO_2. Increasing ETO_2 above 90% is recommended as a threshold value for the adequacy of preoxygenation (Langeron et al., 2018; Tanoubi et al., 2009).

Mask oxygen, BVM, NHFO or NIV are generally used for preoxygenation in patients with or without acute respiratory failure in intensive care. Among these, mask oxygen can be shown as the simplest and easiest method to apply. It is performed by inhaling 12 L/min of oxygen with a face mask for 3-5 minutes. If the flow provided by the mask oxygen, which is the method that requires the least cooperation of the patient, lags behind the patient's inspiratory flow rate, the room air mixes with the breathing air and the preoxygenation time is prolonged and even the target cannot be reached.

Another recommended method is a heated humidified high flow nasal cannula oxygen therapy. Although it is included as a mode in intensive care ventilators, there are also special NHFO devices produced for this purpose. It provides high oxygen flows at 37°C temperature, which can generally be increased up to 60L/min and 100% FiO_2. With NHFO, carbon dioxide is removed with the scavenging effect in the upper airways and the dead space is reduced. When the patient's mouth is kept closed, a continuous positive pressure of about 5cmH_2O is created and the functional residual capacity is increased. In addition, apneic oxygenation can be achieved by continuing the application in the apneic period after anesthesia induction. Patient compliance and comfort are good due to the lack of a mask that puts pressure on the face and the use of a soft cannula. The heated humidified gas is delivered to the patient through a nasal cannula, and gas flow rates are generally higher than the patients peak inspiratory flow rate the adjusted FiO_2 remains stable independent from the patient effort. However if the patient effort is increased due to dispnea, especially when breathing through the mouth room air may be entrained and applied FiO_2 may decrease. In a study conducted with healthy adults, heated, humidified high-flow nasal oxygen was compared with mask oxygen as a preoxygenation method. Mask oxygen was applied at 12L/min for 3 minutes and NHFO at 60L/min. In this study, it was concluded that NHFO is not superior to mask oxygen (Hanouz et al., 2019).

Balloon-valve-mask system stands out as the most commonly used method in preoxygenation in intensive care. There is a valve in the system that prevents re-inhalation of expired gas. When connected to oxygen and the reservoir is attached, it provides a FiO_2 close to 100% to the patient. When using a facemask that does not leak and does not mix the room air, the desired FiO_2 can be achieved due to its reservoir even in patients with high flow requirement. Previously, explaining the procedure to be performed with a good communication with the patient may increase the patient's cooperation, but in patients with severe respiratory distress, it may not be possible to keep the mask tightly attached to the patient's face due to anxiety. Its use is simple and cheap, making this method widely used.

Noninvasive ventilation is a preoxygenation method that can be applied with devices for this purpose as well as through conventional intensive care ventilators. Modes such as CPAP, PSV, BIPAP can be applied. By adjusting PEEP, the alveoli are kept open and the shunt is reduced. As a result of recruitment of atelectatic areas, the improvement in the ventilation-perfusion ratio and reaching a higher FRC provides an increase in oxygen reserve. When the BIPAP mode is used, it is possible to continue ventilation with sufficient tidal volumes until the patient is fully curarized. Preoxygenation performed with a tight-fitting facemask with 100% FiO_2 has been found superior to other methods in many clinical studies (Baillard et al., 2018; Fong et al., 2019; Vourc'h et al., 2019).

While receiving NHFO or NIV treatment due to acute respiratory failure, when the decision to intubate is made at some point of the treatment, generally this decision is made due to failure in improving hypoxemia or respiratory distress, with low oxygen saturation. The intubation of all these hypoxemic and dyspneic patients is a high risk procedure due to the severe lung disease that the patients have. The preoxygenation method to be applied becomes important as these patients may rapidly desaturate during the apnea period due to their very low lung reserves. It should be aimed to minimize hypoxemia and related complications with effective and correct preoxygenation method.

When the decision of intubation is made for a patient who is being treated with NHFO due to acute respiratory failure and who cannot be applied NIV for any reason, it seems that the most appropriate preoxygenation method to be applied is to continue with NHFO. In addition, it can be used during intubation with apneic oxygenation after induction. In the research conducted by Guitton et al, it was concluded that preoxygenation with NHFO with 100% oxygen concentration gave similar results with the BVM. In this randomized controlled trial no difference was found between NHFO and BVM in terms of saturation levels during intubation (Guitton et al., 2019). In this study of intensive care patients with non-severe respiratory failure, 192 patients were randomized. Before induction, BVM (with 15L/min oxygen flow) or heated humidified NHFO (60L/min, FiO_2:1.0) was applied for 4 minutes, after which rapid sequence intubation was performed. In the study, no significant difference was found among the groups in terms of the lowest SpO_2 value. However, when the complications related to intubation were evaluated, it was found that it was seen 3 times more in patients who were preoxygenated with BVM. In the study, it was stated that the NHFO cannula did not interfere with laryngoscopy in almost none of the patients using NHFO, and the cannula was removed because it prevented visualization of the larynx in only one patient. The same team previously compared NHFO and BVM in severe hypoxemic respiratory failure and reported that there was no significant difference (Vourc'h et al., 2015).

Noninvasive ventilation administration would be appropriate for the preoxygenation of intensive care patients with acute respiratory failure who are being treated with NHFO or NIV. In many studies, the effectiveness and complication rates of all these methods were compared and in general, NIV applications were found to be either superior or similar. When adverse events related to hypoxemia are examined, similar results are obtained in NIV and NHFO (Fong et al., 2019; Frat et al., 2019; Jaber et al., 2016). It would be preferred to continue with NIV in the preoxygenation of patients with respiratory failure who are currently being treated with NIV. Some studies have concluded that desaturation is higher in patients who are decided to intubate while NIV is being administered, if preoxygenation is not continued with NIV. In the FLORALI-2 study, in which preoxygenation was evaluated in patients with acute respiratory failure, patients were divided into two groups regardless of the ventilation support applied before the intubation decision. While NIV was applied to one group as a preoxygenation method, NHFO treatment was applied to the other group. When all patients were evaluated, it was concluded that preoxygenation with NIV and preoxygenation with NHFO were not superior to each other in terms of the number of patients whose oxyhemoglobin saturation was below 80%. However, when NIV was used in preoxygenation in patients with moderate to severe hypoxemia ($P/F \leq 200mmHg$), it was observed that the saturation decreased below 80% in fewer patients during the intubation process (Frat et al., 2019). In the study of Baillard et al., (Baillard et al., 2018) published in 2017, the effect of preoxygenation with NIV on organ failure was investigated. NIV and BVM were compared in preoxygenation and no difference was found in the SOFA scores investigated as the primary outcome. In their subgroup evaluations, the researchers found that the patients who were randomized to the BVM group after NIV were performed before the intubation decision, had more adverse events in preoxygenation and intubation. According to the data obtained, they stated that while respiratory failure is being treated with NIV, preoxygenation should be continued with NIV in patients who are decided to intubate.

In the PREOPTIPOP study published by Vourc'h et al., in 2019, preoxygenation assessment was performed in the anesthesia induction of obese patients and 100 patients were included in the study (Vourc'h et al., 2019). In the study comparing NIV and NHFO in preoxygenation, patients in both groups were preoxygenated for 4 minutes, and apneic oxygenation was continued after anesthesia induction in the NHFO group. After intubation, the lowest value of ETO_2 and also the lowest SpO_2 and intubation related complications were recorded. At the end of the study, better ETO_2 values were obtained in the NIV group. In addition, it has been reported that higher SpO_2 values were obtained with NIV and saturation values less than 95% were observed 2.5 times lower. There was no significant difference between NIV and NHFO in terms of intubation-related complications.

In a systematic review published in 2019 evaluating preoxygenation, 959 patients from 7 randomized controlled trials were included (Fong et al., 2019). The efficacy of NIV, NHFO and COT for preoxygenation in patients with respiratory failure for whom intubation was decided was compared. According to the results, the decrease in saturation observed during intubation was the least in patients preoxygenated with NIV. Although the evidence is insufficient, it has been stated that the use of combined NHFO and NIV may also be effective in limiting desaturation. The decrease in saturation below 80% has also occurred at least with NIV. It was stated that despite the low number of patients and insufficient evidence, NHFO combined with NIV might be the best preoxygenation method. Complications associated with intubation were seen least with NIV and NHFO. When evaluated in terms of mortality, it was reported that no method was superior to another.

It is important to evaluate the last respiratory support of each patient and to apply preoxygenation with the most appropriate method. However, although there are conflicting results about apneic oxygenation with NHFO, its combined application with NIV seems to be a method that can be used.

References

Baillard, C., Prat, G., Jung, B., Futier, E., Lefrant, J. Y., Vincent, F., Hamdi, A., Vicaut, E., & Jaber, S. (2018). Effect of preoxygenation using non-invasive ventilation before intubation on subsequent organ failures in hypoxaemic patients: a randomised clinical trial. *Br. J. Anaesth.,* 120(2), 361-367. https://doi.org/10.1016/j.bja.2017.11.067.

De Jong, A., Rolle, A., Molinari, N., Paugam-Burtz, C., Constantin, J. M., Lefrant, J. Y., Asehnoune, K., Jung, B., Futier, E., Chanques, G., Azoulay, E., & Jaber, S. (2018). Cardiac Arrest and Mortality Related to Intubation Procedure in Critically Ill Adult Patients: A Multicenter Cohort Study. *Crit. Care Med.*, 46(4), 532-539. https://doi.org /10.1097/ccm.0000000000002925.

Fong, K. M., Au, S. Y., & Ng, G. W. Y. (2019). Preoxygenation before intubation in adult patients with acute hypoxemic respiratory failure: a network meta-analysis of randomized trials. *Crit. Care*, 23(1), 319. https://doi.org/10.1186/s13054-019-2596-1.

Frat, J. P., Ricard, J. D., Quenot, J. P., Pichon, N., Demoule, A., Forel, J. M., Mira, J. P., Coudroy, R., Berquier, G., Voisin, B., Colin, G., Pons, B., Danin, P. E., Devaquet, J.,

Prat, G., Clere-Jehl, R., Petitpas, F., Vivier, E., Razazi, K., Nay, M. A., Souday, V., Dellamonica, J., Argaud, L., Ehrmann, S., Gibelin, A., Girault, C., Andreu, P., Vignon, P., Dangers, L., Ragot, S., & Thille, A. W. (2019). Non-invasive ventilation versus high-flow nasal cannula oxygen therapy with apnoeic oxygenation for preoxygenation before intubation of patients with acute hypoxaemic respiratory failure: a randomised, multicentre, open-label trial. *Lancet Respir. Med.,* 7(4), 303-312. https://doi.org/ 10.1016/s2213-2600(19)30048-7.

Guitton, C., Ehrmann, S., Volteau, C., Colin, G., Maamar, A., Jean-Michel, V., Mahe, P. J., Landais, M., Brule, N., Bretonnière, C., Zambon, O., & Vourc'h, M. (2019). Nasal high-flow preoxygenation for endotracheal intubation in the critically ill patient: a randomized clinical trial. *Intensive Care Med*., 45(4), 447-458. https://doi.org/ 10.1007/s00134-019-05529-w.

Hanouz, J. L., Lhermitte, D., Gérard, J. L., & Fischer, M. O. (2019). Comparison of pre-oxygenation using spontaneous breathing through face mask and high-flow nasal oxygen: A randomised controlled crossover study in healthy volunteers. *Eur. J. Anaesthesiol*., 36(5), 335-341. https://doi.org/10.1097/eja.0000000000000954.

Jaber, S., Monnin, M., Girard, M., Conseil, M., Cisse, M., Carr, J., Mahul, M., Delay, J. M., Belafia, F., Chanques, G., Molinari, N., & De Jong, A. (2016). Apnoeic oxygenation via high-flow nasal cannula oxygen combined with non-invasive ventilation preoxygenation for intubation in hypoxaemic patients in the intensive care unit: the single-centre, blinded, randomised controlled OPTINIV trial. *Intensive Care Med.*, 42(12), 1877-1887. https://doi.org/10.1007/s00134-016-4588-9.

Langeron, O., Bourgain, J. L., Francon, D., Amour, J., Baillard, C., Bouroche, G., Chollet Rivier, M., Lenfant, F., Plaud, B., Schoettker, P., Fletcher, D., Velly, L., & Nouette-Gaulain, K. (2018). Difficult intubation and extubation in adult anaesthesia. *Anaesth. Crit. Care Pain Med.,* 37(6), 639-651. https://doi.org/10.1016/j.accpm.2018.03.013.

Nimmagadda, U., Salem, M. R., & Crystal, G. J. (2017). Preoxygenation: Physiologic Basis, Benefits, and Potential Risks. Anesth. Analg., 124(2), 507-517. https://doi.org/ 10.1213/ANE.0000000000001589.

Nolan, R. T. (1967). Pre-oxygenation and thiopentone-suxamethonium induction. *Br. J. Anaesth*., 39(10), 794-797. https://doi.org/10.1093/bja/39.10.794.

Tanoubi, I., Drolet, P., & Donati, F. (2009). Optimizing preoxygenation in adults. *Can. J. Anaesth.*, 56(6), 449-466. https://doi.org/10.1007/s12630-009-9084-z.

Vourc'h, M., Asfar, P., Volteau, C., Bachoumas, K., Clavieras, N., Egreteau, P. Y., Asehnoune, K., Mercat, A., Reignier, J., Jaber, S., Prat, G., Roquilly, A., Brule, N., Villers, D., Bretonniere, C., & Guitton, C. (2015). High-flow nasal cannula oxygen during endotracheal intubation in hypoxemic patients: a randomized controlled clinical trial. *Intensive Care Med.*, 41(9), 1538-1548. https://doi.org/10.1007/s00134-015-3796-z.

Vourc'h, M., Baud, G., Feuillet, F., Blanchard, C., Mirallie, E., Guitton, C., Jaber, S., & Asehnoune, K. (2019). High-flow Nasal Cannulae Versus Non-invasive Ventilation for Preoxygenation of Obese Patients: The PREOPTIPOP Randomized Trial. *EClinicalMedicine*, 13, 112-119. https://doi.org/10.1016/j.eclinm.2019.05.014.

Weitzner, S. W., King, B. D., & Ikezono, E. (1959). The rate of arterial oxygen desaturation during apnea in humans. *Anesthesiology*, 20, 624-627. https://doi.org/10.1097/ 00000542-195909000-00013.

In: Non-Invasive Mechanical Ventilation Complications
Editor: Antonio M. Esquinas
ISBN: 978-1-53619-515-6

Chapter 27

INTUBATION-RELATED COMPLICATIONS ASSOCIATED WITH DELAYED INTUBATION AFTER FAILED NIPPV

Carmine Iacovazzo, MD, Claudia Veropalumbo, MD, Maria Vargas*, MD and Giuseppe Servillo

Department of Neuroscience and Reproductive and Odontostomatological Sciences, University of Naples Federico II, Naples, Italy

ABSTRACT

While Noninvasive Positive Pressure Ventilation (NIPPV) has been shown to efficiently reduce the need for endotracheal intubation in various groups of patients with acute respiratory failure, several studies have demonstrated an increase in mortality with delayed intubation after failed NIPPV. Intubation-related complications experienced with delayed endotracheal intubation may partially explain the reason behind the increased mortality seen after failed NIPPV that requires intubation.

Keywords: noninvasive ventilation failure, intubation related complications, delayed intubation, noninvasive ventilation outcome, predictor factors for noninvasive ventilation failure

* Corresponding Author's E-mail: vargas.maria82@gmail.com.

INTRODUCTION

Noninvasive positive pressure ventilation (NIPPV) is now widely used to treat critically ill patients with acute respiratory failure (ARF) across a variety of etiologies.

According to Official ERS/ATS guidelines, NIPPV is strongly recommended in patients with COPD exacerbation (acute-on-chronic respiratory failure): in this clinical setting, NIPPV should be considered either to prevent acute respiratory acidosis or, when a mild to moderate acidosis is already present, to prevent a deterioration such that invasive ventilation would be necessarily taken into account; lastly, NIPPV also plays a role as an alternative to invasive ventilation in patients with severe acidosis and respiratory distress [1].

Furthermore, NIPPV is highly recommended in the treatment of patients with ARF due to cardiogenic pulmonary edema (CPE): in this context, it has the ability to improve respiratory mechanics and facilitate left ventricular work by decreasing left ventricular afterload [1].

In support of this recommendations, there are different trials that showed decreased intubation and mortality rates when performing this ventilation mode, both in COPD exacerbation and CPE [2, 3].

There are additional clinical settings in which NIPPV is suggested to be effective, even if with weaker evidences: early NIPPV after planned extubation should be considered to prevent and treat post-extubation ARF, as it is linked to a decrease in both intubation rate and mortality in patients at high risk of extubation failure (i.e., >65 years old or with underlying cardiac or respiratory disease) [4]. Moreover NIPPV plays a role in postoperative settings: surgery, anesthesia and post-operative pain may all have deleterious effects on the respiratory system; the use of NIPPV may increase lung aeration and decrease the amount of atelectasis during the post-operative period [5].

By contrast, the beneficial effects of NIPPV remain uncertain in patients with *de novo* acute hypoxemic respiratory failure (AHRF), namely non-hypercapnic patients having acute respiratory failure in the absence of a cardiac origin or underlying chronic pulmonary disease, like asthma, pneumonia, ARDS: NIPPV is more likely to fail in these patients [6], and this occurrence is associated with increased mortality [7].

NIPPV FAILURE

NIV failure has been defined as the need for endotracheal intubation (ETI) or death [8]. Its rate greatly varies between 5 and 60%, depending on numerous factors, including the underlying cause of ARF [9]. Unsuccessful NIV was found to be independently associated with death [7].

The range of criteria to declare NIPPV failure and the subsequent need for intubation is wide and includes:

- unremitting respiratory distress with respiratory rate more than 35 breaths/min,
- failing in maintaining a PaO_2/FiO_2 above 100 mmHg,
- inability to correct respiratory acidosis,
- management of profuse tracheal secretions,
- development of conditions which need protection of the airway (coma or seizure disorders),
- hemodynamic instability with no response to fluids and vasoactive agents,
- respiratory or cardiac arrest [8].

As it concerns patients groups that mostly benefit from NIPPV, the percentage of patients with cardiogenic pulmonary edema (CPE) transitioned from NIPPV to Invasive Mechanical Ventilation (IMV) is relatively low (5-9%) [10, 11].

The rate of intubation after a NIPPV trial in patients with COPD exhacerbation is 8,9-18,9% and the subsequent mortality is 23-30%, with a 61% higher odds of death compared to patients directly placed on IMV; furthermore these patients experience a prolonged stay in ICU [9, 12, 13].

In postoperative settings, a retrospective study confirmed that NIPPV could avoid invasive ventilation in some patients, but also showed that the failure rate was high (42%), identifying the strongest predictive factor of failure in the nosocomial-acquired pneumonia causing ARF: if pneumonia is present, NIPPV failure rate could reach 70% [14].

Regarding patients who had respiratory failure after extubation, Esteban et al., conducted a multicenter randomized trial to evaluate the effect of NIPPV on mortality in this clinical setting. The main finding of this study was that noninvasive ventilation did not reduce the need for reintubation among these patients and the mortality rate tended to be higher among the patients assigned to NIPPV than among those assigned to standard medical therapy (supplemental oxygen, respiratory physiotherapy, bronchodilators), and the interval from the development of respiratory failure to reintubation was considerably longer with NIPPV than with standard therapy [15].

Lastly, in patients admitted to ICUs for AHRF, the rate of intubation is notably high, reaching 60%, and their in-ICU mortality, when intubation is delayed by a trial of NIPPV, may exceed 60% [7, 16, 17].

Ultimately, NIPPV is literally a double-edged sword that may improve outcome of patients who succeed in it by avoiding ETI, but may worsen outcome by delaying intubation in those having failed NIPPV. Consequently, there is a need for early recognition of patients at risk for transition from NIPPV to IMV.

Being NIPPV failure in most cases predictable, a careful monitoring of the patient's status should occur to determine if the patient is improving and the ventilatory support is adequate. Confalonieri et al., found that NIPPV most likely fails on patients who had more severe respiratory acidosis, a lower level of consciousness, were older, more hypoxemic and had a higher breathing frequency; thus They identified APACHE II score, Glasgow Coma Scale (GCS), Respiratory Rate (RR) and ABG pH value as predictive factors for NIPPV success or failure and suggest to asses them at the admission and at least after 2 hours of NIPPV. (Table 1)

Table 1. Predictive factors for Moderate and High risk of NIPPV Failure [9]

Factors	Moderate Risk	High Risk
GCS	12-14	≤11
pH	7.25-7.29	≤7.25
RR	30-34	≥35
APACHE II score		≥29

Clinical signs that are doubtful on presentation, become more convincingly predictive of failure if they persist after 2 h of NIPPV. At the admission, the main factor which worsens the outcome is GCS ≤ 11, while after 2 h of NIPPV, the stronger variable is the pH value ≤7.25, which dramatically increases the risk of failure up to 99% [9].

Delayed Intubation-Related Complications

While NIPPV has been shown to decrease the need for ETI in patients with respiratory failure, literature is gaunt regarding the risk of intubation-related complications associated with delayed intubation in patients on whom NIPPV fails. As mentioned before, several studies have demonstrated an increase in mortality with delayed intubation after failed NIPPV in acute respiratory failure and after failed extubation [7, 13, 15, 18].

Given the underlying fragility and the limited physiologic reserve, high risk of hypoxemia, hemodynamic deterioration and even cardiac arrest with intubation in all critically ill patients, these results on the subject of mortality could be partially explained by complications experienced with delayed intubation in these settings.

A multicenter observational study shows that in ICU setting, intubation-related moderate complications (such as difficult intubation, cardiac arrhythmia, esophageal intubation, agitation, aspiration and dental injury) happen in nearly half of the patients, and at least one among severe complications takes place in 28% of cases. The most frequent of them are severe hypotension, frequently needing use of vasopressor, and severe hypoxemia, both with a similar incidence of 25-26%, while cardiac arrest and death are less frequent (0,8-2%). Unsurprisingly, the presence of ARF as a reason for intubation, has emerged as an independent risk factor for the occurrence of the listed complications [19].

In order to avoid or at least reduce the occurrence of hypoxemia, it is crucial to maximize the patient's oxygen stores in the arterial, venous, and tissue beds but, in contrast to elective settings or patients which have their airway secured solely for the purpose of airway protection, it may be difficult to achieve this for patients with ARF like the ones on whom NIPPV failed.

The effectiveness of preoxygenation has been found to be restricted in those with significant cardiopulmonary pathology like congestive heart failure, COPD, pneumonitis and respiratory failure complicated by excessive secretions. In those critically ill patient, despite optimal preoxygenation, the pulse oximetry oxygen saturation (SpO2) may barely reach the 90%; this level of arterial oxygen is situated on the downward slope of the oxyhemoglobin saturation curve, and further desaturation beyond this point may be dramatically rapid. Moreover, hypoxemia may be exaggerated if multiple intubation attempts, esophageal intubation, aspiration, main stem bronchus intubation, or loss of the airway complicate the intervention [20].

Furthermore, profound hypoxemia (SpO2 < 70%) proved to be a primary contributing factor to severe bradycardia and definitively to cardiac arrest during ETI in critical settings, worsening the possible effect of vagotonic stimulation due to vigorous or prolonged laryngoscopy and tracheal manipulation. The reduction in heart rate is typically accompanied by a significant lowering in blood pressure, often requiring aggressive therapy [21].

As already mentioned, postintubation hypotension in the critical setting is the most common of the hemodynamic alterations and may be based on many factors: the application of positive-pressure ventilation and PEEP, plus any vasodilatation and myocardial depression from anesthesia agents, may contribute to postintubation hypotension. This response is accentuated in incidence and intensity in the critically ill patient who is yet struggling with cardiopulmonary deterioration or acid-base imbalance, [22] like in NIPPV failure cases.

Mosier et al., conducted a single-center retrospective cohort study comparing patients intubated after failed NIPPV versus those patients intubated without undergoing a trial of NIPPV, measuring the incidence of a composite complication (desaturation, hypotension or aspiration) as primary outcome, and the odds of death in the ICU following the occurrence of a complication during intubation as secondary outcome.

Notwithstanding patients on whom NIPPV failed had significantly lower severity of illness scores (APACHE II, APACHE IV, and SAPS II) at the admission than the group that was primarily intubated, the results show an increased risk of complications when intubation is delayed due to a trial of NIPPV. (Table 2)

Table 2. Rate of intubation-related complications in primary intubation VS delayed intubation after failed NIPPV trial [23]

	Primary intubation	Failed NIPPV
Hypotension	27.3%	32%
Desaturation	23.6%	32%
Aspiration	1.8%	1.6%
>1 Complication	10%	12.8%

Moreover, when one of these complications occurs, these data show an association with increased odds of death in the ICU [23].

Despite the need for further data desirably from prospective trials, it is plausible that a delay in intubation can cause the increase in the risk of death in patients treated with NIPPV reported in clinical trials, through mechanisms that include complications strictly related to intubation.

REFERENCES

[1] Rochwerg, B., Brochard, L., Elliott, M. W., et al., Official ERS/ATS clinical practice guidelines: noninvasive ventilation for acute respiratory failure. s.l.: *Eur Respir J*, 2017.

[2] Brochard, L., Mancebo, J., Wysocki, M., Lofaso, F., Conti, G., Rauss, A., Simonneau, G., Benito, S., Gasparetto, A., Lemaire, F. et al., Noninvasive ventilation for acute exacerbations of chronic obstructive pulmonary disease. 333, 1995, *New English Journal of Medicine*, pp. 817-822.

[3] Masip, J., Betbese, A. J., Paez, J., Vecilla, F., Canizares, R., Padro, J., Paz, M. A., de Otero, J., Ballus, J. Non-invasive pressure support ventilation versus conventional oxygen therapy in acute cardiogenic pulmonary oedema: a randomised trial. 356, 2000, *Lancet*, pp. 2126-32.

[4] Thille, A. W., Boissier, F., Ben-Ghezala, H., et al., Easily identified at-risk patients for extubation failure may benefit from noninvasive ventilation: a prospective before-after study. 20, s.l.: *Crit Care*, 2016.

[5] Jaber, S., Chanques, G., Jung, B. Postoperative noninvasive ventilation. 112, s.l.: *Anesthesiology*, 2010, pp. 453-461.

[6] Demoule, A., Girou, E., Richard, J. C., Taille, S., Brochard, L. Increased use of noninvasive ventilation in French intensive care units. 32, 2006, *Intensive Care Medicine*, pp. 1747-1755.

[7] Demoule, A., Girou, E., Richard, J. C., Taille, S., Brochard, L. Benefits and risks of success or failure of noninvasive ventilation. 32, 2006, *Intensive Care Medicine,* pp. 1756-1765.

[8] Duan, J., Wang, S., Liu, P., Han, X., Tian, Y., Gao, F., Zhou, J., Mou, J., Qin, Q., Yu, J., Bai, L., Zhou, L., Zhang, R. Early prediction of noninvasive ventilation failure in COPD patients: derivation, internal validation, and external validation of a simple risk score. 108, 2019, *Annals of Intensive Care.*

[9] Confalonieri, M., G. Garuti, M. S. Cattaruzza, J. F. Osborn, M. Antonelli, G. Conti, M. Kodric, O. Resta, S. Marchese, C. Gregoretti, A. Rossi. A chart of failure risk for noninvasive ventilation in patients with COPD exacerbation. 25, 2005, *European Respiratory Journal*, pp. 348-355.

[10] Masip, J., Betbesé, A. J., Páez, J., et al., Non-invasive pressure support ventilation versus conventional oxygen therapy in acute cardiogenic pulmonary oedema: a randomised trial. 356, 2000, *Lancet*, pp. 2126-2132.

[11] Belenguer-Muncharaz, A., Mateu-Campos, L., González-Luís, R., et al., Non-Invasive Mechanical Ventilation Versus Continuous Positive Airway Pressure Relating to Cardiogenic Pulmonary Edema in an Intensive Care Unit. 53, 2017, *Archivos de Bronconeumología*, pp. 561-567.

[12] Steriade, A. T., Johari, S., Sargarovschi, N. et al., Predictors of outcome of noninvasive ventilation in severe COPD exacerbation. 131, 2019, *BMC Pulmonary Medicine.*

[13] Chandra, D., Stamm, J. A., Taylor, B., Ramos, R. M., Satterwhite, L., Krishnan, J. A., et al., Outcomes of noninvasive ventilation for acute exacerbations of chronic obstructive pulmonary disease in the United States, 1998-2008. 185, 2012, *American Journal of Respiratory and Critical Care Medicine*, pp. 152-159.

[14] Wallet, F., et al., Factors associated with noninvasive ventilation failure in postoperative acute respiratory insufficiency: an observational study. s.l.: *European Journal of Anaesthesiology*, 2010, Vol. 27.

[15] Esteban, A., Fernando Frutos-Vivar, Niall D. Ferguson, Yaseen Arabi, Carlos Apezteguía, et al., Noninvasive Positive-Pressure Ventilation for Respiratory Failure after Extubation. 350, 2004, *New English Journal of Medicine*, pp. 2452-2460.

[16] Schettino, G., Altobelli, N., Kacmarek, R. M. Noninvasive positive-pressure ventilation in acute respiratory failure outside clinical trials: experience at the Massachusetts General Hospital. 36, 2008, *Critical Care Medicine*, pp. 441-447.

[17] Rana, S., Jenad, H., Gay, P. C., Buck, C. F., Hubmayr, R. D., Gajic, O. Failure of non-invasive ventilation in patients with acute lung injury: observational cohort study. 2006, *Critical Care Medicine*, Vol. 10.

[18] Carrillo, A., Gonzalez-Diaz, G., Ferrer, M. et al., Non-invasive ventilation in community-acquired pneumonia and severe acute respiratory failure. 38, 2012, *Intensive Care Medicine*, pp. 458-466.

[19] Jaber, S., Jibba Amraoui, Jean-Yves Lefrant, Charles Arich, Robert Cohendy et al., Clinical practice and risk factors for immediate complications of endotracheal intubation in the intensive care unit: a prospective, multiple-center study. 34, 2006, *Critical Care Medicine*, pp. 2355-61.

[20] Mort, T. C. Preoxygenation in critically ill patients requiring emergency tracheal intubation. 33, 2005, *Critical Care Medicine*, pp. 2672-2675.

[21] Mort, T. C. The incidence and risk factors for cardiac arrest during emergency tracheal intubation: a justification for incorporating the ASA Guidelines in the remote location. 16, 2004, *Journal of Clinical Anesthesia,* pp. 508-516.

[22] Klinger, J. R. Haemodynamics and positive end-expiratory pressure in critically ill patients. 1996, *Critical Care Clinics,* Vol. 12, pp. 841-864.

[23] Jarrod, M., Mosier, John C. Sakles, Sage P. Whitmore, Cameron D. Hypes, Danielle K. Hallett et al., Failed noninvasive positive-pressure is associated with an increased risk of intubation-related complications. 5, 2015, *Annals of Intensive Care.*

[24] Antonelli, M., Conti, G., Rocco, M., Bufi, M., De Biasi, R. A., Vivino, G., et al., A comparison of noninvasive positive-pressure ventilation and conventional mechanical ventilation in patients with acute respiratory failure. 339, 1998, *New English Journal of Medicine*, pp. 429-435.

[25] Confalonieri, M., Potena, A., Carbone, G., Porta, R. D., Tolley, E. A., Umberto Meduri, G. Acute respiratory failure in patients with severe communityacquired pneumonia: a prospective randomized evaluation of noninvasive ventilation. 160, 1999, *American Journal of Respiratory and Critical Care Medicine*, pp. 1585-1591.

In: Non-Invasive Mechanical Ventilation Complications ISBN: 978-1-53619-515-6
Editor: Antonio M. Esquinas

Chapter 28

Complications during Non-Invasive Mechanical Ventilation. Weaning Process. Extubation and Re-Intubation

Carmen Pascale, MD, Maria Vargas*, MD and Giueppe Servillo, MD
Department of Neuroscience and Reproductive and Odontostomatological_Sciences, University of Naples Federico II, Naples, Italy

Abstract

Weaning in the clinical history of an intubated and ventilated patient with mechanical ventilation is an extremely delicate moment. Several studies have been performed to understand the appropriate time to wean and how to perform weaning correctly and safely. In this regard, the spontaneous breathing trial has been developed, which makes it possible to understand whether the patient is able to breathe independently or not. This test, together with the overall clinical evaluation of the patient, allows to decide whether to proceed with the extubation. However, a proportion of extubated patients experience respiratory failure and require reintubation. These are usually complex patients with a variety of comorbidities and in 50% of cases, they die. In recent years it is becoming increasingly common to use NIV immediately after extubation, even before any respiratory failure can occur. The use of non-invasive mechanical ventilation seems to significantly reduce the mortality of extubated patients and the risk that they will experience reintubation.

Keywords: non-invasive ventilation, weaning, extubation, re-intubation, failure

* Corresponding Author's E-mail: argas.maria82@gmail.com.

Acute respiratory failure, either as a consequence of an exacerbation of a chronic obstructive pulmonary disease or as an event that occurs following surgery, represents a dramatic event, so much so that it requires the intubation of the patient who must be ventilated mechanically. Invasive mechanical ventilation and hospitalization in intensive care have a strong impact on the patient, so you need a correct evaluation to establish how long the patient must be kept sedated and intubated, in order to avoid all those complications related to hospitalization in ICU. Already after 72 hours of intubation, a possible weaning and extubation could present difficulties. In fact, all major studies have focused on the management of weaning in patients intubated for at least 48-72 hours, in order to prevent a possible improper extubation. It may happen, in fact, that after extubation the patient shows signs and symptoms of acute respiratory failure and that requires, even after 48 hours, a subsequent intubation. For a long time we have been trying to understand what the role of non-invasive mechanical ventilation could be in this slice of patients. Initially it was thought that the NIV only delayed the reintubation and, consequently, had no beneficial effect on the clinical picture of the patient. With more recent studies and a closer analysis of the data collected, it was concluded that NIV performed for at least 72 hours in extubated patients, is able to produce positive effects on patients' life expectancy.

When a patient has acute respiratory failure, invasive mechanical ventilation is essential. Unfortunately, IMV can produce even serious complications such as respiratory muscle weakness, upper respiratory tract disease, pneumonia [1] and sinusitis associated with invasive ventilation. Therefore, as soon as the disease for which intubation and mechanical ventilation have become necessary begins to improve, it becomes of primary importance to understand when to start weaning. Such maneuver, in fact, should be started at an appropriate time, in order to avoid cases of premature extubation with a patient who is not yet able to breathe independently and therefore requires reintubation; or cases of delayed extubation related to all the possible complications encountered with prolonged mechanical ventilation. The main problem is weaning from mechanical ventilation, not from intubation; even though weaning and extubation often tend to coincide, they are overlapping only for patients with less than weekly ventilation. On the basis of what has just been said, it is necessary to set the clinical approach in this way:

- Evaluate if the conditions to extubate the patient are met.
- Evaluate whether the conditions for suspending mechanical ventilation are met, i.e., whether it is foreseeable that the patient will be able to breathe on his own after extubation.

We also emphasize that a possible failed extubation is associated with high mortality, so this manoeuvre should be well considered.

Several studies carried out on this topic have generally considered patients intubated and ventilated for at least 72 hours, and have identified criteria that would allow to consider weaning and extubation. Weaning is considered when the criteria listed are met: cardiovascular stability (hemoglobin $\geq$8 g/dl, no severe arrhythmia), hemodynamic stability (absence of vasopressors or vasopressors in doses $\leq$5 μg/kg/min), gas-exchange stability ($PaO_2 \geq 60$ mm Hg with $SaO_2 \geq 90\%$ and $FiO_2 \leq 40\%$), pulmonary mechanics stability (control of pulmonary edema, atelectases, secretions, and bronchospasm), neurologic stability (GCS, >10), electrolytic stability (control of alkalosis, acidosis, calcium, magnesium, phosphorus, sodium, potassium), preserved cough reflex, rapid and shallow breathing rate (f/TV, ratio of respiratory rate and tidal volume in liters) <105, absence of respiratory infection (defined as a new or progressive pulmonary infiltrate at chest radiograph, temperature <36°C or >37.8°C, leukocytosis (leukocytes >12,000/ml) or leukopenia (leukocytes <4,000/ml)) [2]. The most important moment of weaning is the spontaneous breathing trial, a test to see if the patient will be able to breathe without a mechanical ventilator. It consists of suspending or minimizing ventilatory support. The duration of the test is variable and generally ranges from 30 to 120 minutes. If the patient passes the spontaneous breathing trial, extubation is performed; conversely, if signs and symptoms of respiratory failure appear during the test, intubation is maintained and mechanical ventilation is resumed. The test can be performed in several ways:

- T-tube: remove the mechanical ventilator and connect the tracheal tube to a flow of humidified and oxygen-enriched gas, through a T-tube;
- PS 0 - PEEP 0: get zero support pressure and PEEP, keeping the patient connected to the ventilator;
- CPAP: less than or equal to 5 cm H_2O;
- Support pressure: 5-8 cm H_2O;
- ATC (automatic tube compensation) without inspiratory support: the fan only applies the pressure necessary to cancel the tracheal tube resistances.

These modes are not equivalent [3]. Current guidelines recommend 5-8 cm H_2O support pressure as a strategy to increase the number of successfully extubated patients [4], although the T-tube mode creates a similar workload as after extubation [5]. Let's clarify the concept. It can be hypothesized that an overly prolonged spontaneous breathing trial (120 minutes) such as the T-tube trial will subject patients to excessive stress, "tiring" them unnecessarily. In this regard, in some cases, it was necessary to resume ventilation for one hour and then proceed to extubation. The PS test, on the other hand, requires a shorter duration and shorter effort, so if after 30-60 minutes the test did not fail, you can think of extubating the patient.

However, it should be noted that all studies conducted on spontaneous breathing trials consider only the first attempt. That circumstance gets patients involved (50%) the most easy to treat, with rapid weaning, low mortality and short duration of hospitalization in ICU [6].

Therefore, patients needing particular care are those suffering several failures of spontaneous breath trials and the weaning process is prolonged by days or weeks.

In case the spontaneous breath trial fails, the patient must be kept on the ventilator and the trial can be repeated every day, limiting its duration to 30 minutes, using a limited support pressure in order to make the respiratory work as close as possible to the respiratory work after the extubation. Naturally, extubated patients are only those who successfully pass weaning. However, a part of them (10-20%) [7] will still experience respiratory failure in the following days, sometimes so severe as to require reintubation: weaning failure will be discussed at this point. Several studies have identified the signs and symptoms that can occur in extubated patient from 48-72 hours and that require a new intubation. High-risk patients of reintubation after weaning failure are considered: (a) older than 65 years, cardiac failure as the cause of intubation, or APACHE II score greater than 12 at the time of extubation [8]; (b) more than one of the following: failure of consecutive weaning trials, chronic cardiac failure, arterial pressure of carbon dioxide greater than 45 mm Hg after extubation, more than one noncardiac comorbidity, or weak cough or stridor after extubation not requiring immediate intubation [9]; (c) acute exacerbation of COPD [10]; or (d) history of chronic respiratory disease with ventilation for more than 48 hours and hypercapnia during the spontaneous breathing trial. Reintubation is a dramatic event in the patient's medical history, with high mortality (between 25% and 50%), generally for IMA, VAP, sepsis or MOF. Probably so high mortality is related to a delay in reintubation, due to a slowly and progressive clinical deterioration after extubation, in patients presenting risk factors for a failed extubation: elderly patients, with weak cough, chronic cardiopulmonary disease [11] or chronic obstructive pulmonary disease (COPD) [12] in history. The use of non-invasive mechanical ventilation (NIV), maintained for at least 48 hours, may be included in the treatment of this proportion of patients. NIV may also be used in patients with weaning difficulties after surgery [13]. This would lead to a reduction in the number of reintubations in these patients, as well as a reduction in the risk of pneumonia associated with invasive mechanical ventilation. On this topic several studies in the literature have tried to demonstrate the effectiveness of NIV in extubated patients who do not yet show signs of respiratory failure to prevent the risk of reintubation and reduce hospital mortality. Patients who could benefit from NIV are defined as "frail," i.e., elderly patients (>65 years), extubation hypercapnic patients [14], with heart failure, obese [15], with severe chronic lung disease, with weak cough, and ventilated patients with invasive mechanical ventilation for at least 48-72 hours. NIV post-extubation was compared with simple oxygen therapy to assess the differences in terms of patient outcome and risk reduction of reintubation. Timeliness in the use of NIV after extubation is crucial, especially in patients with chronic and hypercapnic respiratory failure. Non-invasive mechanical ventilation should be established for prophylactic purposes in frail patients even before they can show signs of post-extubation respiratory failure and NIV should be extended as long as possible, as long as 24-48 hours, with average PEEP values around 5 cm H_2O and support pressure around 15 cm H_2O. Although the data provided by the studies from a statistical point of view are not clear, but considering real numbers evaluated, it is clear that post-extubation NIV for prophylactic purposes reduces the risk of reintubation and hospital mortality significantly. Probably good results of NIV is due to immediate application after the planned extubation, it is able to prevent overloading of respiratory muscles, development of atelectasis, ventilation/perfusion ratio disorders, and respiratory distress. It is necessary to stress the concept that the NIV must be immediately applied, because it has been observed that its use after the extubated patient has manifested respiratory distress, it is not able to prevent reintubation.

REFERENCES

[1] Pingleton S. K. Complications of Acute Respiratory Failure. *Am Rev Respir Dis* 1988; 137:1463-93.

[2] Ornico et al., Noninvasive Ventilation Immadiately After Extubation Improves Weaning Outcome After Acute Respiratory Failure: A Randomized Controlled *Trial Critical Care* 2013, 17:R39.

[3] Subirà C., Hernàndez G., Vàzquez A., et al., Effect of Pressure Support vs T-Piece Ventilation Strategies during Spontaneous Breathing Trials on Successful Extubation Among Patients Receiving Mechanical Ventilation: A Randomized Controlled Trial. *JAMA* 2019; 321:2175-21824.

[4] Ouellette D. R. et al., Liberation from mechanical ventilation in critically ill adults: an official American College of Chest Physicians/*American Thoracic Society clinical practice guideline.*

[5] Sklar M. C. et al., Effort to breathe with various spontaneous breathing trial techniques. Aphysiologic meta-analysis. *Am J Respir Crit Care Med* 2017; 195:1477-85.

[6] Bèduneau G., Pham T., Schortgen F., et al., Epidemiology of Weaning Outcome according to a New Definition. The WIND study. *Am J Respir Crit Care Med* 2017; 195:772-783.

[7] Thille A. W. et al., The decision to extubate in the Intensive Care Unit. *Am J Respir Care Med* 2013; 187:1294-1302.

[8] Terrer M., Valencia M., Nicolas J. M., Bernadich O., Badia J. R., Torres A. Early noninvasive ventilation averts extubation failure in patients at risk: a randomized trial *Am J Respir Crit Care Med* 2006, 173:164-17C.

[9] Nava S., Gregoretti C., Fanfulla F., Squadrone E., Grassi M., Carlucci A., Beltrame F., Novalesi: Noninvasive ventilation to prevent respiratory failure after extubation in high-risk patients. *Crit Care Mede* 2005, 33:2465-2470.

[10] Luo I. I., Cheng P., Zhou P. Sequential BiPAP following invasive mechanical ventilation in COPD patients with hypercapnic respiratory failure. *Hunan Yi Ke Da Xue Bao* 2001, 26 563-565.

[11] Winck J. C., Azevedo L. F., Costa-Pereira A., et al., Efficacy and safety of non-invasive ventilation in the treatmente of acute cardiogenic pulmonary edema-a systematic review and meta-analysis. *Crit Care* 2006; 10: R69.

[12] Keenan S. P., Kernerman P. D., Cook D. J., et al., Effect of noninvasive positive pressure ventilation on mortality in patients admitted with acute respiratory failure: a meta-analysis. *Crit Care Med* 1997; 25:1685-92.

[13] Squadrone V., Coha M., Cerutti E., et al., Continuous positive airway pressure for treatment of postoperative hypoxemia: a randomized controlled trial. *J Am Med Assoc* 2005; 293:589-95.

[14] Ferrer M. et al., Non-invasive ventilation after extubation in Hypercapnic patients with chronic respiratory disorders: randomized controlled trial. *Lancet* 2009; 374:1082-8.

[15] El Solh A. A. et al., Noninvasive ventilation for prevention of post-extubation respiratory failure in obese patients. *Eur Respir J* 2006; 28:588-95.

In: Non-Invasive Mechanical Ventilation Complications ISBN: 978-1-53619-515-6
Editor: Antonio M. Esquinas

Chapter 29

Complications during Postoperative Non-Invasive Mechanical Ventilation. Anastomotic Leak. Neurotrauma, Neurosurgery, Thoracic, Cardiac Surgery, Abdominal Surgery and Gastric Bypass

Fátima Espinosa Torre[1,*], MD, Rocío Lombardo Torre[2], MD and Nadia Bouchoucha[3], PhD

[1]Department of Internal Medicine, Hospital Virgen del Rocío, Sevilla, Spain
[2]Department of Anaesthesiology and Resuscitation, Hospital del Henares, Madrid, Spain
[3]Department of Internal Medicine, Medizinische Universitatsklinik, Kantonsspital Baselland Bruderholz, Switzerland

Abstract

Non-invasive ventilation (NIV) allows to mechanically ventilate a patient by means of a full-face or nasal mask instead of an endotracheal tube. The main benefits are decreases in the intubation rate, mortality rate, and number of infectious complications, particularly pneumonia.

In most studies of NIPPV in the ICU setting, the main outcome measure has been the need for tracheal intubation. For those patients who avoid intubation, the main advantage is the avoidance of artificial airway complications. Several studies document a lower infection rate (nosocomial pneumonia and sinusitis) with NIPPV, which may be related to the maintenance of the protective glottic barrier. Other advantages include reduced need for sedative medications. Some NIPPV trials have demonstrated reductions in ICU length of stay, ICU mortality, or in-hospital mortality.

---

* Corresponding Author's E-mail: sync578@hotmail.com.

This chapter is intended to explore the applications and benefits of NIV in postoperative patients, especially in those undergoing neurosurgery, thoracic and abdominal surgery.

Keywords: neurosurgery, NIV, postoperative, critical care, mechanical

INTRODUCTION

The postoperative period is fraught with complications related to the respiratory and cardiovascular systems, especially in the 'at-risk' patient population group. The severity of these complications depends upon the preoperative respiratory status as well as intraoperative factors, such as the type and site of surgery performed and the anaesthesia that the patient is exposed to.

Management begins with careful screening and selection of the at-risk patient, optimising his physiological status in the preoperative period, continuing to provide lung protective ventilation in the intraoperative period and extending optimal respiratory care into the postoperative period [1]. The mainstay of treatment of postoperative respiratory failure so far has been reintubation and mechanical ventilation, which are associated with complications like pneumonia, infections, increased costs, morbidity and mortality. Non-invasive ventilation (NIV) has been used successfully in such instances.

It is important to carefully rule out any of the contraindications to the application of NIV before starting its use. The benefits of NIV have been clearly established in the intensive care unit (ICU) especially in patients with hypercapnic respiratory failure secondary to chronic obstructive pulmonary disease (COPD) or to chest wall deformities, cardiogenic pulmonary oedema and as an aid to facilitate weaning from ventilatory support. The evidence for the beneficial effects of NIV in postoperative patients mainly comes from studies in patients who have undergone major thoracoabdominal or cardiac surgeries. Here, NIV may be applied prophylactically, i.e., in the at-risk postoperative patient to prevent acute respiratory failure from developing, or therapeutically, i.e., to support the patient who has already developed postoperative respiratory failure. In addition, patients at risk of developing acute postoperative pulmonary oedema or postoperative airway obstruction also benefit from trials of NIV.

Each year, more than four million abdominal surgeries are performed in the US and over 250,000 in England. Acute respiratory failure, a common complication that can affect 30% to 50% of people after upper abdominal surgery, can lead to significant morbidity and mortality. Noninvasive ventilation has been associated with lower rates of tracheal intubation in adults with acute respiratory failure, thus reducing the incidence of complications and mortality [2].

Patients in the postoperative period of cardiac surgery have greater risk to develop pulmonary complications.

NIV in the postoperative period of cardiac surgery, compared to standard treatment with oxygen therapy and chest physiotherapy, significantly improved gas exchange without any significant difference in the rate of atelectasia, pneumonia, reintubation rate, and reduced the readmission rate in intensive care [3].

Regarding neurotrauma patients and in order to maintain respiration, optimize oxygenation and protect airway, patients with brain injury usually need Mechanical Ventilation (MV) in ICU. The vast majority of brain injury patients without respiratory problem, when the patient acute physiological disorder has improved, most patients can wean from MV as soon as possible. However, more than 20% of patients still need ventilator support after 21 days. These patients may need tracheotomy or noninvasive ventilation (NIV) for further treatment. Previous studies have shown that long-term mechanical ventilation were associated with a lot of pulmonary complications in patients with severe brain injury, such as ventilator-associated lung injury, pulmonary infection, diaphragm dysfunction, pulmonary embolism and so on, and increased the mortality of disease [4].

In conclusion, NIV has opened up new avenues in the management of respiratory failure in the postoperative patient. The data on the role of NIV for acute respiratory failure in the postoperative setting are selective, with clear evidence in certain patient groups who are undergoing specific surgical procedures.

THE ROLE OF POSTOPERATIVE NON INVASIVE VENTILATION

Postoperative hypoxemia and/or acute respiratory failure (ARF) mainly develop after abdominal and/or thoracic surgery [1]. Anesthesia, postoperative pain, and surgery will induce respiratory modifications: hypoxemia, decrease in pulmonary volume, and atelectasis [1] associated with a restrictive syndrome and a diaphragm dysfunction.

These modifications of the respiratory function occur early after surgery and are more often transient and could lead to ARF. The clinical result (severity of the ARF) is the product of perioperative-related ventilator impairment and severity of the preoperative pulmonary condition. Maintenance of adequate oxygenation in the postoperative period is of major importance, especially when pulmonary complications such as ARF occur. Although invasive endotracheal mechanical ventilation has remained the cornerstone of ventilatory strategy for many years for severe ARF, several studies have shown that mortality associated with pulmonary disease is largely related to complications of postoperative reintubation and mechanical ventilation. Therefore, major objectives are first to prevent the occurrence of postoperative complications and second to ensure oxygen administration and carbon dioxide removal while avoiding intubation if ARF occurs.

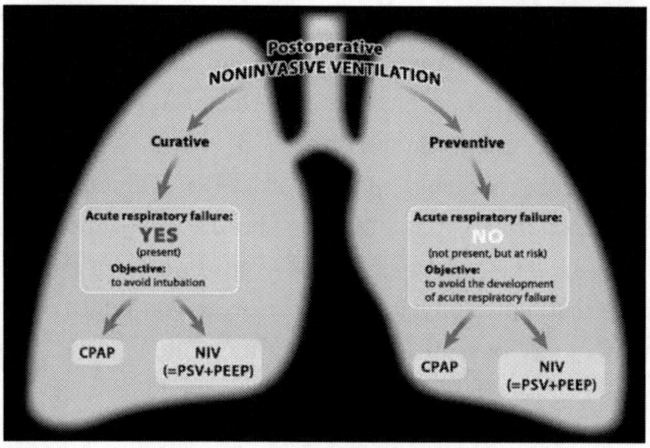

Figure 1. The two main strategy approaches for applying postoperative noninvasive ventilation (NIV). CPAP = continuous positive airway pressure; PSV = pressure support ventilation; PEEP = positive end expiratory pressure. From: *Postoperative Noninvasive Ventilation Anesthesiology*. 2010:112(2):453-461. doi:10.1097/ALN.0b013e3181c5e5f2.

Studies show that patient-related risk factors, such as chronic obstructive pulmonary disease, age older than 60 yr, American Society of Anesthesiologists class of II or higher, obesity, functional dependence, and congestive heart failure, increase the risk for postoperative pulmonary complications. Pulmonary conditions are a key problem for patients who require high-risk surgery for ventilatory function. Then postoperative NIV should be beneficial to these patients at high risk, especially after "aggressive" surgery.

Postoperative NIV improves gas exchange, decreases work of breathing, and reduces atelectasis.

Major changes in respiratory function occur in all patients after thoracic and abdominal surgery because of anesthetic and surgical consequences (more so as the site of the surgery approaches the diaphragm). Anesthetic decreases muscle tone that increases lung retractile forces and thus contributes to atelectasis development [2]. Surgery disrupts abdominal, thoracic, and diaphragmatic muscles forces, reduces phrenic output, and induces pain. Taken together, these changes alter the ventilation/perfusion ratio that leads to hypoxemia. These early and transitory modifications of respiratory function may lead to respiratory failure affecting the "pump" function (respiratory muscles) and the "exchange" function (lungs).

Clinical arguments in favor of postoperative NIV are the same as those for using NIV in postextubation period [5] as well as for the respiratory modifications caused by surgery and anesthesia. NIV should supply pump function and improves gas exchange. The main respiratory modifications are maximum in the first hours after surgery and generally regress after 1–2 weeks [1, 2]. The expected benefit of NIV would be to partially compensate for the affected respiratory function by reducing the work of breathing, by improving alveolar ventilation associated with increased gas exchange, reducing left ventricular afterload with increase of cardiac output, and by reducing atelectasis.

The underlying mechanism by which CPAP exerts its effects is to increase intrathoracic pressure. This way, CPAP prevents airway and alveolar collapse, prevents atelectasis, maintains functional residual capacity, and reduces left ventricular afterload with increase in cardiac output. Moreover, CPAP also permitted to decrease work of breathing by counterbalancing the inspiratory threshold load imposed by intrinsic PEEP in some patients (i.e., chronic obstructive pulmonary disease). Clinical improvements caused *via* an improved cardiac function are sometimes difficult to distinguish from the pulmonary effects of CPAP in postoperative period. PSV is a ventilatory mode in which the patient's spontaneous inspiratory effort triggers the ventilator to provide a variable flow of gas that increases until airway pressure reaches a selected level. Thus, during each spontaneous inspiration, the patient receives a pressure-supported breath.

Initially, the clinical experience reported in postsurgical patients was limited to the use of CPAP alone. Moreover, in these studies, 15 CPAP was used to prevent ARF after surgery (prophylactic use, i.e., immediately after extubation, not waiting for patients to develop respiratory distress) but not to treat ARF once it developed (curative use). 15 However, studies of ARF in the postoperative setting have shown favorable results for both NIV practice PSV + PEEP and CPAP.

NIV Application in Postoperative Period

Postoperative NIV can be proposed in two ways. The first is a preventive or "prophylactic" application to prevent postoperative ARF from developing in patients at risk (elderly, obese, chronic obstructive pulmonary disease, and heart disease) and the second consists of a "curative" application, once ARF occurs, to alleviate respiratory failure while avoiding tracheal intubation, a cause of increased morbidity.

Nevertheless, NIV (PSV+ PEEP or CPAP) should never be initiated in confused patients, those unable to cooperate, or with hemodynamic instability. Moreover, tracheal intubation should never be delayed if respiratory status worsened despite CPAP or PSV + PEEP ventilatory support.

How to Set NIV and Duration of Trial

NIV works best in patients relaxed and prepared. CPAP pressures of 7–10 cm H_2O are required to keep tracheal pressure positive during the entire respiratory cycle and to consistently improve gas exchange. These CPAP pressures are safe, and no adverse hemodynamic effects were observed.

In PSV + PEEP, patient comfort and interface acceptance may be gained by starting with PEEP alone and then slowly increasing the PSV level once the mask is applied

(Figure 3). We recommend starting with a PSV of 3–5 cmH_2O and increasing in increments of 2 cm H_2O to achieve a 6–10 ml/kg expiratory tidal volume, a decrease in the patient's respiratory rate, and a comfort improvement [5]. The PEEP is started at 3–5 cm H_2O and increased as needed to improve oxygenation without adverse hemodynamic effects up to 10 cm H_2O. The insufflation pressure (PSV + PEEP level) applied should be less than 25 cm H_2O. These setting recommendations are based solely on clinical experience without any formal data to support the superiority of one technique over another [6]. A surgical complication arises in nearly half the cases of ARF. The treatment is usually reintervention, management of ARF is only symptomatic, and there is no reason to use NIV to avoid intubation because the patient requires intubation for anesthesia.

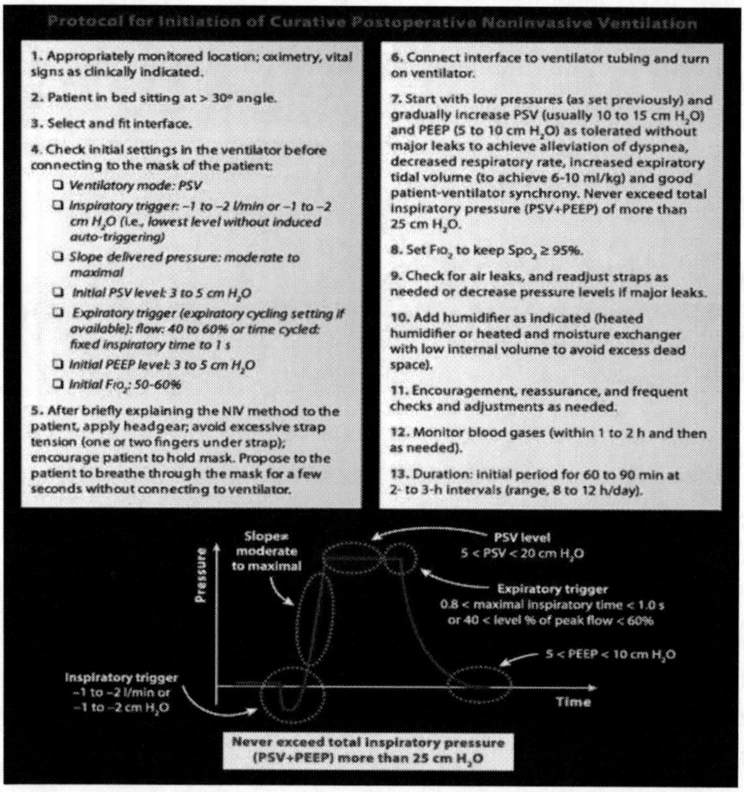

Figure 2. Protocol for initiation of curative postoperative noninvasive ventilation (NIV). PSV = pressure support ventilation; PEEP = positive end expiratory pressure. Fio^2= fraction of inspired oxygen; Spo^2= pulsated oximetry. From: *Postoperative Noninvasive Ventilation Anesthesiology*. 2010:112(2):453-461. doi:10.1097/ALN.0b013e3181c5e5f2.

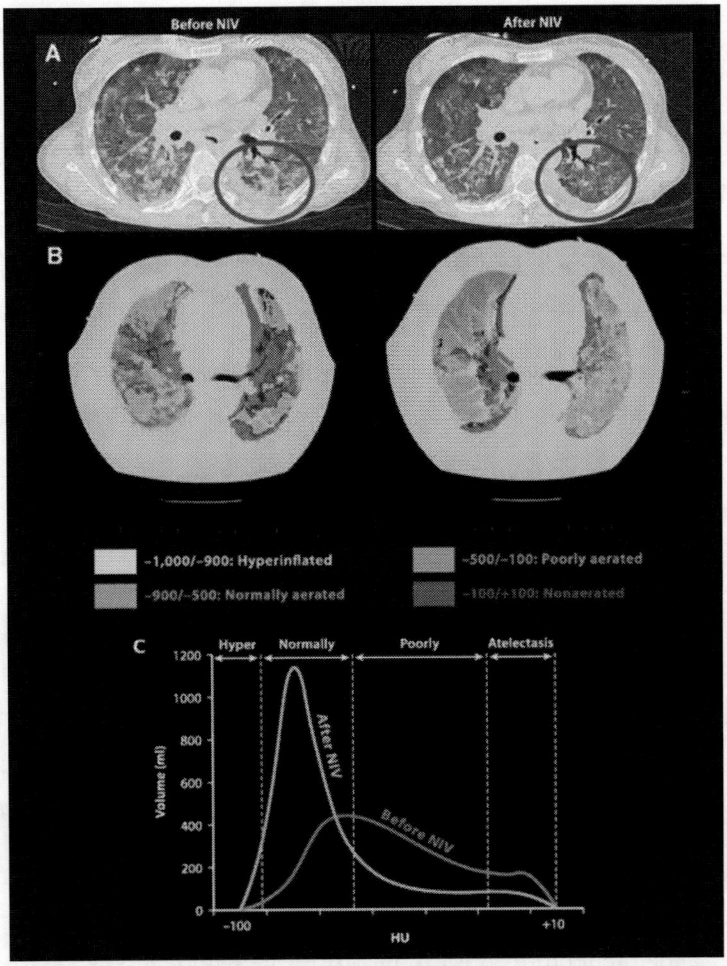

Figure 3. Effects of postoperative noninvasive ventilation (NIV) on computed tomography (CT) lung volumes in patients with acute respiratory failure after abdominal surgery. (A) Representative CT slices of the lung obtained before NIV in spontaneous breathing (left panel) and after 30 min of NIV (PSV 15 cm H^2O and PEEP 5 cm H^2O) (right panel). (B) A color encoding analysis is applied for both CT images obtained before (left panel) and after 30 min of NIV (right panel). Nonaerated voxels (CT attenuation between −100 and +100 Hounsfield Units [HU]) were colored in red, poorly aerated voxels (CT attenuation between −500 and −100 HU) in orange, and normally aerated voxels (CT attenuation between −500 and −900 HU) in green. Overinflated voxels (CT attenuations between −900 and −1,000 HU) were colored in yellow. NIV induced alveolar recruitment as shown by the decrease in poorly (orange) and nonaerated (red) lung regions and an increase in normally aerated lung parenchyma (green). (C) Volumetric quantification of lung aeration and collapse. Histograms show the normalized lung volume for HU ranging from −1,000 to 100. aeration categories (hyperinflated −1,000 and −900 HU, normally aerated −900 and −500, poorly aerated −500 and −100 HU, nonaerated or atelectasis −100 and +100 HU). The red curve was obtained before NIV and the yellow curve was obtained after NIV. Note that the curve obtained after NIV showed a decrease in poorly and nonaerated lung regions and an increase in normally aerated lung parenchyma. From: *Postoperative Noninvasive Ventilation Anesthesiology*. 2010:112(2):453-461. doi:10.1097/ALN.0b013e3181c5e5f2.

Evidence to guide duration of NIV trial is lacking; hence, the recommendations are based largely on practitioner experience. In postoperative area, we recommended "sequential" use wherein periods of use alternate with lengthy ventilatorfree periods, and total daily use ranges between 3 and 12 h depending on the type of application (curative or prophylactic use).

An interface that fits properly is crucial in minimizing air leaks and maximizing NIV efficiency. Recommendations for evaluating different sizes and types of masks at the bedside are important to select the best fit for each patient. The first few minutes should be used to fit the mask and familiarize the patient with the equipment. To date, there is no evidence to support the use of particular patient interface devices in surgical context. Then, practitioners should try different mask sizes and types in an effort to enhance patient comfort.

NEUROTRAUMA/NEUROSURGERY

NIV has become a common alternative to invasive ventilation at present, several studies have shown that NIV weaning strategy was superior to invasive weaning strategy in hypercapnic respiratory failure patients, and it could significantly reduce the re-intubation rate, the incidence of ventilator associated pneumonia (VAP), duration of mechanical ventilation, and the ICU and hospital length of stay [7]. But there were few studies and literatures demonstrated the benefits of NIV in acute hypoxemic respiratory failure, especially in the brain injury patients. Lack of research has caused considerable confusion to clinical workers: could NIV improve the prognosis of patients who accepted brain injury surgery?

In the observational cohort study of Mailing Dong et al. [4], patients were divided into NIV group and tracheotomy group according to whether NIV or tracheotomy was performed after invasive mechanical ventilation during ICU stay.

The incidence of postoperative pulmonary infection in NIV group was lower than tracheotomy group (54.5% vs.84.1%, $P < 0.05$), and the duration of invasive mechanical ventilation was shorter than tracheotomy group ($P < 0.05$). In addition, the length of ICU and hospital stay in the NIV group were also shorter than tracheotomy group. NIV group showed a higher GCS score at discharge ICU and GCS score difference between admission and discharge ICU. This suggested that NIV may accelerate the recovery of consciousness in brain injury surgery patients.

When patients do not meet the MV withdrawal criteria, some medical workers may choose tracheotomy and some may choose early NIV intervention. There still are some controversies about the possible benefits of NIV compared with tracheotomy. The strength of mechanical ventilation support is generally low in patients with brain injury, however, due to disturbance of consciousness or damage of brain stem, airway protective reflexes such as cough and swallow weakened or disappeared, and artificial airway continue to be needed to maintain airway unobstructed [8]. But for patients without other mechanical ventilation indications, people who need respiratory support and artificial airway may be different. For patients who only need respiratory support, the complications caused by artificial airway cannot be ignored [9]. Early and timely application of NIV can reduce complications of artificial airway, avoid delayed extubation and related complications, and shorten length of ICU and hospital stay, leading to improve the prognosis of patients. Coplin et al. found that 48% (29/60) of patients with GCS score < 8 had delayed extubation compared with 10.5% (8/76) of patients with GCS > 8 ($P < 0.05$) [10]. Particularly interesting was the fact that there was almost no difference in consciousness on the day when the extubation criteria were met and the day of extubation in the delayed extubation patients. At the same time, the study also found that patients with swallow reflex and cough reflex disappeared or weakened could also extubated successfully. These findings challenge the conventional indicators of airway protection (such as swallow reflex, cough reflex, GCS score).

Compared with patients underwent tracheotomy, the patients who accepted NIV has a lower incidence of postoperative pulmonary infection, shorter duration of invasive mechanical ventilation, higher GCS score at discharge ICU, as well as significant GCS score difference between ICU admission and discharge. Researches about the impact of noninvasive ventilation and tracheotomy on the prognosis of neurosurgery patients are necessary in the future. Furthermore, the effect of NIV in those patients still requires more efforts.

THORACIC/CARDIAC SURGERY

Cardiac Surgery

The restrictive syndrome consecutive to cardiac surgery is generally less severe than that observed after thoracic or abdominal surgery. However, the incidence of diaphragm dysfunction is higher [11]. Early studies mainly compared CPAP with standard treatment (oxygen, physiotherapy). Most of these studies reported improved oxygenation and ventilation parameters. None of these studies found any reduction in the incidence of atelectasis in the groups treated by NIV, in fact mostly CPAP, except for Jousela et al. Gust et al. obtained a reduction in extravascular lung water when NIV was applied with CPAP alone or with PSV (PSV + PEEP). Matte et al. in a study including 96 patients, evaluated "preventive" NIV in the first 2 days after surgery. Various strategies were compared in three randomized groups. The first group received 1 h of NIV with two pressure levels every 3 h with an average assistance level of 12 cm H2O of PSV and 5 cm H_2O of PEEP. The second group received a 1-h session of CPAP at 5 cm H_2O every 3 h, and a third group had 20 min of incentive spirometry every 2 h. Using NIV whether at one or two pressure levels permitted improved oxygenation and a lower reduction of lung volumes. However, atelectasis incidence was similar (12–15%) in all three groups.

Pasquina et al. compared the effect of systematic application of a 30-min trial of 5 cm H_2O CPAP with NIV (PSV 10 and PEEP 5) in two groups of 75 patients. The NIV group had improved radiologic scores (meaning less marked atelectasis) on standard chest radiograph. There was no significant difference in oxygenation parameters. Zarbock et al. reported in a prospective randomized study included 500 patients scheduled for elective cardiac surgery, the interest of prophylactic nasal CPAP of 10 cm H_2O (study) for at least 6 h/day after surgery in comparison with standard treatment (control) including 10 min of intermittent nasal CPAP at 10 cm H_2O every 4 h. In the study group, CPAP improved arterial oxygenation, reduced the incidence of pulmonary complications including pneumonia and reintubation rate, and reduced readmission rate to ICU or intermediate care unit.

However, according to the systematic review and meta-analysis of Suzimara Monteiro Pieczkoski et al. [11], no difference between the use of prophylactic NIV and conventional physiotherapy or oxygen therapy could be found in patients during the postoperative period of cardiac surgery, in relation to mortality rate and pulmonary complications such as atelectasis, pneumonia, reintubation rate, time spent in the ICU, length of hospital stay and mechanical ventilation time, with an improvement in oxygenation. Therefore, due to the low methodological rigor of the included articles and small sample size, new RCTs should be carried out to corroborate this information.

There have been only a few studies reporting the use of NIV for treatment of respiratory failure following cardiac surgeries. Olper et al. studied 85 patients who received NIV for treatment of respiratory failure following cardiac surgery and reported that NIV was a safe and feasible solution for postoperative acute respiratory failure, even when applied after discharge from the ICU.

Thoracic Surgery

Preventive NIV

In a physiologic study, Aguilo et al. studied the effects of a 1-h NIV trial after pulmonary resection in 10 patients. NIV was applied without any complications due to the technique and allowed improved oxygenation without increasing leaks around thoracic drains in the study group compared with a control group who did not receive NIV [25]. Perrin et al. reported in a prospective randomized clinical trial the benefits of NIV administered pre- and postoperatively. Patients were required to follow standard treatment without or with NIV during 7 days at home before surgery and during 3 days postoperatively. In this study, 2 h after surgery, oxygenation and lung volumes values were significantly better in the NIV group. On days 1, 2, and 3, oxygenation was significantly improved in the NIV group. The hospital stay was significantly longer in the control group than in the NIV group. This first prospective randomized study showed that prophylactic use of NIV in a pre- and postoperative manner significantly reduces pulmonary dysfunction after lung resection.

Curative NIV

In an observational study, Rocco et al. described their experience of NIV after lung transplant in 21 patients who developed ARF. Tolerance of NIV was good for all patients. Eighteen of the 21 patients treated were able to avoid reintubation. In a prospective randomized study including 24 patients in each group, Auriant et al. showed the efficiency of NIV in ARF after lung resection. In this trial, NIV was delivered by a nasal mask using a single circuit ventilator and compared with standard treatment (oxygen, physiotherapy, bronchodilators), reducing the need for invasive mechanical ventilation (21% *vs.* 50%) and mortality (13% *vs.* 38%). Lefebvre et al. confirmed in an observational prospective survey the feasibility and efficacy of early NIV in ARF after lung resection. During a 4-yr period, among 690 patients at risk of severe complications after lung resection, 16% experienced ARF, which was initially managed by NIV. The overall success rate of NIV was 85% [12].

ABDOMINAL SURGERY / GASTRIC BYPASS

Preventive NIV

Hypoxemia complicates the recovery of 30–50% of patients after abdominal surgery, even among those undergoing uneventful procedures. Stock et al. showed that applying a CPAP in patients having cholecystectomy by laparotomy permitted a significant improvement in number of atelectasis compared with treatment by incentive spirometry. After bariatric surgery (gastroplasty) for morbid obesity, Joris et al. demonstrated a significant reduction of the restrictive syndrome and significant improvement in oxygenation evaluated by oximetry (SpO_2) with NIV applied for two-thirds of the first postoperative 24 h. Compared with the control group, forced vital capacity was improved significantly only with a moderately high PSV level of 12 cmH_2O, because another group treated with a PSV level of 8 cmH_2O did not have a significant improvement of functional residual capacity. This finding remains important today, given the sharp increase in the rate of obesity surgery nationwide. Kindgen-Milles et al. studied the effect of a systematic CPAP of 10 $cmH_2O$for 12–24 h a day after thoracoabdominal surgery (aneurysm of thoracoabdominal aorta cure). The group of patients receiving CPAP had significantly improved oxygenation and a shorter ICU and hospital stay than those in the control group. A large Italian study was stopped early because of improvements in intubation related to CPAP therapy in hypoxemic patients after abdominal surgery. This randomized study included 209 patients in two groups: one group received CPAP and a control group receiving oxygen *via* a facial mask. The patients receiving CPAP had significantly lower intubation, pneumonia, and sepsis rates than the control group.

Curative NIV

Patients suffering from postoperative ARF have been included among other types of patients in studies evaluating NIV to treat ARF of multiple causes. In these studies, no comparison has been made between patients presenting with ARF of medical causes and those with postoperative ARF, probably because of the heterogeneity and small numbers of patients included. Varon et al. reported the feasibility of NIV in postoperative ARF in cancer patients (25 digestive, 15 urogenital, and 6 lung). Intubation was avoided in 70% of included patients in this study. Kindgen-Milles et al. in a noncontrolled prospective study, showed that CPAP rapidly improved oxygenation and avoided intubation in 18 of 20 patients treated after abdominal and/or thoracic surgery. Jaber et al. reported in an observational study their experience over a 2-yr period using NIV in 72 patients with severe ARF after digestive surgery.

In this prospective trial, intubation was avoided in 66% of patients. This study demonstrated feasibility, good tolerance, and safety of NIV for the treatment of ARF after digestive surgery. More severe initial hypoxemia and lower improvement of $PaCO_2$ after NIV were predictive of NIV failure. The results obtained in the study by Jaber et al. was confirmed by a recent study that included 72 patients who developed ARF after abdominal surgery and 42 patients avoided intubation (58%). Conti et al. in a match-controlled study compared the efficacy of NIV delivered by a helmet interface and a facial mask in patients with ARF after abdominal surgery. These authors reported an NIV success rate of 80% in the helmet group and of 52% in the facial mask group. Antonelli et al. showed in a controlled randomized trial that in organ transplant recipients with hypoxemic ARF, NIV reduced the rate of intubation, the incidence of fatal complications, and ICU mortality compared with the provision of supplemental oxygenation alone. More recently, Michelet et al. compared in a case-control study the efficacy of NIV with conventional treatment in 36 patients who developed postoperative ARF after planned esophagectomy.

They showed that the use of NIV was associated with a lower intubation rate, frequency of acute respiratory distress syndrome, anastomotic leakage, and a reduction in ICU length of stay [12].

According to Debora A S Faria et al. compared to oxygen therapy, CPAP or bilevel NPPV may reduce the rate of tracheal intubation (risk ratio (RR) 0.25; 95% confidence interval (CI) 0.08 to 0.83; low quality evidence) with a number needed to treat for an additional beneficial outcome of 11. This systematic review included two trials involving 269 participants; there was very low quality evidence that the intervention may also reduce ICU length of stay, it found no differences for mortality (low quality evidence) and hospital length of stay [2].

Anastomotic Leak

There was insufficient evidence to be certain that CPAP or NPPV had an effect on anastomotic leakage, according to Debora A S Faria [2] et al. systematic review.

In the meta-analysis of Michele Carron et al. [13], regarding perioperative noninvasive ventilation in obese patients, NIV-related anastomotic leakage was not reported.

P. Michelet et al. [14] carried out a case–control study to compare the efficacy of non-invasive positive pressure ventilation (NPPV) with conventional treatment in patients who develop postoperative acute respiratory failure (ARF) after oesophagectomy. Anastomotic leakage was less common in patients receiving NPPV (two versus ten; P = 0,027). These patients also showed a greater improvement in gas exchange in the first 3 days after onset of ARF (P = 0,013). For that reason, they concluded that the use of NPPV for the treatment of postoperative ARF may decrease the incidence of endotracheal intubation and related complications, without increasing the risk of anastomotic leakage after oesophagectomy.

The absence of gastric distension might be explained by the limitation of inspiratory pressure to below 25 cmH_2O, a level at which distension is unlikely. Moreover, nasogastric drainage was employed throughout the postoperative period. These results seem to indicate that CPAP or NPPV in patients with postoperative hypoxaemia favours the protective effect of improvement of oxygenation over a hypothetical anastomotic leakage risk.

References

[1] Mathai AS. Non-invasive ventilation in the postoperative period: Is there a role? *Indian J Anaesth*. 2011;55(4):325-333. doi:10.4103/0019-5049.84829.

[2] Faria DA, da Silva EM, Atallah ÁN, Vital FM. Noninvasive positive pressure ventilation for acute respiratory failure following upper abdominal surgery. *Cochrane Database Syst Rev*. 2015 Oct 5;(10):CD009134. doi: 10.1002/14651858.CD009134.pub2. PMID: 26436599.

[3] Pieczkoski, Suzimara Monteiro, Margarites, Ane Glauce Freitas, & Sbruzzi, Graciele. (2017). Noninvasive Ventilation during Immediate Postoperative Period in Cardiac Surgery Patients: Systematic Review and Meta-Analysis. *Brazilian Journal of Cardiovascular Surgery*, *32*(4), 301-311.

[4] Dong, M., Zhou, Y., Yang, J. et al. Compare the effect of noninvasive ventilation and tracheotomy in critically ill mechanically ventilated neurosurgical patients: a retrospective observe cohort study. *BMC Neurol* 19, 79 (2019). https://doi.org/10.1186/s12883-019-1297-3.

[5] Jaber S, Delay J, Sebbane M, Chanques G, Jacquet E, Souche B, Perrigault P, Eledjam J: Outcomes of patients with acute respiratory failure after abdominal surgery treated with noninvasive positive-pressure ventilation. *Chest* 2005; 128:2688 –95.

[6] International consensus conferences in intensive care medicine. Noninvasive positive pressure ventilation in acute respiratory failure. *Am J Respir Crit Care Med* 2001; 163: 283–9.

[7] Ferrer M, Sellares J, Valencia M, Carrillo A, Gonzalez G, Badia JR, et al. Non-invasive ventilation after extubation in hypercapnic patients with chronic respiratory disorders: randomised controlled trial. *Lancet* (London, England). 2009;374(9695):1082–8.

[8] Lazaridis C, DeSantis SM, McLawhorn M, Krishna V. Liberation of neurosurgical patients from mechanical ventilation and tracheostomy in neurocritical care. *J Crit Care*. 2012;27(4):417.e1–8.

[9] Girou E, Schortgen F, Delclaux C, Brun-Buisson C, Blot F, Lefort Y, et al. Association of noninvasive ventilation with nosocomial infections and survival in critically ill patients. *Jama*. 2000;284(18):2361–7.

[10] Coplin WM, Pierson DJ, Cooley KD, Newell DW, Rubenfeld GD. Implications of extubation delay in brain-injured patients meeting standard weaning criteria. *Am J Respir Crit Care Med*. 2000;161(5):1530–6.

[11] Pieczkoski, Suzimara Monteiro, Margarites, Ane Glauce Freitas, & Sbruzzi, Graciele. (2017). Noninvasive Ventilation During Immediate Postoperative Period in Cardiac Surgery Patients: Systematic Review and Meta-Analysis. *Brazilian Journal of Cardiovascular Surgery*, 32 (4), 301-311. https://doi.org/10.21470/1678-9741-2017-0032.

[12] Jaber S, Chanques G, Jung B. Postoperative noninvasive ventilation. *Anesthesiology*. 2010 Feb;112(2):453-61. doi: 10.1097/ALN.0b013e3181c5e5f2. PMID: 20068454.

[13] Carron M, Zarantonello F, Tellaroli P, Ori C. Perioperative noninvasive ventilation in obese patients: a qualitative review and meta-analysis. *Surg Obes Relat Dis.* 2016 Mar-Apr;12(3):681-691. doi: 10.1016/j.soard.2015.12.013. Epub 2015 Dec 10. PMID: 26948450.

[14] Michelet P, D'Journo XB, Seinaye F, Forel JM, Papazian L, Thomas P. Non-invasive ventilation for treatment of postoperative respiratory failure after oesophagectomy. *Br J Surg*. 2009 Jan;96(1):54-60. doi: 10.1002/bjs.6307. PMID: 19108006.

In: Non-Invasive Mechanical Ventilation Complications ISBN: 978-1-53619-515-6
Editor: Antonio M. Esquinas

Chapter 30

DELIRIUM - SEDATION AS COMPLICATIONS OF NON-INVASIVE VENTILATION

Marra A.*[1,*]*, MD, PhD, Vargas M.*[1]*, MD and Servillo G.*[1]*, MD

[1]Department of Neurosciences,
Reproductive and Odontostomatological Sciences,
University of Naples "Federico II",
Naples, Italy

ABSTRACT

Non-invasive ventilation is currently one of the most commonly used support methods in hypoxaemic and hypercapnic acute respiratory failure. Data suggests that the prevalence of delirium it is higher in the subset of patients requiring NIV for acute respiratory failure than in a population of general medical inpatients. The development of agitation and the deterioration of mental status, such as in delirious patients, decreases the ability to cooperate and tolerate NIV, potentially increasing the risks for NIV failure and subsequent intubation.

Agitation, intolerance, and patient–ventilator asynchrony are factors implicated in NIV failure for which judicious sedation is recommended. Sedation during NIV should be performed with no/minimal respiratory depression and no/minimal impairment of the upper airway.

Keywords: sedation, delirium, agitation, respiratory failure, non-invasive ventilation

---

* Corresponding Author's E-mail: dottmarraannachiara@gmail.com.

Non-invasive ventilation (NIV) is currently one of the most commonly used support methods in hypoxaemic and hypercapnic acute respiratory failure (ARF). With advancing technology and increasing experience, indications for NIV are getting broader and more severe patients are treated with NIV. Depending on disease type and clinical status, NIV can be applied both in the general ward and in high-dependency/intensive care unit settings with different environmental opportunities.

Delirium constitutes one of the most frequent complications in hospitalized patients. Delirium is defined in the American Psychiatric Association's (APA) as a disturbance of consciousness and cognition that develops over a short period of time (hours to days) and fluctuates over time [1]. Delirium can be categorized into subtypes according to psychomotor behavior. Hyperactive delirium (CAM positive, RASS positive range) is associated with a better overall prognosis and it is characterized by agitation, restlessness, and emotional lability [2]. Hypoactive delirium (CAM positive, RASS negative range), which is very common and often more deleterious in the long term, is characterized by decreased responsiveness, withdrawal, and apathy and remains unrecognized in 66 to 84% of hospitalized patients [3]. Despite evidence shows that delirium is a strong predictor of increased length of mechanical ventilation, longer ICU stays, increased cost, long-term cognitive impairment, and mortality [4-6] delirium is still underdiagnosed [7, 8]. Several methods have been developed and validated to diagnose delirium in ICU patients but the Intensive Care Delirium Screening Checklist (ICDSC, Figure 1A) and the Confusion Assessment Method for the Intensive Care Unit (CAM-ICU, Figure 1B) are the most frequently employed tools for this purpose. The ICDSC checklist is an eight-item screening tool (one point for each item) that is based on DSM criteria and applied to data that can be collected through medical records or to information obtained from the multidisciplinary team.

The CAM-ICU is composed by four features 1) acute onset of mental status changes or fluctuating course; 2) inattention; 3) disorganized thinking; and 4) altered level of consciousness. The patient is considered CAM positive and, so delirious, if he/she manifests both features 1 and 2, plus either feature 3 or 4 [9].

Data suggests that the prevalence of delirium seems to be higher in the subset of patients requiring NIV for acute respiratory failure (37%) than in a population of general medical inpatients (10 – 31%) in the published literature [10]. The development of agitation and the deterioration of mental status, such as in delirious patients, decreases the ability to cooperate and tolerate NIV, potentially increasing the risks for NIV failure and subsequent intubation. The risk ratio of NIV failure in delirious patients was 2.12 as compared to that of nondelirious patients [10]. Elderly patients are particularly at risk of developing delirium and therefore routine screening for delirium would be beneficial, in addition to severity illness score. Numerous risk factors for delirium have been identified, including preexisting cognitive impairment, advanced age, use of psychoactive drugs, mechanical ventilation, untreated pain, and a variety of medical conditions such as heart failure, prolonged immobilization, abnormal blood pressure, anemia, sleep deprivation, and sepsi [3, 11]. Many studies have reported that disease severity, low level of consciousness, increased respiratory rate and decreased oxygenation were associated with NIV failure [12]. As poor prognosis in delirium patients, prevention of delirium was needed. Pain relief, early mobilization, improvement of sleep quality and minimized noise were the promising methods to reduce delirium in NIV patients.

Intensive Care Delirium Screening Checklist Worksheet (ICDSC)	No 0	Yes 1
1. Altered Level of Consciousness		
Deep sedation/coma over entire shift [SAS= 1, 2; RASS = -4,-5] = Not assessable Agitation [SAS = 5, 6, or 7; RASS= 1-4] at any point = 1 point Normal wakefulness [SAS = 4; RASS = 0] over the entire shift = 0 points Light sedation [SAS = 3; RASS= -1, -2, -3]: = 1 point (if no recent sedatives) = 0 points (if recent sedatives		
2. Inattention		
Difficulty following instructions or conversation, patient easily distracted by external stimuli . Will not reliably squeeze hands to spoken letter A: SAVEA HAART		
3. Disorientation		
In addition to name, place, and date, does the patient recognize ICU caregivers? Does patient know what kind of place they are in?		
4. Hallucination, delusion, or psychosis		
Ask the patient if they are having hallucinations or delusions. (e.g. trying to catch an object that isn't there). Are they afraid of the people or things around them?		
5. Psychomotor agitation or retardation		
Either: a) Hyperactivity requiring the use of sedative drugs or restraints in order to control potentially dangerous behavior (e.g. pulling IV lines out or hitting staff) OR b) Hypoactive or clinically noticeable psychomotor slowing or retardation		
6. Inappropriate speech or mood		
Patient displays: inappropriate emotion; disorganized or incoherent speech; sexual or inappropriate interactions; is either apathetic or overly demandi		
7. Sleep-wake cycle disturbance		
Either: frequent awakening/< 4 hours sleep at night OR sleeping during much of the day		
8. Symptom Fluctuation		
Fluctuation of any of the above symptoms over a 24 hr period.		
Total shift score (0-8)		

Normal 0; Delirium4-8: Subsyndromal Delirium 1-3

Score your patient over the entire shift. Components don't all need to be present at the same time. Components 1 through 4 cannot be completed when the patient is deeply sedated or comatose (ie. SAS = 1 or 2; RASS = -4 or -5); Components 5 through 8 are based on observations throughout the entire shift. Information from the prior 24 hrs should be obtained for components 7 and 8.

Adapted from: Bergeron et al. Intens Care Med 2001;27:859-64; Ouimet et al. Intens Care Med 2007;33:1007-13.

(A)

Figure 1. (Continued)

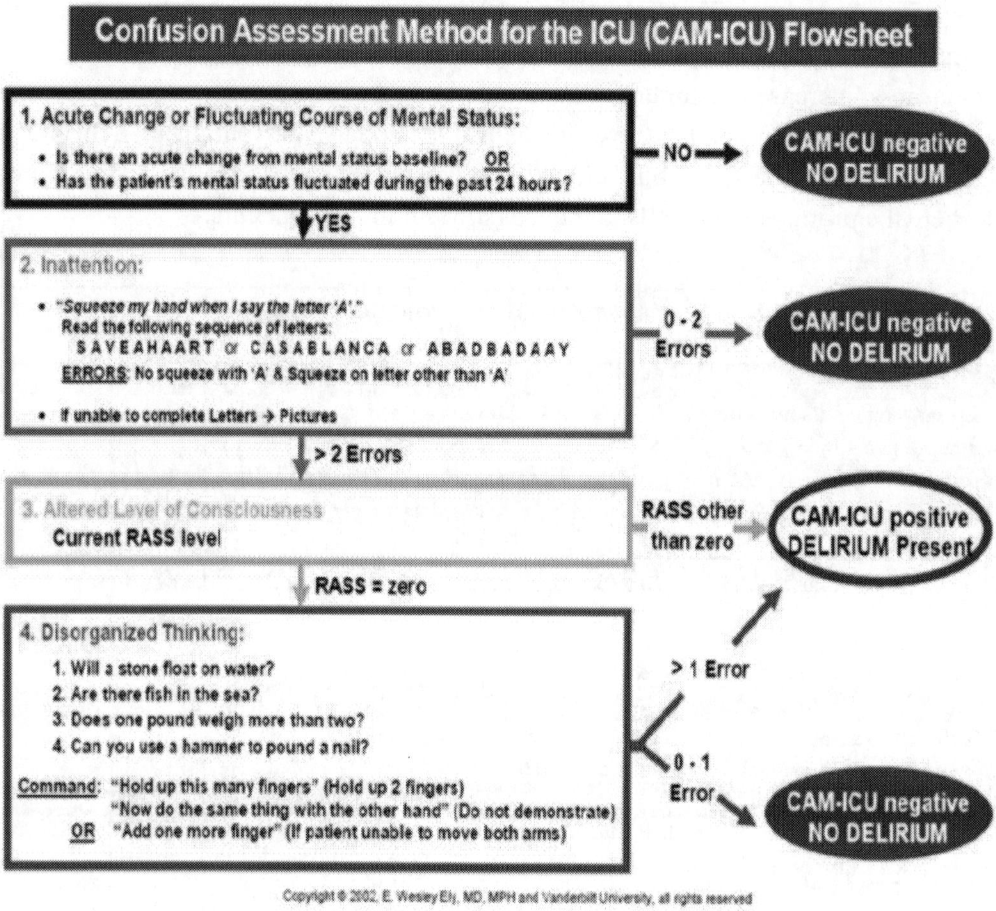

(B)

Figure 1. (A) Intensive Care Delirium Screening checklist (ICDSC). (B) Confusion Assessment Method for the ICU (CAM-ICU).

The use of sedation in patients receiving respiratory support from NIV is an area of critical and intensive care medicine where there are limited, if any, robust data to guide the development of best practice and where local custom appears to exert a strong influence on patterns of care. Agitation, intolerance, and patient–ventilator asynchrony are factors implicated in NIV failure for which judicious sedation is recommended. Any decision to start sedation must be taken as the last stage in a careful evaluation of the causes of discomfort [13] (Figure 2). The goals of sedation for a cooperative patient in the ICU are to provide analgesia and comfort, preserve day/night cycles (including natural sleep) and avoid nuisances such as ambient light and noise. Additional goals include haemodynamic stability, preservation of metabolic homeostasis, muscular relaxation, preservation of diaphragmatic function and attenuation of the stress/immune response, as well as considerations such as programmed withdrawal from sedation: they should be no different during NIV [13].

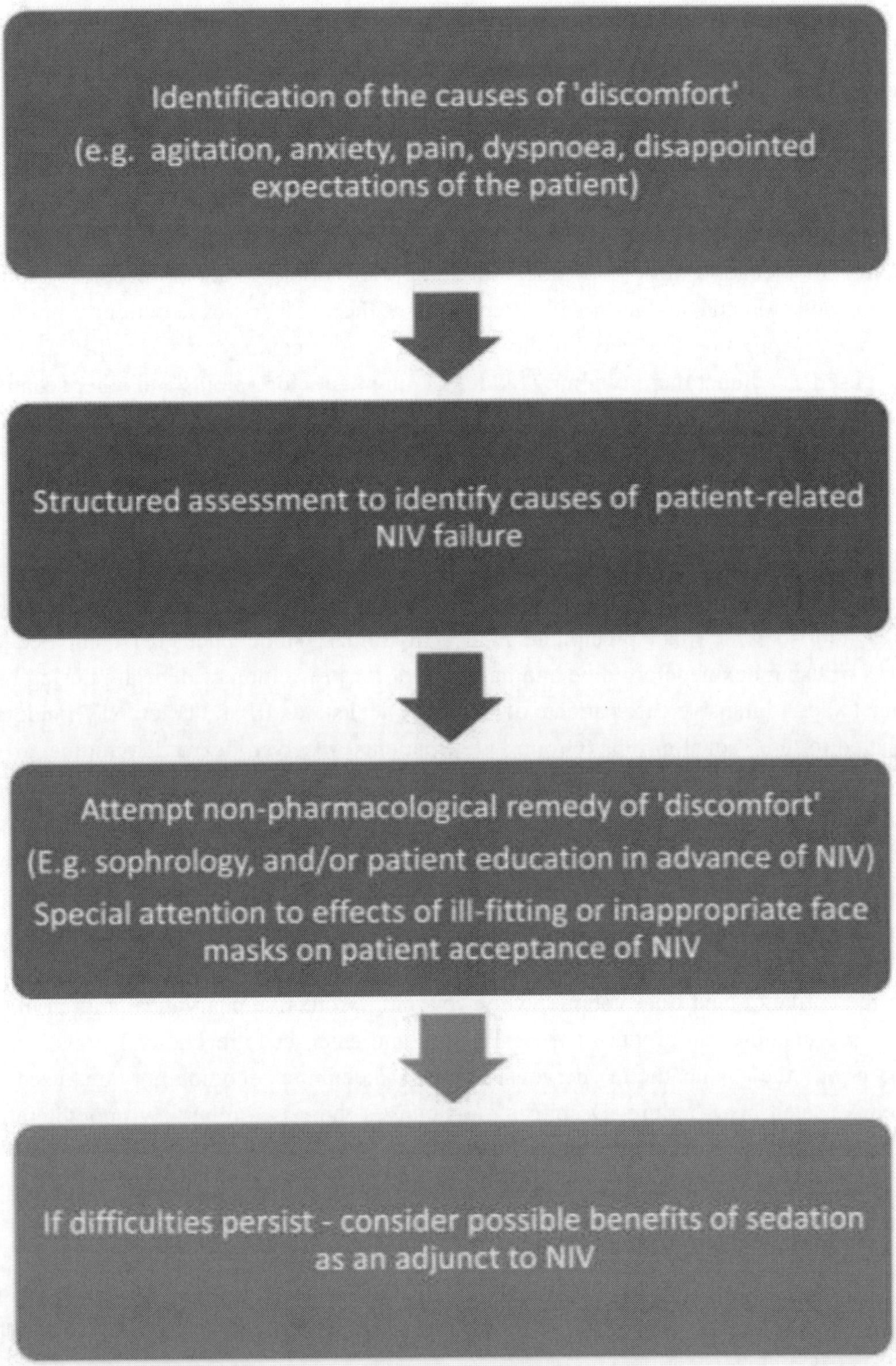

Figure 2. Clinical reasoning pathway for the use of sedation in NIV (Longrois et al. *Multidisciplinary Respiratory Medicine*, 2014 Nov. 4; 9(1):56 [13]).

In addition, sedation during NIV should be performed with no/minimal respiratory depression and no/minimal impairment of the upper airway [13]. Benzodiazepines and opioids have effects on airways patency and respiratory drive the timing. Moreover, sometimes could also be difficult to titrate their pharmacologic effects because they may accumulate with repeated dosing. Benzodiazepines may also be associated with a greater risk of delirium and cognitive impairment [14]. Propofol has also been shown to increase the collapsibility of the upper airway in a dose/concentration dependent manner [13]. Among the sedative drugs, dexmedetomidine, an alpha 2 adrenoreceptor agonist, provides sedation and analgesia with attenuation of the stress response with no significant respiratory depression and has no direct effects on the patency of the upper airways. When used as adjunct therapy it may reduce requirements for opioids and other sedatives and so reduce the likelihood of opioid-induced compromise of the upper airways. Haloperidol is a D2 receptors antagonist. Blockade of D2 receptors may result in improvement of hallucination and delusions. The use of haloperidol can also reduce the need for sedative and analgesic drugs in ventilated patients. Haloperidol has a number of side effects, including extrapyramidal manifestations and rarely neuroleptic malignant syndrome but the most dangerous adverse effect is prolongation of the corrected QT (QTc) interval which can precipitate fatal arrhythmias. Abdelgalel [15] compared the effects of using dexmedetomidine and haloperidol for prevention of delirium during NIV in ninety adult intensive care patients of ASA physical status III and IV on NIV randomly allocated to three equal groups (Group D (30 patients) received dexmedetomidine, group H (30 patients) received haloperidol, and group P (30 patients) received normal saline infusion). They showed that dexmedetomidine was more effective than haloperidol for prevention of delirium during NIV with lower incidence of endotracheal intubation and shorter ICU and hospital stay [15]. Ketamine does not cause respiratory depression at doses given for analgesia or procedural sedation. Furthermore, it decreases airway resistance, improves dynamic compliance and preserves functional residual capacity, minute ventilation and tidal volume, while retaining protective pharyngeal and laryngeal reflexes. Ketamine can produce hypersalivation and emergence reactions. Because of its effects on the sympathetic nervous system, ketamine should not be used in decompensated heart failure. Despite its advantages there is a relatively poor literature concerning the use of ketamine during NIV.

No single sedative agent is currently available that fulfils the criteria for an ideal agent and here are no robust data to favor any one drug, class of drugs or protocol over all others.

Sleep disruption was identified as a factor in late NIV failure. In mechanically ventilated patients, ventilator asynchrony may adversely affect sleep and there is evidence that in NIV patients, sleep is associated with more asynchrony and blood-oxygen desaturations than the awake state [16]. Environmental factors, mechanical ventilation, critical illness itself, and medication play an important role in sleep disruption in critically ill patients. Multiple studies indicated that impaired secretion of melatonin was observed in critically ill patients, which may be associated with the development of sleep deprivation and delirium.

The subject of sleep disruption in ICU patients and its relation with delirium has attracted much research in recent years Although the relationship between sleep disturbance and delirium has not been well established, the literature suggests that both phenomena share similarity of mechanisms, such as neurohormonal changes, imbalances in neurotransmitters, and similar sites of action in the central nervous system. Clinical characteristics associated with delirium, such as inattention, fluctuating mental status and cognitive dysfunction may also be present in patients with disrupted sleep. Moreover, the risk factors for the development of sleep deprivation in critically ill overlap with those of delirium. The administration and the sudden discontinuation of many medications can influence the wake–sleep-regulatory system by a direct effect on neurotransmitter and hormone activity. Benzodiazepines and opioids can reduce both SWS and REM sleep via GABA type A and opioid □ receptor stimulation, respectively. Additionally, opioids can cause delirium by decreasing acetylcholine and increasing dopamine and glutamate activity. Propofol suppresses the REM sleep stage and further worsens the poor sleep quality of these patients, and might be associated with short-term (delirium) and long-term (post-traumatic stress disorder, PTSD) effects in critically ill patients.

Pharmacological treatment of sleep disturbances of patients in critical care units is problematic, both in terms of drug efficacy and adverse effects, specially upon the architecture of normal sleep [17]. The efficacy of exogenous melatonin to improve sleep in critically ill patients has been studied in a variety of doses and preparations. Selective melatonin receptor agonists have been used for the treatment of insomnia and circadian rhythm. Currently, 2 agents, Ramelteon and Tasimelteon, are available in the United States and a third agent, Agomelatine has been used in Europe for the treatment of major depressive episodes due to its additional serotonin 5HT-2C antagonist properties. Ramelteon is the only agent that has been studied in the ICU setting, and it appears to enhance sleep by shortening sleep latency and extending the total duration of sleep through diminishing arousal signals generated by the suprachiasmatic nucleus (SCN). Ramelteon has been shown to have no abuse potential, less sedating effects, and minimal cognitive impairment effects.

There is limited published data available regarding delirium in NIV. From this limited data, delirium is associated with NIV failure and the risk of this is 112% more than that in nondelirious patients [10]. Historically, delirium is understudied, underreported, and underappreciated despite the profound impact on patients [10]. Without a diagnosis of delirium, predisposing risk factors cannot be modified as recommended.

Delirium can be managed by pharmacological and nonpharmacological methods and this may improve NIV success.

Adequate sedation, can not rescue a poorly configured or inappropriate NIV but can improve patient comfort in specific situations and help in avoid NIV failure.

REFERENCES

[1] APA. *Diagnostic and Statistical Manual of Mental Disorders* (5th Ed.); 2013.

[2] Pun, B. T., Ely, E. W. The Importance of Diagnosing and Managing ICU Delirium. *Chest,* 2007. https://doi.org/10.1378/chest.06-1795.

[3] Marcantonio, E. R., Goldman, L., Mangione, C. M., Ludwig, L. E., Muraca, B., Haslauer, C. M., Donaldson, M. C., Whittemore, A. D., Sugarbaker, D. J., Poss, R., Haas, S., Cook, E. F., Orav, E. J., Lee, T. H. A Clinical Prediction Rule for Delirium After Elective Noncardiac Surgery. *JAMA, J. Am. Med. Assoc.,* 1994. https://doi.org/10.1001/jama.1994.03510260066030.

[4] Ely, E. W., Baker, A. M., Dunagan, D. P., Burke, H. L., Smith, A. C., Kelly, P. T., Johnson, M. M., Browder, R. W., Bowton, D. L., Haponik, E. F. Effect on the Duration of Mechanical Ventilation of Identifying Patients Capable of Breathing Spontaneously. *N. Engl. J. Med.,* 1996. https://doi.org/10.1056/ NEJM199612 193352502.

[5] Ely, E. W., Shintani, A., Truman, B., Speroff, T., Gordon, S. M., Harrell, F. E., Inouye, S. K., Bernard, G. R., Dittus, R. S. Delirium as a Predictor of Mortality in Mechanically Ventilated Patients in the Intensive Care Unit. *J. Am. Med. Assoc.,* 2004. https://doi.org/10.1001/jama.291.14.1753.

[6] Marra, A., Ely, E. W., Pandharipande, P. P., Patel, M. B. The ABCDEF Bundle in Critical Care. *Crit. Care Clin.,* 2017, 33 (2). https://doi.org/10.1016/ j.ccc.2016.12.005.

[7] Morandi, A., Piva, S., Ely, E. W., Myatra, S. H., MD, Salluh, J. I. F., Amare, D., Azoulay, E., Bellelli, G., Csomos, A., Fan, E., Fagoni, N., Girard, T. D., La Calle, G. H., MD, Inoue, S., Lim, C. M., Kaps, R., Kotfis, K., Koh, Y., Misango, D., Pandharipande, P. P., Permpikul, C., Tan, C. C., Wang, D. X., Sharshar, T., Shehabi, Y., Skrobik, Y., Singh, J. M., Slooter, A., Smith, M., Tsuruta, R. and Latronico, N. Worldwide Survey of the "Assessing Pain, Both Spontaneous Awakening and Breathing Trials, Choice of Drugs, Delirium Monitoring/ Management, Early Exercise/Mobility, and Family Empowerment" (ABCDEF) Bundle. *Crit. Care Med.,* 2017.

[8] Marra, A., Kotfis, K., Hosie, A., MacLullich, A. M. J., Pandharipande, P. P., Ely, E. W., Pun, B. T. Delirium Monitoring: Yes or No? That Is the Question. *American Journal of Critical Care,* 2019. https://doi.org/10.4037/ajcc2019874.

[9] Ely, E. W., Inouye, S. H., Bernard, G. R., Gordon, S., Francis, J., May, L., Truman, B., Speroff, T., Gautam, S., Margolin, R., Hart, R. P., Dittus, R. Delirium in

Mechanically Ventilated Patients: Validity and Reliability of the Confusion Assessment Method for the Intensive Care Unit (CAM-ICU). *J. Am. Med. Assoc.,* 2001. https://doi.org/10.1001/jama.286.21.2703.

[10] Charlesworth, M., Elliott, M. W., Holmes, J. D. Noninvasive Positive Pressure Ventilation for Acute Respiratory Failure in Delirious Patients: Understudied, Underreported, or Underappreciated? A Systematic Review and Meta-Analysis. *Lung,* 2012. https://doi.org/10.1007/s00408-012-9403-y.

[11] Inouye, S. K., Charpentier, P. A. Precipitating Factors for Delirium in Hospitalized Elderly Persons: Predictive Model and Interrelationship with Baseline Vulnerability. *J. Am. Med. Assoc.,* 1996. https://doi.org/10.1001/jama.275.11.852.

[12] Nava, S., Hill, N. Non-Invasive Ventilation in Acute Respiratory Failure. *The Lancet,* 2009. https://doi.org/10.1016/S0140-6736(09)60496-7.

[13] Longroi, S. D., Conti, G., Mantz, J., Faltlhauser, A., Aantaa, R., Tonner, P. Sedation in Non-Invasive Ventilation: Do We Know What to Do (and Why)? *Multidisciplinary Respiratory Medicine,* 2014. https://doi.org/10.1186/2049-6958-9-56.

[14] Pandharipande, P. P., Shintani, A., Peterson, J., Pun, B. T., Wilkinson, G. R., Dittus, R. S., Bernard, G. R., Ely, E. W. Lorazepam Is an Independent Risk Factor for Transitioning to Delirium in Intensive Care Unit Patients. *Anesthesiology,* 2006. https://doi.org/10.1097/00000542-200601000-00005.

[15] Abdelgalel, E. F. Dexmedetomidine versus Haloperidol for Prevention of Delirium during Non-Invasive Mechanical Ventilation. *Egypt. J. Anaesth.,* 2016. https://doi.org/10.1016/j.egja.2016.05.008.

[16] Fanfulla, F., Taurino, A. E., Lupo, N. D. A., Trentin, R., D'Ambrosio, C., Nava, S. Effect of Sleep on Patient/Ventilator Asynchrony in Patients Undergoing Chronic Non-Invasive Mechanical Ventilation. *Respir. Med.,* 2007. https://doi.org/10.1016/j.rmed.2007.02.026.

[17] Marra, A., McGrane, T. J., Henson, C. P., Pandharipande, P. P. Melatonin in Critical Care. *Critical Care Clinics,* 2019. https://doi.org/10.1016/ j.ccc.2018.11.008.

In: Non-Invasive Mechanical Ventilation Complications
Editor: Antonio M. Esquinas
ISBN: 978-1-53619-515-6

Chapter 31

COMPLICATIONS OF NON-INVASIVE VENTILATION IN THE EMERGENCY DEPARTMENT: KEY PRACTICAL ISSUES

***Manjush Karthika*[1,*] *and Jithin K Sreedharan*[2]**
[1]Department of Health and Medical Sciences, Khawarizmi International College, Abu Dhabi, United Arab Emirates
[2]Department of Respiratory Care, Prince Sultan Military College of Health Sciences, Dammam, Kingdom of Saudi Arabia

ABSTRACT

The utility of non-invasive ventilation (NIV) in the emergency departments (ED) may reduce mortality and morbidity, provided the right approach for the right patient at the right time. More important is the balance between clinical outcome and prevention of untoward complications, which decides the success of NIV in the ED. Complications in the initial hours of stabilization are mostly related to patient-NIV asynchrony, interfaces, and high airflows. Fatal complications, like barotraumas and pulmonary aspiration are few and may occur rarely. ED clinicians are expected to balance the cart of physiological homeostasis by understanding the patients' clinical demand against the potential complications of NIV, which are preventable.

Keywords: non-invasive ventilation, emergency department, complications

* Corresponding Author's E-mail: manjushnair@hotmail.com.

Introduction

Emergency departments (EDs) play a pivotal role in the hospital and healthcare system, providing care for the patients with acute illness or injury, including triage, stabilization, and route the care plan as per the patient's presentation. One of the cardinal symptoms of patients presenting to ED is dyspnea, which is the subjective inability to breathe comfortably. Any acute decompensated systemic presentation will reflect on the respiratory system as dyspnea; however, some common causes include pneumonia, decompensated heart failure, chronic obstructive pulmonary disease (COPD), asthma, and pulmonary embolism. Stabilization of airway, breathing, and circulation is considered the primary objective, including respiratory support with oxygen supplementation. Oxygen delivery in such patients is accomplished by various oxygen delivery devices, including nasal cannula, face masks, and gets stepped up to high flow nasal cannula (HFNC) and mechanical ventilation with either invasive or non-invasive approaches. Existing literature supports that non-invasive ventilation (NIV) avoids the need for endotracheal intubation and its related complications, as well as mortality in specific patient populations [1]. Timely initiation, selecting the right device, accessories, and interface, and most importantly, selecting the right patients are considered as the critical indicators for a successful outcome in NIV. Although NIV is well tolerated by most of the patients in the ED, the caregivers should anticipate potential adverse effects and complications related to NIV. Such are classified as patient, device, and caregiver related complications. As the authorized people to use such a lifesaving equipment, we are responsible for anticipating and understanding various processes related to the safe practice of NIV, to prevent any untoward events to our patients. Some of those complications related to NIV in ED settings are as narrated below.

Patient Related Complications

Patient-related complications with NIV are never to be ignored in ED, as in most of the acutely symptomatic patients, NIV trials are found to be beneficial, and the ED clinicians will give their best to utilize that window period to prevent endotracheal intubation. Hence the benefits of NIV need to be weighed against the adverse effects, and close surveillance is required to prevent complications like gastric distension, eye irritation, barotraumas, agitation, hemodynamic instability, and patient-ventilator asynchrony.

Gastric Distension and Aspiration

Aerophagia is not rare in patients on NIV, and eventual gastric distension/ insufflation is reported in up to 40% of patients but is tolerable [2]. Aerophagia depends on respiratory mechanics, lower esophageal sphincter pressure, head position, and inspiratory flow. Gastric distention compresses the lungs and induces high intrathoracic pressures, resulting in high inspiratory pressure to ventilate the lung [3]. If the positive airway pressure delivered by the NIV exceeds the lower esophageal sphincter pressure, i.e., approximately 20–25 cmH_2O, it results in the entry of air into the gastrointestinal tract, resulting in gastric insufflation. The scenario worsens if abdominal compliance is greater than the chest. Ongoing distention of the stomach may also lead to regurgitation of the gastric contents, resulting in pulmonary aspiration. Even though gastric distention is considered a minor complication, if unresolved, the resultant will be abdominal compression on the thorax, leading to intra-abdominal hypertension, and the possibility of abdominal compartment syndrome cannot be excluded [4]. In the ED, the prime objective of NIV is to relieve the acute cardiopulmonary symptoms thereby improving oxygenation-ventilation status. Emergency admissions are unplanned; clinicians are expected to focus on balancing the pressures to avoid untoward events like gastric distention and consequent pulmonary aspiration, which may later turn fatal in extreme cases. Some of the practices to avoid complications related to gastric distention include insertion of an open ended naso-gastric tube and encouraged sitting position post meal. Other strategies include pharmacological adjuncts to accelerate intestinal motility and titration of NIV pressures, balancing the benefit and risks.

Barotrauma

Another important complication seen in ED is barotrauma associated with NIV. Barotrauma is an umbrella term defined as the abnormal collection of air in the extra-alveolar spaces, such as pneumothorax, pneumopericardium, pneumomediastinum, pneumoperitoneum, or extensive subcutaneous emphysema due to the over-inflation of lungs caused by high distending pressure. In a typical ED scenario, all the acute cardiorespiratory presentations, regardless of the causes like COPD, asthma, pneumonia, or pulmonary edema, are initially trialed with NIV if the patients meet the criteria. Sound knowledge of titrating the NIV pressures balancing the symptoms of the patients is vital here. Patients presenting with similar diagnosis and clinical presentations might vary in their lung mechanics like compliance and resistance. Many anecdotal experiences of pneumothorax, pneumocephalus, bilateral tympanic rupture and subconjunctival emphysema sets an important reminder of the potential for barotrauma associated with different modes of NIV [5]. Barotrauma related to NIV is controllable, provided if the clinicians adopt approaches like titration of inspiratory pressures (less than 30 cm H20) in patients with poor lung compliance as seen in parenchymal and interstitial disorders, optimization of inspiratory and expiratory times to provide sufficient expiratory time to prevent air trapping and auto-PEEP and avoidance of patient-ventilator asynchrony. Permissive hypercapnia (pH up to 7.2 to 7.25) is accepted, while attempts are made to balance ventilation and inspiratory pressures [6]. Nevertheless, the risk of barotrauma observed in NIV patients is less than those of patients who are on invasive mechanical ventilation [7].

Hemodynamic Instability

NIV application, especially continuous positive airway pressure (CPAP), is hemodynamically beneficial for patients with pulmonary congestion and left ventricular systolic dysfunction as it increases the cardiac output. This effect is ascribed by the increased intrathoracic pressure and subsequent reduction in the left ventricular afterload, thereby improving the systolic function [8]. Contradictory to this, if pulmonary hypertension is present, positive pressure ventilation is associated with unfavorable hemodynamic effects. The application of CPAP will increase the intrathoracic pressure and right-ventricular after-load and reduce pre-load, causing hypotension in a susceptible patient [8]. It is not uncommon that patients may present to the ED with symptoms that directly reflect pulmonary hypertension or complaints related to the underlying conditions, which contribute to pulmonary hypertension such as acute exacerbation of chronic obstructive pulmonary disease or asthma, or unrelated complaints of a coexisting illness. Hence it is suggested that patients with pulmonary hypertension need to be extra cautiously monitored in the ED while on NIV.

Discomfort and Intolerance

Patients who are presenting to the ED are symptomatic, and they expect immediate relief. Understanding the morbidity and associated mortality of presenting complaints, ED clinicians prefer to start NIV over endotracheal intubation. The transition from the atmospheric pressure to positive pressure application through a mask may cause transient discomfort for the patients already symptomatic. Discomfort levels with NIV can be related to anxiety, interface, pressure or flow, or the entire system itself. The success of an NIV trial is defined as patient's tolerance to it and the avoidance of endotracheal intubation. Intolerance to NIV is a frequently occurring patient-centered complication in the ED and may result in NIV failure. Even though the clinical characteristics, predictors, and outcomes of NIV intolerance are unclear, the multifactorial causes include underlying pathology, caregiver's expertise, patient-ventilator asynchrony, interface compliance, and agitation [9, 10]. Age, heart rate, and respiratory rate are considered the independent risk factors of NIV intolerance [9]. Interface-related NIV intolerance is studied many times, and observed that patient's comfort and compliant levels are a better indicator of interface tolerance [11, 12]. Patients presenting with acute respiratory failure are more found to be intolerant to NIV, and the factors predisposed included worsened distress, induced dyspnea, and intolerable flow or pressure [9]. These factors are relatable to the aforementioned causes like underlying pathology, caregiver's expertise, patient-ventilator asynchrony, and interface compliance. Since there is a paucity of literature supporting an optimal target pressure, achieving the required inspiratory pressure based on comfort and tolerance is suggested.

Patient-Centered Asynchrony

Another critical challenge faced by the ED clinicians is patient-NIV asynchrony when the ventilator does not meet the patient's respiratory efforts. Asynchrony is the mismatch between the patient's and ventilator assisted breaths and/or when ventilator flow delivery is inadequate to match the patient's ventilatory flow demand despite a matched inspiratory time. Interestingly, the patient-ventilator asynchrony can be quantified by the asynchrony index [13]. Asynchrony index is expressed as the number of asynchrony events divided by the total respiratory rate computed as the sum of the number of ventilator cycles (patient-triggered) and wasted efforts; i.e., asynchrony index (%) = number of asynchrony events/total respiratory rate (ventilator cycles + ineffective triggering) × 100. For instance, 43% of patients presenting with an acute respiratory failure are reported to have asynchrony with the NIV, with a severe asynchrony index of > 10% [14]. As previously mentioned, the patients presenting to the ED require urgent attention to stabilize their clinical presentation, and NIV is a clinically proven tool for acute cardiorespiratory symptoms. However, many times, some of the patient-centered factors and NIV-centered factors, if not identified, may result in patient-NIV asynchrony. The underlying pathology, low respiratory drive, weak inspiratory muscles, or dynamic hyperinflation resulting in trapped air and auto positive end-expiratory pressure are some of the patient-centered factors of asynchrony. Some of the device centered causes include expiratory and inspiratory air leak, inadequate or excessive pressure support, types of interface, and improper humidification, which points toward inspiratory triggering mechanism, breath delivery pattern, and cycling mechanisms. This to an extent can be controlled with a sound knowledge of underlying physiology and operational aspects of the machine.

Several approaches like using ventilators with algorithms for air-leak detection and compensation [15], titration of the pressure according to patient tolerance [16], and choice of the appropriate interface and proper seal may limit the number of asynchronies during NIV.

Machine Related Complications

The choice of a ventilator is crucial in NIV success in the acute setting. An ideal NIV machine will essentially have sufficient leak compensation, uninterrupted monitoring of all parameters including exhaled tidal volume and respiratory rate, oxygen blenders to guarantee continuous oxygen delivery, different levels of adjustment of the trigger, and cycling to manage patient-ventilator asynchrony. A typical NIV machine should have sophisticated monitoring and alarm functions. These allow clinicians to assess scalar graphics and monitor pressures (high and low), breathing frequency, tidal volumes, and degree of the leak. Hypothetically, this should improve patient-ventilator synchrony and safety. New generation critical care ventilators have options for NIV. In the presence of leaks, most ICU ventilators, but not all, required adjustments to maintain synchrony. It is essential to know that the power source must be ideally connected to the NIV machine since most NIV machines have significant battery life variability, and some may not even have a battery backup. Any un-intentional disconnection is deemed to be catastrophic [17].

Interface Related Complications

Interfaces are devices that connect the ventilator tubing to the patient's face. Oronasal masks, full face masks, and helmets are the frequently used interfaces in the ED because patients with acute respiratory failure in the ED are mainly mouth breathers. Therefore nasal masks are not suitable for ED use. Oronasal masks cover the nasal bridge, go around the nose, and form a seal around the chin and the patient's mouth. Basically, for this reason, oronasal masks are the most appropriate type for ED use, even though there is a risk of claustrophobia and skin lesions [12]. It is essential to trace the exhalation port, reassure its patency, and check the compatibility of the circuit and mask before starting NIV. Finding the best strap tension is challenging; however, always maintain an even distribution of pressure across the mask's circumference, allowing for both a good seal and low pressure on the skin.

On the other hand, full face masks will increase the dead space and cause rebreathing of carbon dioxide. When a helmet mask is used, there is a high risk of rebreathing carbon dioxide, especially if the patient's respiratory rate is high [18]. The helmet is also very noisy, and it may hinder communication and potentially have a high occurrence of claustrophobia, hence not routinely used in the ED.

Circuit Related Complications

It is essential to be aware of which circuit is used before the interface is selected. If a ventilator with a single lumen circuit is selected, then the exhalation port must be at the end of the circuit or on the mask, whereas if a double-lumen circuit is chosen, then there must be no exhalation port on the mask. For instance, the wrong combination, a non-vented mask in an open single-limb system, and no exhalation port in the system can be fatal. Likewise, an exhalation port should never be obstructed intentionally (e.g., taping up the holes in the mask) to decrease leakage. In critical care ventilators, dual limb circuits are used separately for the inspiratory gas and the expiratory gas movement [19]. Appropriate precautions are necessary when NIV is used for patients with highly contagious respiratory infections due to leak port exposure and the potential of exposure of healthcare providers to contaminants in the exhaled gas of the patient.

Leakage and Associated Complications

One of the leading causes of NIV failure in the ED is a leak. The ventilators are not uniform to perform adequate leak compensation, and the amount of compensated air leak is highly variable; hence the ED clinicians and Respiratory Therapists must understand the leak compensation capabilities of their devices [19]. Deciding on the appropriate interface will enhance the patient's comfort and eliminate the complications related to the straps' excessive tightening. An intentional leak is acceptable, which is imperative for patient-ventilator synchrony and the success of NIV [16].

Machine Centered Asynchrony

Ineffective triggering, double-triggering, auto-triggering, premature cycling, and delayed cycling are the different types of asynchrony. The leak from the interface is one of the key factors associated with asynchrony [13]. When the clinician sets the trigger sensitivity too high, ineffective triggering will occur. Ineffective triggering may also happen due to high intrinsic PEEP, generalized weakness of the patient, inappropriate ventilator sensitivity settings, and ventilator dysfunction. As per the nature of patient presentation, double triggering is seen frequently in the ED due to too short inspiratory time, too low inspiratory flow and tidal volume, and cough/hiccups. The leak will cause auto triggering, and when the ventilator is triggered differently from the patient's respiratory effort [20]. In the incidence of a profound leak in NIV, the cycle criteria may need to be adjusted to a higher percentage to allow the breath to cycle to expiration. Cycling criteria may be auto-adaptive on bi-level ventilators and require no adjustment, but in the presence of a profound leak, auto-adaptive algorithms may fail to cycle the breath to exhalation, leading to premature or delayed cycling phenomena [19].

Contamination from the Equipment

Patients requiring NIV in the ED settings are usually acutely ill and are often managed with a provisional diagnosis of their respiratory failure. It is ideal to use disposable mask and circuit for patients requiring NIV. The mask, circuit, and other NIV accessories, if reusable, are classified as semi-critical items and necessary to clean and sterilize before its reuse. The manufacturer's directives of disinfection must be checked for compatibility of the instrument or equipment [17]. Considering the dispersion of aerosols or droplets generated from NIVs, care must be taken to avoid the transmission of infections to the caregivers.

Conclusion

NIV is essential in the ED settings, proven to decrease the need for endotracheal intubation and invasive ventilation and its related complications. Nevertheless, care must be taken to avoid various complications that can occur with instituting and ongoing NIV in acutely ill patients. The success of NIV primarily depends on the selection of the appropriate device, interface, accessories, and, most importantly, the right selection of the patients.

References

[1] Göksu E, Kılıç D, İbze S. Non-invasive ventilation in the ED: Whom, When, How? *Turk. J. Emerg. Med.* 2018;18(2):52-56.

[2] Summers R L, Patch J, Kolb J C. Effect of the initiation of noninvasive bi-level positive airway pressure on haemodynamic stability. *Eur. J. Emerg. Med.* 2002; 9: 37–41 98.

[3] De Luca A, Sall F S, Khoury A. Leak Compensation Algorithms: The Key Remedy to Noninvasive Ventilation Failure? *Respir. Care.* 2017;62(1):135-136.

[4] De Keulenaer B L, De Backer A, Schepens D R, Daelemans R, Wilmer A, Malbrain M L. Abdominal compartment syndrome related to noninvasive ventilation. *Intensive Care Med.* 2003;29(7):1177-1181.

[5] Cross A M. Review of the role of non-invasive ventilation in the emergency department. *J. Accid. Emerg. Med.* 2000;17(2):79-85.

[6] Davidson A C, Banham S, Elliott M, Kennedy D, Gelder C, Glossop A, et al. BTS Standards of Care Committee Member, British Thoracic Society/Intensive Care Society Acute Hypercapnic Respiratory Failure Guideline Development Group, On behalf of the British Thoracic Society Standards of Care Committee. BTS/ICS guideline for the ventilatory management of acute hypercapnic respiratory failure in adults. *Thorax.* 2016 Apr;71 Suppl 2:ii1-35. doi: 10.1136/thoraxjnl-2015-208209. Erratum in: *Thorax.* 2017;72 (6):588.

[7] Carron M, Freo U, BaHammam A S, Dellweg D, Guarracino F, Cosentini R, Feltracco P, Vianello A, Ori C, Esquinas A. Complications of non-invasive ventilation techniques: a comprehensive qualitative review of randomized trials. *Br. J. Anaesth.* 2013;110(6):896-914.

[8] Bento A M, Cardoso L F, Tarasoutchi F, Sampaio R O, Kajita L J, Lemos Neto P A. Hemodynamic Effects of Noninvasive Ventilation in Patients with Venocapillary Pulmonary Hypertension. *Arq. Bras. Cardiol.* 2014;103(5):410-417.

[9] Liu J, Duan J, Bai L, Zhou L. Noninvasive Ventilation Intolerance: Characteristics, Predictors, and Outcomes. Respir Care. 2016;61(3):277-284.

[10] Dres M, Demoule A. Noninvasive Ventilation: Do Not Tolerate Intolerance. *Respir. Care.* 2016;61(3):393-394.

[11] Antonelli M, Conti G, Pelosi P, Gregoretti C, Pennisi M A, Costa R, et al. New treatment of acute hypoxemic respiratory failure: noninvasive pressure support ventilation delivered by helmet: a pilot controlled trial. *Crit. Care Med.* 2002;30(3):602–608.

[12] Roy B, Cordova F C, Travaline J M, D'Alonzo G E Jr., Criner G J. Full face mask for noninvasive positive-pressure ventilation in patients with acute respiratory failure. *J. Am. Osteopath. Assoc.* 2007;107(4):148–156.

[13] Kondili E, Prinianakis G, Georgopoulos D: Patient-ventilator interaction. *Br. J. Anaesth.* 2003, 91: 106-119.

[14] Longhini F, Colombo D, Pisani L, et al. Efficacy of ventilator waveform observation for detection of patient-ventilator asynchrony during NIV: a multicentre study. *ERJ Open Res.* 2017;3(4):00075-2017.

[15] Carteaux G, Lyazidi A, Cordoba-Izquierdo A, et al. Patient-ventilator asynchrony during noninvasive ventilation: a bench and clinical study. *Chest* 2012; 142: 367–376.

[16] Vignaux L, Vargas F, Roeseler J, et al. Patient-ventilator asynchrony during non-invasive ventilation for acute respiratory failure: a multicenter study. *Intensive Care Med.* 2009; 35: 840–846.

[17] Scott J B. Ventilators for Noninvasive Ventilation in Adult Acute Care. *Respir. Care.* 2019;64(6):712-722.

[18] Brill A, How to avoid interface problems in acute noninvasive ventilation. *Breathe.* 2014;10(3):230-242.

[19] Gay P C. Complications of noninvasive ventilation in acute care. *Respir. Care.* 2009;54(2):246-257;

[20] Carron, M, Freo, U, BaHammam, A, Dellweg, D, Guarracino, F, Cosentini, R, Feltracco, P, Vianello, A, Ori, C. and Esquinas, A. Complications of non-invasive ventilation techniques: a comprehensive qualitative review of randomized trials. *British Journal of Anaesthesia*, 2013;110(6):896-914.

In: Non-Invasive Mechanical Ventilation Complications ISBN: 978-1-53619-515-6
Editor: Antonio M. Esquinas

Chapter 32

Complications during Nasal High Flow Oxygen Neonatology-Pediatrics

Mohanchandra Mandal[1,*], MD and Suman Chattopadhyay[2,†]
[1]Professor, Department of Anaesthesiology,
Nil Ratan Sircar Medical College and Hospital, Kolkata, West Bengal, India
[2]Professor and Head of Department,
Post Graduate Department of Anaesthesiology and Critical Care,
Midnapore Medical College, Midnapore, West Bengal, India

Abstract

High flow nasal oxygen therapy (HFNO) through specially designed nasal cannula is a novel non-invasive breathing device that has caught the imagination of intensivists worldwide. This device is being used in many acute and chronic situations with further emerging fields of application including pediatric population. However, with wider usage various problems are coming into our purview - the most worrisome of which is generation of unpredictable pharyngeal pressure with alveolar over distension. The safe practitioner should be thorough about every nitty-gritty while applying these devices - from looking at the evidence regarding its use in a particular scenario, diligently monitoring the patient parameters and device function throughout duration of therapy, and act judiciously when problems arise including escalation of therapy or on the other hand abandoning this therapy altogether for an alternate therapy as the situation demands. Some problems are relatively minor while others are really life-threatening, and can develop during short term as well as at long term use of these devices. This article highlights the vital practice points and important complications of HFNO from published articles till date.

Keywords: high flow, nasal cannula, oxygen therapy, pediatric, neonate, complications

* Corresponding Author's E-mail: drmcmandal@gmail.com.
† Corresponding Author's E-mail: sumanc24@gmail.com.

INTRODUCTION

High flow nasal oxygen (HFNO) therapy using high flow nasal cannula (HFNC) device is a novel non-invasive respiratory support which can be thought of as a 'bridge therapy' between conventional low-flow oxygen therapy and noninvasive ventilation (NIV) in terms of the level of support, and may reduce the need for nasal continuous positive airway pressure (nCPAP) or intubation [1]. HFNC delivers heated and humidified gas (air-oxygen mixture) through a specially designed nasal cannula at a high flow which usually exceeds the peak inspiratory flow rate of patient. HFNC is not merely a device for oxygen enrichment; rather it is something more owing to beneficial effects such as washout of nasopharyngeal dead space and producing a positive distending pressure at the pharynx [2-4]. Although initially it was introduced for treatment in mild to severe bronchiolitis in neonates and children, the popularity of its use is increasing day by day to include respiratory distress syndrome, apnea of prematurity, etc. which usually warrants this therapy for comparatively long period in days rather than hours [4, 5]. The triad of humidity, compliance and high FiO_2 that HFNC devices offer is probably the reason for its popularity and application for a wide variety of clinical scenarios [6]. However, there may be unpredictable and fluctuating positive pressure generation which may be a limiting factor while using this device. This chapter intends to describe common indications for short-term and long-term use of HFNC therapy. The reason of unpredictable pressure is described. The factors influencing the occurrence of unwanted effects and the practice points (regarding problems and precautions) intended to minimize such adverse events have been elicited. The chapter also depicts some reported and potential complications of HFNC therapy during short term and long term use of such device in neonates and pediatric population.

INDICATIONS: SHORT-TERM AND LONG-TERM USE

Although HFNC therapy has gained popularity in treating both type I and type II acute respiratory failure, it is used more commonly in acute care settings for treatment of non-hypercapneic de novo hypoxemic failure owing to various disease processes [3, 7, 8]. The short-term use of HFNC are also being reported for other conditions such as pneumonia, croup, asthma, during transport of critically ill children from emergency department to PICU, for pre- and peri-oxygenation during intubation and bronchoscopy, for respiratory support in the post-extubation phase in ICU or following surgery [9]. HFNC are being used as an alternative to intubation in patients who are immunocompromised or those with a 'do-not-intubate' status. Long-term use has also been reported for chronic airway diseases and for palliative care in wards and at home.

Other indications of long-term therapy with HFNC may be idiopathic pulmonary fibrosis [4, 10], tracheomalacia [11] and atypical CHARGE syndrome [12], etc.

However, as opposed to CPAP and other modes of NIV, no monitoring of pressure or volume is available for patients breathing with HFNC at present [13]. Hence, implementation of this technique in emergency department, respiratory ward or ICU warrants proper selection of right patients and intense monitoring by experienced care giver to detect early signs of failure and adverse events to prevent or minimize complications.

A Major Problem of HFNC- Generation of Unpredictable Pressure

HFNC is able to increase end-expiratory pressure despite being an open ventilation system. Unlike nasal CPAP, the HFNC prongs are not designed to occlude the nares avoiding the creation of a seal for generating positive pressure. The generated pharyngeal pressure is however affected by delivered flow, size of nasal prong and position of mouth (opening or closing). Usually a pharyngeal pressure of less than 5 cm H_2O is produced. However, the pressure is not predictable or sustained, and is higher with HFNC therapy compared with CPAP at comparative flow [14]. For example, flows as low as 2L/min can generate pressure as high as 6 cm H_2O, while with a flow of 8 L/min pressure of >120 cm H_2O was detected at the level of prongs, this pressure was significantly more than the approximate 30 cm H_2O with CPAP [15, 16]. Artificial lung model studies [17] have also reported dangerously high airway pressures with minimal leaks in HFNC.

The flow driver in a traditional CPAP setup delivers flows only during child's inspiration through Coanda effect during expiration. In contrast, during HFNC the flows are delivered continuously during both inspiration and expiration [16]. High flow of gas though nasal cannula can alter the intrinsic breathing patterns into periodic breathing especially in neonates and infants compared with older children. During HFNC therapy in infants with highly compliant lungs a larger tidal volume may be delivered for the same inspiratory effort compared with spontaneous breathing. Sometimes, complete delivery of a large inspiratory flow can occur with resultant alveolar overdistension [18]. This may create a large fluctuation in pressure and can result in alveolar overdistension leading to volutrauma, barotraumas and the so-called 'air leak syndromes' [18]. These are more common with the use of inappropriate-sized prongs obstructing the nostril lumen.

Practice Points (Precautions and Problems) during HFNC Use

The widespread use of HFNC has occurred in the absence of a strong evidence base. No comprehensive guideline exists for initiation of flow or FiO_2 [18]. Hence, this therapy should be used with caution and with an awareness of potential adverse effects.

Cannula size varies by age and body weight. Choosing the appropriate sized cannula is of utmost importance for the success of HFNC therapy. When larger nasal cannula is used, the occlusion of nasal passages is greater, thereby higher pressures are achieved in the nasopharynx even with the same flow rate [19]. Manufacturers recommend that the cross-sectional area of the cannula be no more than 50% of the nares to prevent unexpected elevations in airway pressure and subsequent risk of air leak. This translates into the fact that the appropriate outer diameter of the cannula would be no more than the two-thirds of the nares [20].

Flow rate is started at the lowest recommended flow (1 L/kg/min) and is increased to meet the child's demand. The most supported flow rate is 2 L/kg/min for infants and 1 L/kg/min for older children [21-25]. Flows >2 L/min has been reported with a higher rate of discomfort (in verbal children) and with a longer stay in PICU. This flow (>2 L/min) can cause unpredictable positive airway pressure and should be used with caution in neonates [21, 24, 26, 27].

Fractional inspired oxygen (FiO_2) is to be increased until satisfactory oxygen saturation is achieved. However, we should be aware that if a high FiO_2 is used, oxygen saturation may be maintained despite development of hypercapneic failure. Rapid deterioration of oxygen saturation as evidenced by pulse oximetry or noticeable increased work of breathing should raise suspicion of pneumothorax. $FiO_2 \leq 0.4$ is a simple and advantageous predictor [28] of successful separation from HFNO and does not require any calculation from multiple parameters at the bedside, unlike Respiratory Rate Oxygenation (ROX) index [29].

Temperature is set initially at 37 degree Celsius. Some authors have recommended initial setting at 1-2 degree Celsius below body temperature and to adjust as needed for patient comfort [22].

Patency of ventilation slots and filters is a very important practical point. The room air enters through a ventilation slot which must be patent. This slot should not be kept covered with linen or be stuck to wall. The air-intake filter must be clean for adequate entry of air to the turbine [19].

Tubing position of the ventilator tubing should be always below the patient so that water condensation can be prevented from entering the airway. Moreover, it would minimize the pressure injuries to nasal mucosa [19].

Periodic cleaning of mucus is required for proper nasal mucosal hygiene. Hot and humidified gas results in vasodilation of nasal mucosa and copious mucus production which may compromise the tolerance and effectiveness of the therapy. Runny nose and blocked nasal cannula are distinct possibilities [19].

Movement of the child gets restricted because of the fact that the patient needs to be connected with the device constantly, a problem similar to NIV. During transfer or during diagnostic or therapeutic procedures HFNC must not be ceased without prior consultation with the treating consultant. This restriction of movement has serious impact on quality of life with decrease in autonomy [19].

Noise level while using this device can reach to about 80 dB. The decibel level is correlated with flow rate, and it may be higher than other CPAP systems [26, 30]. Claustrophobia and noise taken together can lead to intolerance.

Alteration of smell, feeling hot and suffocation are also complained by verbal children owing to intense entry of constant air associated with difficulty in expiration [19]. Neonates can't express suffocation but will suffer if pressure builds up unpredictably.

Continuous close monitoring of heart rate, respiratory rate and pulse oximetry is essential. The following signs assessed within 1 to 2 hours of HFNC initiation usually indicate about no response to treatment (i.e., negative prognostic signs) predicting a higher risk of HFNC failure): persistent hypoxemia (SpO_2 < 88-90%) despite high FiO_2 and high gas flow, persistent increased respiratory rate (>35 breaths/min), frequent incidences of apnea or bradycardia, use of accessory muscles of respiration, presence of thoraco-abdominal asynchrony [3, 9, 22]. The verbal children may express concern about increasing respiratory distress and discomfort.

Failure to improve within 48 hours warns about considerable lung injury. Lung imaging such as chest radiography and ultrasound could play an important role in early identification of patients with extensive lung opacities or pleural effusion who may eventually be non-responders to HFNC therapy [31]. Also it should be borne in mind that cardiac failure and respiratory failure may have similar manifestations in children with cardiac disease, thereby creating confusion in treatment modality. The high flows can affect pulmonary and systemic circulation which has important implication during HFNC therapy in children with cardiac disease [32].

Risk of delayed endotracheal intubation is one of the major concerns of HFNC therapy. Overall a higher ICU mortality has been observed in 'late-intubated' group (patients intubated 48 hours after HFNC initiation, median duration of HFNC support for 126 hours) compared with 'early-intubated' group (intubated within 48 hours, median duration of HFNC support for 10 hours) [33]. Early review between 60 to 120 minutes after the initiation of therapy is essential to detect failure of therapy which needs escalation of respiratory support to minimize morbidity and mortality [9].

Last but not the least, we should be always aware of contraindications of HFNC use. Severe nasal obstruction, considerable nasal bleeding, fracture involving base of the skull, recent trauma or surgery involving nose and nasopharynx can all be considered as potential contraindications for the use of HFNC therapy. Critically ill infants and children or those with decreased level of consciousness (Glasgow Coma Scale <8 points with no upper airway reflexes) requiring immediate escalation of respiratory support such as NIV or intubation should not be treated with HFNC. Similarly, the children suffering from central apnea or having upper airway obstruction should not receive HFNC therapy [34].

Complications Associated with HFNC

Serious adverse events are extremely rare. In a retrospective study Baudin et al. [35] reported major complications of HFNC were only 0.9 per 100 HFNC treatment days in pediatric ICU. The complications associated with use of HFNC therapy in pediatric population can be broadly classified into two broad groups depending on the onset of problem as early and late complications. The complications can also be varied from mild to very severe. Some of the common problems associated with HFNC use have been discussed in the previous section.

Early Complications

Irritation to nasal mucosa leads to nasal mucosal abrasion. It can be minimized by choosing the correctly sized cannula and proper stabilization of the patient to prevent tube traction. Poor placement of cannula can place its tip against nasal mucosa results in cannula obstruction, patient discomfort, mucosal injury and bleeding. The nasal cannula has a pad to improve patient comfort and is attached to the patient's head using a harness.

Gastric distension leading to aspiration is an ever present risk associated any non-invasive ventilation mode.

Air leak syndromes (pneumothorax and / or pneumomediastinum, pneumo-encephalus) have been documented. Cases of pulmonary 'air leak syndromes' (such as, pneumothorax or pneumomediatinum) have been reported in older children receiving HFNC therapy [36]. However, a case of pneumo-encephalus has been reported in a premature neonate [37]. These adverse events actually put emphasis about proper use of HFNC by allowing ample gas leak between the prongs and the surrounding nostrils. There must be some clearance between the prong and the wall of nostril. The HFNC is an 'open system' which must ensure that the nasal cannula prongs are non-occlusive, thereby should reduce the risk of sudden increase in airway pressure as a result of inadvertent obstruction [22]. Hegde and Prodhan [36] reported three cases of serious air leaks related to HFNC therapy. First, a right-sided pneumothorax developed in a 2-month baby with bronchiolitis receiving HFNC therapy at 8 L/min. Second, incidence of pneumomediatinum was reported in a 16-year old male with cerebral palsy receiving HFNC therapy started at a flow of 4 L/min, then increased to 8 L/min, 15 L/min and finally to 20 LPM to optimize the support. Lastly, an incidence of right-sided pneumothorax developed after 5 hours of post-extubation support using HFNC at a flow of 6 LPM in a 22-month-old male with subdural hematoma. The above case reports indicate that the adverse events might be due to unpredictable pressure generated owing to use of arbitrary titration of flow rate to the clinical effects. However, an overall low rate of barotrauma (1%) has been reported [35]. In a randomized clinical trial comparing

HFNC and nasal CPAP, comparable incidence of pulmonary air leak has been observed in vulnerable preterm neonates [38].

Epistaxis of clinical significance has been reported in 0.6% of cases emphasizing proper placement of HFNC inside the nasal passage [35].

Pressure injury leading to mucosal injury is another possible complication, commoner in premature neonate and infant whose skin is especially susceptible to injury from nasal prongs of HFNC devices. Injury can occur at the nares, intranasal septum, columella (the anterior tip of nasal septum), or philtrum [39]. The incidence of skin breakdown has been reported to be lower with HFNC compared with nCPAP owing to the fact that the latter requires pressure on to the skin surface to create an occlusive seal while the former is an 'open system' warranting some leak for proper application.

Late Complications

Gastrointestinal complications are associated with gastric insufflations. Apart from gastric distension, major risk from gastric insufflations is gastrointestinal perforation and necrotizing enterocolitis which is more frequently observed during face-mask NIV compared to HFNC devices in neonates [40].

Decubitus ulcers occur inside the nasal cavities, in the occipital region or around the auricle in patients with prolonged HFNC therapy. It may be especially important if the child has facial anomalies (any syndrome) or previous surgeries or trauma involving the face, nose or airways thus preventing proper placement of nasal cannula [19]. Misalignment or improper fixation of nasal prongs can result in nasal snubbing and circumferential distortion (widening) of nares, especially if therapy continues for more than a few days [40].

Increase in the rates of broncho-pulmonary dysplasia (BPD) and longer stay in hospital are also reported. In a retrospective study involving premature infants (<30 weeks of gestational age, or <1500g body weight) over 7 years period (2010-2016), it was found that utilization of HFNC can lead to an increase in the rates of broncho-pulmonary dysplasia (BPD) and longer stay in hospital among premature infants. The consistent continuous positive pressure provided by modes such as nasal CPAP is claimed to be more beneficial to premature lung development than the washout provided by HFNC [41, 42].

Increased rate of retinopathy of prematurity is another serious concern. The weaning of patients from CPAP to HFNC was associated with longer duration of respiratory support and increased rate of retinopathy of prematurity (ROP) in neonates in age-group between 24 to 32 weeks of gestation [43]. The inconsistent pressure generation during HFNC can lead to progressive atelectasis which may contribute to prolonged duration of respiratory support. Generalized poor health status, background presence of BPD, and associated higher oxygen exposure in those utilizing HFNC all might contribute to occurrence of such adverse events [44]. While increased rates of BPD and/or longer duration of respiratory support are associated with HFNC, there are conflicting associations between HFNC use and rates of ROP [43, 45].

In the recent past, a questionnaire-based nationwide survey [27] has been performed involving 226 pediatric clinics of which 67 clinics responded, revealing complications of HFNC and the practice patterns in Germany. HFNC was applied in the age group of 8 to 14 years in 42% and between 14 to 18 years in 33% of the clinics. It was found that applied flow rate varied considerably between the clinics. Seventy percent of clinics have used HFNC outside the established indications. Severe complications such as pneumothorax have been reported by 17.9% of the clinics. Other adverse events were non-adherence to therapy or failure of therapy, conjunctivitis, problems with feeding and vomiting.

To conclude, although the HFNC is widely accepted as a non-invasive respiratory support owing to its several advantages such as improved patient comfort and compliance, preservation of heat and humidification, ease of application, etc. the therapy should be intensely monitored continuously, and especially during the first few hours after initiation for better titration and early detection of non-responders. No therapy is immune to adverse events. The wisdom and trained eyes can prevent the complications. Strict adherence to the appropriate cannula size for the age is essential. A comprehensive guideline regarding flow rate is also warranted in this regard and till then the enthusiasm for rampant 'off-label' use of HFNC should be curtailed.

References

[1] Spoletini G, Hill NS. High-flow nasal oxygen versus noninvasive ventilation for hypoxemic respiratory failure: Do we know enough? *Ann Thorac Med* 2016;11(3):163-6.

[2] Díaz-Lobato S, Alonso JM, Carratalá JM, Mayoralas S. High-flow nasal oxygen is not an oxygen therapy device. [Letter to the Editor]. *Revista Portuguesa de Pneumologia* (English Edition) 2017;23(1):51-52.

[3] Mauri T, Wang YM, Dalla Corte F, Corcione N, Spinelli E, Pesenti A. Nasal high flow: physiology, efficacy and safety in the acute care setting, a narrative review. *Open Access Emerg Med* 2019;11:109-120.

[4] Spoletini G, Alotaibi M, Blasi F, Hill NS. Heated humidifed high-flow nasal oxygen in adults: mechanisms of action and clinical implications. *Chest* 2015;148(1):253-261.

[5] Díaz-Lobato S, Alises SM. High-flow nasal cannula can be used outside the ICU. *Chest*. 2015;148(4):e127. doi: 10.1378/chest.15-1212.

[6] Ashraf-Kashani N, Kumar R. High-flow nasal oxygen therapy. *BJA Education* 2017;17(2):63-67.

[7] Spicuzza L, Schisano M. High-flow nasal cannula oxygen therapy as an emerging option for respiratory failure: the present and the future. *Ther Adv Chronic Dis.* 2020;11:2040622320920106. doi: 10.1177/2040622320920106.

[8] Frat JP, Coudroy R, Marjanovic N, Thille AW. High-flow nasal oxygen therapy and noninvasive ventilation in the management of acute hypoxemic respiratory failure. *Ann Transl Med* 2017;5(14):297. doi: 10.21037/atm.2017.06.52.

[9] Ischaki E, Pantazopoulos I, Zakynthinos S. Nasal high flow therapy: a novel treatment rather than a more expensive oxygen device. *Eur Respir Rev* 2017;26:170028 https://doi.org/10.1183/16000617.0028-2017.

[10] Santos PS, Cravo J, Esquinas AM. New perspectives for the use of high-flow nasal oxygen [Correpondence]. *Rev Port Pneumol.* 2016;22(6):368. http://dx.doi.org/10.1016/j.rppnen.2016.06.008.

[11] Hatipoglu Z, Esquinas AM, Ozcengiz D. Can high flow nasal cannula be used in a pediatric patient with tracheomalacia? [Letter to the Editor] *Pediatr Pulmonol* 2018;53(1):9. doi: 10.1002/ppul.23914.

[12] Sato A, Hamada S, Ishigami T. Effect of long-term domiciliary high-flow nasal cannula use in a child with atypical CHARGE syndrome. *Arch Bronconeumol* 2019;55(4):219-220.

[13] Dres M, Demoule A. What every intensivist should know about using high-flow nasal oxygen for critically ill patients. *Rev Bras Ter Intensiva* 2017;29(4):399-403. doi: 10.5935/0103-507X.20170060.

[14] Nishimura M. High-flow nasal cannula oxygen therapy in adults: physiological benefits, indication, clinical benefits, and adverse effects. *Respir Care* 2016;61(4):529-41.

[15] Hasan RA, Habib RH. Effects of flow rate and airleak at the nares and mouth opening on positive distending pressure delivery using commercially available high-flow nasal cannula systems: a lungmodel study. *Pediatr Crit Care Med* 2011;12(1):e29-e33.

[16] Chang GY, Cox CA, Shaffer TH. Nasal cannula, CPAP, and high-flow nasal cannula: effect of flow on temperature, humidity, pressure, and resistance. *Biomed Instrum Technol* 2011;45:69-74.

[17] Sivieri EM, Gerdes JS, Abbasi S. Effect of HFNC flow rate, cannula size, and nares diameter on generated airway pressures: an in vitro study. *Pediatr Pulmonol* 2013;48:506-514.

[18] Piper L, Stalets EL, Statile AM. Clinical Progress Note: High flow nasal cannula Therapy for bronchiolitis outside the ICU in infants. *J Hosp Med* 2020;1;49-51. Published Online First November 20, 2019. doi:10.12788/jhm.3328.

[19] Díaz-Lobato S, Perales JMC, Íñigo JMA, Alises SM, Segovia B, et al. Things to keep in mind in high flow therapy: as usual the devil is in the detail. *Int J Crit Care Emerg Med* 2018; 4:048. doi. org/10.23937/2474-3674/1510048.

[20] Kwon JW. High-flow nasal cannula oxygen therapy in children: a clinical review. *Clin Exp Pediatr* 2020;63(1):3-7. doi:10.3345/kjp.2019.00626.

[21] Yurtseven A, Saz EU, Hennes H. Safety and Efficacy of High-flow Nasal Cannula Therapy in the Pediatric Emergency Department. *J Pediatr Emerg Intensive Care* Med 2019;6:121-129.

[22] Slain KN, Shein SL, Rotta AT. The use of high-flow nasal cannula in the pediatric emergency department. *J Pediatr (Rio J)* 2017;93:36-45.

[23] Er A, Çağlar A, Akgül F, Ulusoy E, Çitlenbik H, Yılmaz D, Duman M. Early predictors of unresponsiveness to high-flow nasal cannula therapy in a pediatric emergency department. *Pediatr Pulmonol* 2018;53(6):809-815.

[24] Mayfield S, Bogossian F, O'Malley L, Schibler A. High-flow nasal cannula oxygen therapy for infants with bronchiolitis: pilot study, *J Paediatr Child Health* 2014;50:373-378.

[25] Metge P, Grimaldi C, Hassid S, Thomachot L, Loundou A, Martin C, et al. Comparison of a high-flow humidified nasal cannula to nasal continuous positive airway pressure in children with acute bronchiolitis: experience in a pediatric intensive care unit. *Eur J Pediatr* 2014;173:953-958.

[26] Milési C, Boubal M, Jacquot A, Baleine J, Durand S, Odena MP, Cambonie G. High-flow nasal cannula: recommendations for daily practice in pediatrics. *Ann Intensive Care* 2014;4:29. doi: 10.1186/s13613-014-0029-5.

[27] Schmid F, Olbertz DM, Ballmann M. The use of high-flow nasal cannula (HFNC) as respiratory support in neonatal and pediatric intensive care units in Germany - A nationwide survey. *Respir Med* 2017;131:210-214. doi: 10.1016/j.rmed.2017. 08.027.

[28] Rodriguez M, Thille AW, Boissier F, Veinstein A, Chatellier D, Robert R, et al. Predictors of successful separation from high-fow nasal oxygen therapy in patients with acute respiratory failure: a retrospective monocenter study. *Ann. Intensive Care* 2019;9:101. https://doi.org/10.1186/s13613-019-0578-8.

[29] Roca O, Caralt B, Messika J, Samper M, Sztrymf B, Hernández G, et al. An index combining respiratory rate and oxygenation to predict outcome of nasal high-flow therapy. *Am J Respir Crit Care Med* 2019;199(11):1368-1376.

[30] König K, Stock EL, Jarvis M. Noise levels of neonatal high-flow nasal cannula devices--an in-vitro study. *Neonatology* 2013;103(4):264-267. doi:10.1159/ 000346764.

[31] Koga Y, Kaneda K, Mizuguchi I, Nakahara T, Miyauchi T, Fujita M, et al. Extent of pleural effusion on chest radiograph is associated with failure of high-flow nasal cannula oxygen therapy. *J Crit Care* 2016;32:165-9.

[32] Inata Y, Takeuchi M. Complex effects of high-flow nasal cannula therapy on hemodynamics in the pediatric patient after cardiac surgery. *J Intensive Care* 2017;5:30. doi: 10.1186/s40560-017-0227-y.

[33] Kang BJ, Koh Y, Lim CM, Huh JW, Baek S, Han M, et al. Failure of high-flow nasal cannula therapy may delay intubation and increase mortality. *Intensive Care Med* 2015;41(4):623-32.

[34] Nishimura M. High-flow nasal cannula oxygen therapy in adults. *J Intensive Care* 2015 Mar 31;3(1):15. doi: 10.1186/s40560-015-0084-5.

[35] Baudin F, Gagnon S, Crulli B, Proulx F, Jouvet P, Emeriaud G. Modalities and complications associated with the use of high-flow nasal cannula: experience in a pediatric ICU. *Respir Care* 2016;61(10):1305-10. doi: 10.4187/respcare.04452.

[36] Hegde S, Prodhan P. Serious air leak syndrome complicating high-flow nasal cannula therapy: a report of 3 cases. *Pediatrics* 2013;131:939-944.

[37] Jasin LR, Kern S, Thompson S, Walter C, Rone JM, Yohannan MD. Subcutaneous scalp emphysema, pneumo-orbitis and pneumocephalus in a neonate on high humidity high flow nasal cannula. *J Perinatol* 2008;28(11):779-81.

[38] Kotecha SJ, Adappa R, Gupta N, Watkins WJ, Kotecha S, Chakraborty M. Safety and Efficacy of High-Flow Nasal Cannula Therapy in Preterm Infants: A Meta-analysis. *Pediatrics* 2015;136(3):542-553.

[39] Ward JJ. High-flow oxygen administration by nasal cannula for adult and perinatal patients. *Respir Care* 2013;58(1):98-122.

[40] DiBlasi RM. Neonatal noninvasive ventilation techniques: do we really need to intubate?. *Respir Care*. 2011;56(9):1273-1297. doi:10.4187/respcare.01376.

[41] Abdel-Hady H, Shouman B, Aly H. Early weaning from CPAP to high flow nasal cannula in preterm infants is associated with prolonged oxygen requirement: a randomized controlled trial. *Early Hum Dev* 2011;87(3):205-208.

[42] Sasi A, Malhotra A. High flow nasal cannula for continuous positive airway pressure weaning in preterm neonates: a single-centre experience. *J Paediatr Child Health* 2015;51(2):199-203.

[43] Hoffman SB, Terrell N, Driscoll CH, Davis NL. Impact of high-flow nasal cannula use on neonatal respiratory support patterns and length of stay. *Respir Care* 2016;61(10):1299-304.

[44] Healy LI, Corcoran P, Murphy BP. High-flow nasal cannulae, bronchopulmonary dysplasia and retinopathy of prematurity. *Ir Med J* 2019;112(8):985.

[45] Heath Jeffery RC, Todd DA. Heated Humidified High-Flow Nasal Cannula: Impact on Neonatal Outcomes. *Respir Care* 2016;61(10):1428-1429. doi:10.4187/respcare.05151.

In: Non-Invasive Mechanical Ventilation Complications
Editor: Antonio M. Esquinas
ISBN: 978-1-53619-515-6

Chapter 33

General Non-Invasive Ventilation Complications in Acute and Chronic Paediatric Applications

Paula Santos Herraiz * ***and María Herrera López***
Department of Paediatric Intensive Care,
Toledo University Hospital, Toledo, Spain

Abstract

Complications of Non-Invasive Ventilation are similar both in paediatric and adult patients. The real incidence is still unknown, it varies between 10 - 20% according to previous papers, being skin lesions the most common.

Major complications are serious yet very uncommon: barotrauma, aspiration pneumonia or hemodynamic effects. Minor complications are more frequent: skin and mucosal lesions, gastric distention, and irritative conjunctivitis.

Keywords: non-invasive ventilators, paediatric, complications, noninvasive ventilation, critical care

Abbreviation

Non Invasive Ventilation	NIV

* Corresponding Author's E-mail: pau@isobox.es.

Introduction

Complications of Non-Invasive Ventilation (NIV) are adverse events that appear after its application and are exclusively attributed to its use. In this chapter, we will not talk about technical problems (such as auto-cycling or desynchronization), this topic will be addressed in other chapters of this manual.

The majority of the information gathered in this chapter comes from adult-based studies, however complications are almost the same in children, so they can be extrapolated.

The incidence in adult patients ranges between 10% and 20%, being cutaneous necrosis due to interface pressure the most reported, while gastric distension, pneumothorax or aspiration pneumonia are infrequent complications [1].

In a Spanish prospective study that included 72 asthma episodes treated with NIV in children, 11 cases developed irritative dermatitis, 4 cases presented gastric distension and there were one barotrauma and one upper tract bleeding cases [2].

We will discuss separately the most frequent major and minor complications [3]. In addition, other less common adverse effects are also listed. Preventive measures are also explained in order to minimize the risk of appearance.

Major Complications

Major complications are infrequent, but can become serious for the patient and have an impact on the effectiveness of NIV.

1. *Barotrauma.* The risk of barotrauma or air leakage is low, the same as pneumothorax, pneumomediastinum, or subcutaneous emphysema. In the previously cited study in paediatric patients, 3% [2] were affected and in adults the range reported is between 1% and 10%.
   Barotrauma should be expected and suspected before respiratory conditions get worse. To avoid this situation, continuous monitoring of the patient becomes essential (minimum heart rate and oxygen saturation levels), and adjust ventilator parameters to achieve the patient needings, using the least aggressive measures possible (use the minimum positive pressures needed).
2. *Aspiration pneumonia.* Patients who maintain oral or nasogastric tube feeding, are at risk of vomiting and pulmonary aspiration, especially in those using a facial interface. The risk is also increased when high pressures are programmed. Prophylactic measures to decompress the stomach (such as indicating naso / oro-gastric tubes) can also increase vomiting risk and should be avoided if possible. In some cases, nausea can be treated with antiemetics. Although pulmonary

aspiration cases have been reported, this is an infrequent complication as long as VIN is avoided in patients with altered neurological status, absence of protective airway reflexes, or difficulty managing secretions [3].
In chronic patients who require NIV, the use of nasal interfaces become a good option because of the lower pulmonary aspiration risk.

3. *Hemodynamic instability.* Deteriorating cardiac output secondary to a reduction in preload due to positive pressure ventilation has been described [4].
Nevertheless, this is an uncommon complication even more if we follow NIV indications and assess the patient frequently and diligently, avoiding delayed intubation in shock patients who do not respond quickly to fluids reposition and inotropic drugs.

Minor Complications

Minor complications generally do not interfere with the effectiveness of NIV and can be easily resolved to make the patient feel more comfortable.

1. *Skin lesions.* Dermatitis, pressure ulcers and skin necrosis have been one of the most frequent reported complications in patients who require continuous NIV.
There is a distinct correlation between the occurrence of this condition and patients undergoing NIV. Skin lesions can occur at any location where the interface lean on, typically in the nasal bridge of patients using nasal or oronasal interfaces. In a study including 25 pediatric patients using the facial interface, 5 patients developed skin ulcers in those areas where the mask leaned on [5]
Skin lesions can be prevented by using specially designed dressings and introducing regularly rotation of the interface. This is essential for chronic patients undergoing home NIV.
2. *Lesions of the nasal mucose.* Mainly related to the use of nasal masks or nasal cannulas and olives. There is an induced mucosal hypersecretion which can obstruct the nostrils.
When oral leaks are present, the absence of humidity increase nasal resistance and decrease both tidal volume and patient comfort [6]. Furthermore, the absence of humidification can dry out the mucosa and even result in epistaxis. That's why air humidification is recommended in all patients undergoing NIV.
3. *Gastric distention.* Gastric distention usually appears when inspiratory pressures are higher than 25cmH2O.
Nevertheless, in neuromuscular patients gastric distention can occur with pressures below 20cmH2O due to diaphragmatic muscles and lower esophageal sphincter weakness.

This distention can possibly induce vomiting, leading to aspiration problems, especially in patients using a facial interface.

Keeping patients calm, using sedation to achieve this goal if necessary, and adjusting ventilator parameters to ensure the minimum support needed, can also be helpful preventing gastric distention. In children wearing gastric tubes, regular opening may be useful. However, prophylactic decompression through the placement of a naso- or oro-gastric tubes could induce vomiting or increase risks and it's not recommended.

4. *Irritant conjunctivitis.* Ocular trauma or corneal ulcers can potentially occur if the edges of the mask are in contact with the ocular surface. In the case of nasal or oro-nasal interfaces, air leakage through the edges can cause conjunctival irritation and even corneal ulcers.

   In both cases, prevention and treatment essentially consists of proper adjustment of the mask or change of interface position to the one that best suits the patient.

OTHER COMPLICATIONS

Several complications have been reported in the literature, but are infrequent or very uncommon [6].

1. *Maxillary hypoplasia.* Patients undergoing home NIV with nasal interface for long periods have been associated with underdevelopment of the malar massif and secondary malocclusion.
2. *Vertebrobasilar ischemia.* Excessive restraint with straps can cause ischemic brain lesions by compression of the basilar circulation due to bone plasticity in newborn patients.
3. *Axillary vein thrombosis.* The "Helmet" type interface is fixed with straps below the armpits, this can potentially increase the risk of thrombosis.

   There are several models designed for infants, for instance, specific harness that supports the diaper area to avoid this complication.

REFERENCES

[1] Esquinas, A. *Fundamentos de metodología y organización hospitalaria en Ventilación Mecánica No Invasiva.* 3ª edición. [*Fundamentals of methodology and hospital organization in Non-Invasive Mechanical Ventilation.*]

[2] Mayordomo-Colunga, J., Medina, A., Rey, C. et al. Non-invasive ventilation in pediatric status asthmaticus: A prospective observational study. *Pediatr. Pulmonol.,* 2011; 46:949.

[3] Uptodate.

[4] Teague, W. G. Non-invasive positive pressure ventilation: Current status in paediatric patients. *Paediatr. Respir. Rev.*, 2005; 6:52.

[5] Yañez, L. J., Yunge, M., Emilfork, M. et al. A prospective, randomized, controlled trial of noninvasive ventilation in pediatric acute respiratory failure. *Pediatr. Crit. Care Med.*, 2008; 9:484.

[6] Pons, M., Balaguer, M. *Complicaciones y problemas técnicos de la ventilación no invasiva.* En: Medina, A., Pons, M., Martinón-Torres, F. *Ventilación No Invasiva en Pediatría.* 2ª Edición. Madrid: Ergon; 2009. p. 85 - 90. [*Non-Invasive Ventilation in Pediatrics*.]

[7] Padman, R., Lawless, S. T., Kettrick, R. G. Noninvasive ventilation via bilevel positive airway pressure support in pediatric practice. *Crit. Care Med.,* 1998; 26:169.

[8] Akingbola, O. A., Hopkins, R. L. Pediatric noninvasive positive pressure ventilation. *Pediatr. Crit. Care Med.,* 2001; 2:164.

[9] Carroll, C. L., Zucker, A. R. Barotrauma not related to type of positive pressure ventilation during severe asthma exacerbations in children. *J. Asthma,* 2008; 45:421.

[10] Chynkiamis, N., Armstrong, M., Manifield, J. et al. Hemodynamic effects of portable non-invasive ventilation in healthy men. *Respir. Physio. Neurobiol.*, 2019 Oct.; 268:103248.

In: Non-Invasive Mechanical Ventilation Complications ISBN: 978-1-53619-515-6
Editor: Antonio M. Esquinas

Chapter 34

Complications during Non-Invasive Mechanical Ventilation. Malar Hypoplasia

María Ana Pasquali de Sidi-Said*, MD
Pediatrician, PhD in Medicine and Surgery, Chief of the Intermediate Care Unit, Misericordia Nuevo Siglo Hospital, Córdoba, Argentina

Abstract

Non-invasive mechanical ventilation (NIV) at home has been widely used since 1981 to date in both children and adults. There are several complications reported in the literature, the most frequent being conjunctivitis and skin lesions, the rarest being malar hypoplasia. There are several theories to explain this complication in pediatrics. When using NIV for chronic pediatric patients, it should be kept in mind that children's faces are in process of development. The treatment involves a multidisciplinary team of pediatricians, dentists, surgeons, and speech therapists.

Keywords: malar hypoplasia, non-invasive mechanical ventilation, complication, children

The use of non-invasive home mechanical ventilation (NIHMV), has been widely used in both the adult and child at home, with a good response, the first publications date from 1981 [1].

The chronic use of NIHMV, leads to various complications, the most common are skin lesions, conjunctivitis. The rarest being maxillary hypoplasia.

---

* Corresponding Author's E-mail: marianapa428@yahoo.com.

Hypoplasia of the upper jaw is a very rare complication in pediatric patients. In the medical literature, there are only a few cases described [2].

Maxillary hypoplasia or in other words, a lack of development of the upper jaw bones. This results in the patient having half of the face with a sunken appearance and the lower jaw protruding much more than normal.

It is important to be aware of the possible theories of jaw growth control according to Proffit. It is true that growth depends significantly on genetic factors, but it can also be greatly affected by the role played by the environment, in the form of nutritional level, amount of physical activity, health status and other factors.

In the last few years, three important theories have tried to explain the factors that determine craniofacial growth: 1. The bone, like other tissues; is the main factor that determines its own growth (Sicher). 2. Cartilage is the main factor that determines bone growth, while bone responds in a secondary and passive way (Scott). 3. The soft tissue matrix in which the skeletal elements are found is the main determinant of growth and both bone and cartilage are secondary followers (Melvin Moss).

Supporters of Scott's (cartilage theory) postulate that the nasal cartilaginous septum acts as a regulator of other facets of jaw growth. The cartilage is located so that its growth could easily produce an anteroinferior displacement of the upper jaw.

However, the decline in growth in experimental animals is remarkable enough to suggest that septal cartilage has some innate growth potential. This theory is very important, considering that the nasal interface is the most used in NIHMV, this would lead to compression of the nasal septum, producing a decrease in bone tissue and resulting in maxillary hypoplasia.

By age 4, 60% of the adult face has been developed. It has been shown that the growth in width of the jawbone in the middle suture continues until the juvenile stage, between approximately 17 and 18 years of age and parallel to the growth curve in height [3].

This complication was reported in 68% of the cases and 37% presented alteration in dental occlusion, with different degrees, in patients using chronic non-invasive ventilation (NIV) [4].

When using NIV chronically in pediatric patients, it should be kept in mind that children's faces are in the process of development.

The use of NIHMV is more frequent in children with craniofacial malformations, trisomy 21, obesity, neuromuscular diseases (Figure 1), Wiedemann-Beckwith syndrome, cleft palate, obstructive sleep apnea 2. These pathologies are strongly associated with hypoplasia, but not the type of mask, age or gender of the child [5-6]. In a univariate and multivariate analysis, it was found association with retropulsion of the lower jaw when using more than 10 hours per day [7].

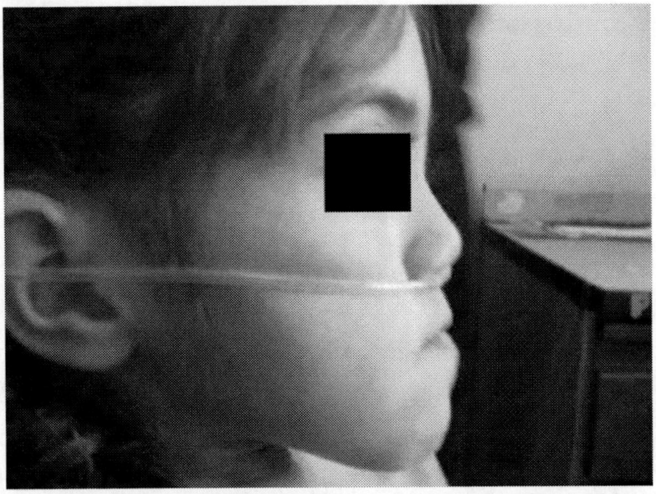

Figure 1. Maxillary hypoplasia with pseudo prognathism of the lower jaw.

At first sight, aesthetically it can influence in an important way the patient's daily life but it can also cause problems to eat therefore the sooner it is diagnosed and treated, better results and better quality of life will be obtained.

A comprehensive evaluation should be performed along with maxillofacial surgery. The complementary methods have been changing over the years, from x-rays, through pantomography and finally the computed tomography (Figure 2), which allows us to measure the different angles needed to perform the appropriate treatment.

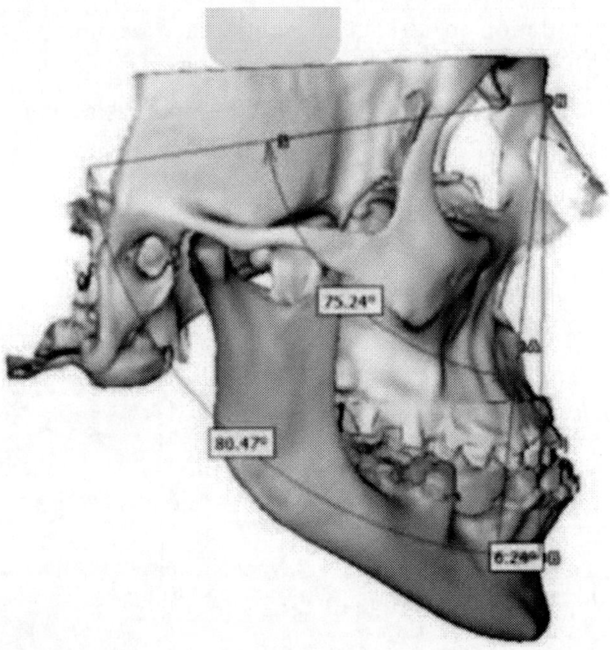

Figure 2. Maxillary Hypoplasia CT.

The procedure consists of dental treatment, bone advancement surgery, as well as some refinements of soft structures, which may or may not be accompanied by rhinoplasty. The ideal age is 17 years old or older, having undergone medical treatment with the orthodontist [8].

REFERENCES

[1] Sullivan C. E., Berthon-Jones M., Isa F. G. Reserva lof obstructive sleep apnea by continous positive airway presure applied through the nose. *Lancet* 1981:1:862-863.

[2] Li K. K., Riley R. W., Guilleminault C. An unreported risk in the use of home nasak continuous poistive airway pressure and home nasal ventilation in children. *Chest* 2000; 117:916-918.

[3] Sorolla J. P. *Anomalías craneofaciales.* RMCLC doi: https://10.1016/S0716-8640 (10)70500-9.

[4] Villa M. P., Pagani J., Ambrosio R. et al., Mid-face hipoplasia after long-term nasal ventilation. *Am J Respir Crit Care Med* 2002; 166:1142-1143.

[5] Fauroux B., Lavis J. F., Nicot F., et al., Facial side effects during noninvasive positive pressure ventilation in childre. *Intensive Care Med* 2009; 31 (7):965-9.

[6] Fauroux B., Lavis J. F., Nicot F. et al., Facial side effects during noninvasive positive pressure ventilation in children. *Intensive Care Med* 2005, 31:965-9.

[7] Castro-Codesal M. L., Olmstead D. L., MacLean J. E. Mask intefaces for home non-invasive ventilation in infants and children. *Paediatric Respiratory Reviews,* https://doi.org/10.1016/j.prrv2019.03.004.

[8] Rodríguez González L. Tratamiento de la hipoplasia anteroposterior maxilar. *Medicentro Electrónica* 2020, 24(1): 29-32.

In: Non-Invasive Mechanical Ventilation Complications ISBN: 978-1-53619-515-6
Editor: Antonio M. Esquinas

Chapter 35

Complications during Long Term Non-Invasive Mechanical Ventilation

Oktay Demirkiran * ***and Olcay Dilken***
Istanbul University - Cerrahpasa, Cerrahpasa Medical School,
Department of Anaesthesiology and Intensive Care, Istanbul, Turkey

Abstract

Noninvasive ventilation has been used as a short term adjunct to the main therapy in acute critical settings like pneumonia, postoperative hypoxemia or acute exacerbation of chronic obstructive pulmonary disease. In these cases, typically, a short trial of NIV is commonly applied. Subsequently, careful evolution of the patient is required to assess the positive (or negative) effects of the treatment to continue the NIV or not. However, NIV can also be employed for longer durations as in sleep apnea, chronic obstructive pulmonary disease and neuromuscular disorders. NIV improves daytime sleepiness, lung functions and gas exchange in Obstructive Sleep Apnea Syndrome and. End stage Chronic Obstructive Pulmonary Disease (COPD) patients commonly develop hypercapnic respiratory failure. Eventually, fatigue, daytime headache, dyspnea and impaired Quality of Life (QoL) is encountered. Long term NIV application may partially alleviate these symptoms and improves QoL and reduce mortality improves oxygenation, decreases dyspnea and increases walking distance. Neuromuscular Disorders (NMDs) are heterogeneous group of diseases and their response to NIV differs. Commonly, Work of Breathing (WoB) is significantly increased at the expense of already weakened respiratory muscles. The imbalance between the WOB and the muscle capacity elicits a typical pattern of rapid shallow breathing. Some disorders such as Spinal Muscular Atrophy or mitochondrial diseases requires very early respiratory support. On the other hand, respiratory failure may develop slowly and gradually or they may never require respiratory support during the course. Air leaks and pressure wounds due to interfaces can be encountered in long term NIV. In conclusion, long term NIV therapy is a

* Corresponding Author's E-mail: odemirkiran@yahoo.com.

significant burden both to the patient and to the caregivers. Its success relies on a collaboration between the patient, the caregiver and the clinician.

Keywords: non-invasive ventilation, long term, complications, apnea, neuromuscular

Non-invasive ventilation (NIV) has been increasingly used in a wide array of diseases. It is commonly employed during episodes of hypoxemia, hypercarbia, weaning and end-of-life care settings. Usually, a trial of NIV is applied to the patient and after a pre-set time, a careful evolution of the patient is required to assess the positive (or negative) effects of the treatment [1]. This pre-set time can be as short as half an hour, such as in spontaneous breathing trials. It can extend to several hours as in hypoxemia or a few days as in hypercarbia. However, NIV can also be employed for longer durations as in sleep apnea, chronic obstructive pulmonary disease and neuromuscular disorders.

Physiological Effects of NIV

NIV applies a positive pressure to the airways and lungs via an interface. The primary effect of NIV is to maintain oxygenation and removal of carbon dioxide, while offloading respiratory muscles. While effects of NIV are close to invasive ventilation in many aspects, there are important differences. Appliance of NIV is prone to substantial air leaks and this can prevent reaching target pressure and volume. Leaks can also cause triggering and patient ventilator asynchrony. NIV can also cause gastric distention if high enough pressures are applied to the upper airways. This makes patients prone to aspiration from distended stomach. However, there are also many advantages of NIV. Patients are able to talk and swallow during therapy intervals which greatly improves patient comfort and reduce the need for sedation. It also maintains upper airway opening. All of these effects make NIV an ideal choice for patients suffering from obstructive sleep apnea, obesity hypoventilation syndrome and chronic obstructive pulmonary disease (COPD) [2].

NIV enhances tidal volumes by increasing pressure and flow. Minute ventilation is also increased, unless there is a significant increase in dead space. Eventually, additional O_2 is provided to the alveoli and excess CO_2 is removed. However, positive pressure breaths provided by the mechanical ventilator are distributed to highly compliant and low resistance alveoli. This may create regional overdistention albeit normal tidal volumes. In this manner, NIV can also lead to ventilator-induced lung injury [3]. High tidal volumes and pressures excessively stretch alveoli and if applied for prolonged intervals, increases the risk of parenchymal damage. Diffuse alveolar damage ensues and proinflammatory cytokines are released which subsequently has systemic effects. Lung protective settings reduces the risk of VILI. However, even in the absence of high volumes or pressures, rigorous patient effort can also increase transpulmonary pressures and lead to lung injury.

Diaphragm is the primary muscle of ventilation. It consists of fatigue resistant type I muscle fibres, and has increased mitochondrial and capillary density compared to limb muscles. Thus, it can extract O_2 several folds more compared to the latter. However, intrinsic positive pressure, as seen in COPD patients, flattens the diaphragm, displacing it to an unfavourable length-tension curve. Additional malnutrition, anemia or hypoxemia only worsens the muscle failure. Ventilatory muscle failure is associated with alveolar hypoventilation and results in to hypercarbia. Additionally, high resistive loads due to COPD or high elastance due to parenchymal lung diseases imposes an even higher workload to inspiratory muscles. NIV can reduce muscle fatigue by unloading respiratory muscles and reducing the neural respiratory drive by improving ventilation. Resting of the overloaded muscles during NIV also improves muscle function when NIV is not in use [4].

NIV can recruit collapsed alveoli by providing PEEP. As a result, ventilation/perfusion mismatch and gas exchange improve. Also, alveoli are protected from atelectotrauma. However, it can also over distend or poorly recruit the alveoli [5]. Thus, optimizing PEEP requires a balance between these two circumstances.

Apart from its effects on the lungs, NIV can be either detrimental or beneficial to the heart. As positive pressure is applied to the lungs, the intrathoracic pressure is also increased which impedes venous return to the right atrium. This can decrease pulmonary perfusion and increase right ventricular afterload. However, it also improves left ventricular function due to reduced left ventricular afterload. Consequently, patients with left ventricular failure may benefit from NIV treatment and removal of NIV can lead to alveolar flooding [6].

NIV for OSAS and OHS

Obstructive Sleep Apnea Syndrome (OSAS) is characterized by partial or complete obstruction of the airways during sleep which results in desaturation, daytime sleepiness and eventually left and right ventricular dysfunction. It is commonly manifested as obesity-hypoventilation syndrome (OHS). 90% of the patients with OHS have sleep apnea. Hypotonia of the respiratory muscles, i.e., intercostal muscles, and reduced lung volume due to atelectasis leads to nocturnal desaturation and hypercapnia. Additionally, fat accumulates around the lateral aspect of the pharynx facilitating collapse and apnea [7]. Treatment includes weight loss, upper airway surgery and implementation of CPAP during sleep. The duration of treatment with NIV or CPAP is lifelong.

Administering positive airway pressure to the upper airways substantially increase sleep quality and subsequent day time performance. NIV reduces mechanical load on the respiratory muscles and allows them to work more efficiently during daytime after a night long treatment. CPAP is also effective as it prevents repetitive collapse of the upper airways. However, more severe patients eventually require NIV, mostly in the form of bilevel positive airway pressure. NIV also recruits atelectasis which results in a greater functional lung volume.

Short term effects of CPAP include an improvement in gas exchange in a period of 1 to 3 months. Long term effects include improved lung function, and a less blunted CO_2 response. Treatment failure of CPAP is defined as daytime $PaCO_2$ >45 mm Hg, sustained desaturation during sleep. Although both CPAP and NIV improves sleep quality, NIV can achieve greater improvement in terms of lung function. In a retrospective study with a follow-up duration of 8 ± 4.8 years, Baseline Body Mass Index (BMI), FEV_1/FVC, Supplemental oxygen requirement and weight gain during the study follow-up were associated with CPAP failure [8]. Additionally, in a randomized controlled trial comparing NIV to lifestyle changes, NIV was associated with a significantly greater reduction in $PaCO_2$ and improvement in Quality of Life (QoL) assessments [9]. Finally, OHS patients are at increased risk of mortality. In a retrospective study comparing OHS and OSAS patients, OHS patients mainly died from heart failure and respiratory failure was infrequent among both groups [10]. These results show that CPAP effectively provides the patency of the upper airway. On the other hand, NIV should be started in patients suffering from daytime hypercarbia as opposed to CPAP alone. However, introducing mandatory breaths during sleep time can lead to asynchronies with the patient effort. Polysomnography, ventilator software and pulse oximetry are used to assess the efficacy of the treatment. Increases in upper airway resistance and inappropriate interfaces and subsequent leaks are other events that can reduce the effectiveness of CPAP and NIV. Switching interfaces in such cases can be beneficial.

NIV for COPD

Chronic Obstructive Pulmonary Disease (COPD) is the fourth most common cause of mortality around the world [4]. Patients frequently have exacerbations during the course of the disease and the long-term mortality following acute exacerbation is quite high. Patients discharged after such an exacerbation face increased risk of readmission and eventually, death. End stage COPD patients commonly develop hypercapnic respiratory failure. Eventually, fatigue, daytime headache, dyspnea and impaired QoL is encountered.

Long-term NIV relieves patient symptoms and improves QoL and reduce mortality improves oxygenation, decreases dyspnea and increases walking distance [11, 12]. NIV achieves these effects by unloading respiratory muscles and reducing work of breathing (WOB) by alleviating intrinsic PEEP. PEEP (or Expiratory positive airway pressure –

EPAP), might reduce dynamic hyperinflation which facilitates triggering supportive breaths. Combination of these effects relieves dyspnea and improves exercise induced hyperlactatemia. Long term NIV reduces readmissions in hypercapnic COPD patients [13]. Additionally, two RCTs showed reduced mortality with NIV use in stable COPD patients [14]. A metanalysis of six RCTs showed significant reduction in $PaCO_2$ and a trend towards improved survival in those with initial hypercapnia. Current guidelines suggest long term nocturnal NIV use in chronic stable hypercapnic COPD [4, 15]. Although long-term NIV use is rising, the survival remains poor. In a recent cohort of 1746 patients, 5 year survival after home NIV initiation was 58% [16]. Adherence to treatment, i.e., NIV use >4 hours per night, was associated with increased survival.

COPD patients may also have other comorbidities, namely ischaemic cardiac disease. Airway pressures are relatively lower in NIV, compared to invasive ventilation. However, excess positive airway pressures may jeopardise cardiovascular function and reduce the cardiac output. In a study among advanced stage COPD patients, an IPAP of 16 cm H_2O improved stroke volume. However, stroke volume and cardiac output were reduced in a subgroup of patients with severe dynamic hyperinflation [17]. In another study, long-term NIV did not have an adverse effect on cardiac performance [18]. Nevertheless, a thorough evaluation of cardiac function is necessary prior to long term NIV therapy. Older age is also associated with poor prognosis in long term NIV. Additionally, mental disability, cachexia and lack of sufficient caregivers can reduce the effectiveness of NIV in this group of patients.

COPD patients require extended periods of NIV therapy, such as 6 hours per day. Selection of the correct interface is critical. Long term NIV can be delivered by nasal, oronasal or full-face masks. Although patients have more comfort with nasal masks, they are prone to leaks, which results in reduced alveolar ventilation. Currently, there is no evidence to confirm greater benefit among interfaces. As a result, interfaces should be chosen to patient needs.

NIV for Neuromuscular Disorders

Neuromuscular diseases affect a number of structures including the motor nerves, neuromuscular junctions or the muscles [19]. Spinal cord traumas, demyelinating diseases, amyotrophic lateral sclerosis (ALS), spinal muscular atrophy, myasthenia gravis, lambert-eaton syndrome, corticosteroids, muscular dystrophies and metabolic disorders such as glycogen storage diseases or Pompe's, all affect the neuromuscular system. Ultimately, they cause respiratory insufficiency albeit with different mechanisms. Their onset and progression can be quite variable.

Table 1. Neuromuscular Disorders with Respiratory Failure

Rate of respiratory failure occurrence	Disease
Certain	Duchenne Muscular Dystrophy Amyotrophic Lateral Sclerosis
Frequent	Spinal Muscular Atrophy- Type 2 Myotonic Dystrophy Guillain-Barré syndrome Myasthenia Gravis
Infrequent	Becker Muscular Dystrophy Inflammatory Myopathies Spinal Muscular Atrophy- Type 3
Rare	Chronic inflammatory demyelinating polyneuropathy

Respiratory muscle weakness is the inability of the rested muscles to generate adequate pressure and flow during inspiration and expiration [20]. Ventilatory muscle strength is diminished in most cases. A reduction in vital capacity greater than 19% implies diaphragm weakness. Patients with diaphragm weakness may feel dyspnea while lying flat, such as during the night. Initially, muscle weakness and subsequent respiratory failure can only be nocturnal. Coughing is also impaired and is caused by both the inspiratory and expiratory muscle weakness. Deterioration of the coughing function exposes patients to recurrent infections, hypoxemia and hypercarbia. A cough peak flow less than 160 L/min indicates inadequate clearance of secretions. Bulbar involvement of the diseases also impairs coughing function. Sleep disorders are also common and worsens with disease progression. In addition to the muscle weakness that results in hypoventilation, drive to breath can also be impaired especially in myotonic and muscular dystrophies. Finally, respiratory system compliance is markedly reduced in these patients. Loss of respiratory system volume, atelectasis and increased chest wall rigidity can be the underlying reason. Whatever the reason is, WOB is significantly increased at the expense of already weakened respiratory muscles. The imbalance between the WOB and the muscle capacity elicits a typical pattern of rapid shallow breathing.

NMDs are heterogeneous group of diseases and response to NIV also differs. Some disorders such as SMA or mitochondrial diseases requires very early respiratory support. On the other hand, respiratory failure may develop slowly and gradually or they may never require respiratory support during the course (Table 1) [20]. However, aims in this patient population are common and can be listed as relieving symptoms, reducing hospital admission and increasing quality of life.

NIV significantly improves survival in Duchenne Muscular Dystrophy and can be beneficial in ALS [21]. In this groups, NIV should be initiated in patients with nocturnal hypoventilation. CPAP is not appropriate because the essential problem in these patients is hypoventilation in which CPAP is ineffective. Another indication for NIV in ALS patients is reduction of FVC < 50% [22]. However, most ALS patients demand initiation of NIV therapy at the onset of respiratory symptoms, such as dyspnea. Again, nasal masks, oronasal masks and face masks can be used. Nasal masks can lead to significant air leakage if the mouth remains open during sleep. Air leakages cause asynchrony and loss of efficacy of NIV therapy [23]. A chin strap can help in this situation. Interchanging masks reduces the risk of skin ulcerations. Unfortunately, if the disease is progressive, day time NIV use and eventually invasive ventilation or tracheostomy is needed. Additionally, patients with bulbar involvement will transit to invasive ventilation earlier due to unmanageable sialorrhea or emotional lability.

Conclusion

Long-term NIV and CPAP use has been rising steadily in the last decades. Air leaks and pressure wounds due to interfaces can be encountered. These can be addressed by changing interfaces. However, bulbar dysfunction and cognitive impairment are key determinants of NIV compliance. The bottom line is that, long term NIV therapy is a significant burden both to the patient and to the caregivers [21]. Its success relies on a collaboration between the patient, the caregiver and the clinician. Therefore, all aspects of the therapy, i.e., tracheostomy or withdrawal of support, should be discussed before initiation.

References

[1] Thille A. W., Frat J. P. Noninvasive ventilation as acute therapy. *Curr Opin Crit Care.* 2018; 24(6):519-24.

[2] MacIntyre N. R. Physiologic Effects of Noninvasive Ventilation. *Respiratory Care.* 2019 Jun 1; 64(6):617-28.

[3] Grieco D. L., Menga L. S., Eleuteri D., Antonelli M. Patient self-inflicted lung injury: implications for acute hypoxemic respiratory failure and ARDS patients on non-invasive support. *Minerva Anestesiol.* 2019 Sep; 85(9):1014-23.

[4] Macrea M., Oczkowski S., Rochwerg B., Branson R. D., Celli B., Coleman J. M., et al., Long-Term Noninvasive Ventilation in Chronic Stable Hypercapnic Chronic Obstructive Pulmonary Disease. An Official American Thoracic Society Clinical Practice Guideline. *Am J Respir Crit Care Med.* 2020 Aug 15; 202(4):e74-87.

[5] Kacmarek R. M. Noninvasive Respiratory Support for Postextubation Respiratory Failure. *Respir Care.* 2019 Jun; 64(6):658-78.

[6] Bello G., De Santis P., Antonelli M. Non-invasive ventilation in cardiogenic pulmonary edema. *Ann Transl Med.* 2018 Sep; 6(18):355.

[7] Ramírez-Molina V. R., Gómez-de-Terreros F. J., Barca-Durán J., Masa J. F. Non-invasive Positive Airway Pressure in Obesity Hypoventilation Syndrome and Chronic Obstructive Pulmonary Disease: Present and Future Perspectives. *COPD.* 2017 Aug; 14(4):418-28.

[8] de Llano L. P., Castro-Añón O., Castro-Cabana L., Méndez Marote L., Golpe R. Long-term effectiveness of CPAP in patients with severe obesity-hypoventilation syndrome. *Sleep Breath*. 2020 Aug 26;

[9] Masa J. F., Corral J., Caballero C., Barrot E., Terán-Santos J., Alonso-Álvarez M. L., et al., Non-invasive ventilation in obesity hypoventilation syndrome without severe obstructive sleep apnoea. *Thorax.* 2016 Oct; 71(10):899-906.

[10] Castro-Añón O., Llano L. A. P. de, Sánchez S. D. la F., Golpe R., Marote L. M., Castro-Castro J., et al., Obesity-Hypoventilation Syndrome: Increased Risk of Death over Sleep Apnea Syndrome. *Plos One*. 2015 ub; 10(2):e0117808.

[11] Vitacca M., Ambrosino N. Non-Invasive Ventilation as an Adjunct to Exercise Training in Chronic Ventilatory Failure: A Narrative Review. *Respiration.* 2019; 97(1):3-11.

[12] Duiverman M. L. Noninvasive ventilation in stable hypercapnic COPD: what is the evidence? *ERJ Open Res* [Internet]. 2018 Apr 9 [cited 2020 Sep 13]; 4(2). Available from: https://www.ncbi.nlm.nih.gov/pmc/articles/PMC5890025/.

[13] Ankjærgaard K. L., Maibom S. L., Wilcke J. T. Long-term non-invasive ventilation reduces readmissions in COPD patients with two or more episodes of acute hypercapnic respiratory failure. *Eur Clin Respir J.* 2016; 3:28303.

[14] Gantzhorn E. K., Prior T. S., Hilberg O. Long-term non-invasive ventilation for stable chronic hypercapnic COPD. *Eur Clin Respir J.* 2019; 6(1):1644893.

[15] Ergan B., Oczkowski S., Rochwerg B., Carlucci A., Chatwin M., Clini E., et al., European Respiratory Society guidelines on long-term home non-invasive ventilation for management of COPD. *Eur Respir J.* 2019 Sep; 54(3):1901003.

[16] Patout M., Lhuillier E., Kaltsakas G., Benattia A., Dupuis J., Arbane G., et al., Long-term survival following initiation of home non-invasive ventilation: a European study. *Thorax.* 2020 Sep 7; thoraxjnl-2019-214204.

[17] Duiverman M. L., Maagh P., Magnet F. S., Schmoor C., Arellano-Maric M. P., Meissner A., et al., Impact of High-Intensity-NIV on the heart in stable COPD: a randomised cross-over pilot study. *Respir Res.* 2017 02; 18(1):76.

[18] Funk G. C., Breyer M. K., Burghuber O. C., Kink E., Kirchheiner K., Kohansal R., et al., Long-term non-invasive ventilation in COPD after acute-on-chronic respiratory failure. *Respir Med.* 2011 Mar; 105(3):427-34.

[19] Benditt J. O. Respiratory Care of Patients with Neuromuscular Disease. *Respir Care.* 2019 Jun; 64(6):679-88.

[20] Racca F., Vianello A., Mongini T., Ruggeri P., Versaci A., Vita G. L., et al., Practical approach to respiratory emergencies in neurological diseases. *Neurol Sci.* 2020; 41(3):497-508.

[21] Crimi C., Pierucci P., Carlucci A., Cortegiani A., Gregoretti C. Long-Term Ventilation in Neuromuscular Patients: Review of Concerns, Beliefs, and Ethical Dilemmas. *Respiration.* 2019 Jan 25; 97(3):185-96.

[22] Thakore N. J., Lapin B. R., Pioro E. P., Aboussouan L. S. Variation in noninvasive ventilation use in amyotrophic lateral sclerosis. *Neurology.* 2019 16; 93(3):e306-16.

[23] Fiorentino G., Annunziata A., Gaeta A. M., Lanza M., Esquinas A. Continuous noninvasive ventilation for respiratory failure in patients with amyotrophic lateral sclerosis: current perspectives. *Degener Neurol Neuromuscul Dis.* 2018 Sep 4; 8:55-61.

In: Non-Invasive Mechanical Ventilation Complications ISBN: 978-1-53619-515-6
Editor: Antonio M. Esquinas

Chapter 36

Non-Invasive Mechanical Ventilation Complications. Mortality, Determinants, Prevention and Treatment

Anna Annunziata*, MD, Maurizia Lanza, MD and Giuseppe Fiorentino, MD
Unit of Respiratory Physiopathology, Monaldi Hospital, Naples, Italy

Abstract

Non-invasive ventilation is more utilised in acute respiratory failure to prevent endotracheal intubation and invasive ventilation, however, failure rates of NIV include selection of patients, intervention, careful monitoring and a skilled team. The pathophysiology of NIV failure is difficult to prevent and some cases early diagnosis are important for example Patient–ventilator asynchrony, Upper airway disorerders, secretions and bronchial aspiration are key determinants

Keyword: noninvasive ventilation, mortality complications, prevention

Introduction

Non invasive ventilation (NIV) is more utilised in acute respiratory failure, for example, in patients with exacerbation of chronic obstructive pulmonary disease or acute heart failure [1]. A fundamental goal of NIV is to prevent endotracheal intubation and thereby decrease the complications related to invasive ventilation [1]. But, failure rates of NIV range within 5 and 50% [2]. Several factors have been identified that impact the

* Corresponding Author's E-mail: anna.annunziata@gmail.com.

failure rate of NIV and mortality. These determinants include particular selection of patients, accurately timed intervention, a comfortable and well-fitting interface, coaching and motivating of patients, careful monitoring, and a skilled and motivated team [1]. NIV is connected with numerous uncomfortable or even life-threatening adverse effects, and patients should be wholly screened previously to diminish potential critical complications. Now, the pathophysiology of NIV failure is imperfectly recognised. A significant discrepancy in the utilisation of NIV versus invasive ventilation is, apparently, the relationship with the upper airway. During invasive ventilation, the endotracheal tube avoids the upper airway, and the cuff of the endotracheal tube gives an air-tight seal in the trachea. In opposition, during NIV, the upper airway might represent a role in the performance of delivered ventilation. Positively, ventilator settings during NIV affect the patency of the upper airway [3]. This consequence suggests that abnormal function of the upper airway may play a part in the failure of NIV.

Patient–Ventilator Asynchrony

Different examples of asynchrony and dyssynchrony within the patient's neural drive and ventilator support have been recognised [4]. Suboptimal synchrony among the patient and the ventilator may be determined by respiratory mechanics, the breathing pattern, neural drive, ventilator settings, the type of interface and the amount of air leakage. The importance of patient-ventilator asynchrony is inadequately known, but a high incidence of asynchrony is correlated with extended duration of NIV and NIV failure [5]. During NIV, it is also essential that the ventilator acts in synchrony among the upper airway muscles. Glottic narrowing during inspiration improves upper airway stability and may limit adequate ventilation.

Upper Airway

The upper airway includes the nose, oral cavity, pharynx and larynx. The upper airway is included in chewing, swallowing, speech and smell, and its principal functions are to act as a conduit of air, to humidify and warm the inspired air and prevent foreign materials from entering the tracheobronchial tree. The nose and oral cavity are mostly static in their conducting function, whereas the pharynx and larynx predominantly are muscular structures and thus may alter the patency of the upper airway [6]. Opperman et al., have determined that management of the upper airway is complex and regulated by NIV. The latter findings are mostly based on animal data. Knowledge of the laryngeal reactions through various modes and settings of NIV in patients will be crucial to determine whether diminished upper airway patency offers to NIV failure.

Secretions and Bronchial Aspiration

NIV does not concede direct access to the airways. A weak cough reflex beginning to ineffective clearance of excessive secretions from airways is a frequent cause of immediate NIV failure [7]. The incapacity to spontaneously eliminate secretions is considered a relative contraindication for NIV, particularly in patients with damaged consciousness and depressed cough. Specific "manual" or "mechanical" physiotherapeutic techniques may increase mucociliary clearance during NIV and that NIV can still be used in these circumstances [8]. The patient suffering from neuromuscular pathology may have the aspiration of saliva or food residues that can stagnate in the oral cavity due to an modification of the post-swallowing phase, with vallecular stagnation. This can cause post-swallowing ab ingestiis and in any circumstances, respiratory arrest if not recognised early and managed.

Pneumonia

The rate of NIV failure in patients with pneumonia is generally variable, being lower in controlled clinical trials (21-26%) [9] than observational studies (33-66%), probably due to variety criteria of patients. M. Carron et al., described that NIV-associated pneumonia occurred in 5.7% (67/1172) of patients. In their meta-analysis of pneumonia incidence in NIV vs standard medical care revealed no clear statistical relationship within NIV treatment and pneumonia in different medical conditions. NIV was associated with particularly lower mean pneumonia ORs vs standard therapy for failure in hypoxic acute respiratory failure (ARF) (RR 0.89, CI: 0.82–0.95, P¼0.0025) and postoperative ARF (RR 0.94, CI: 0.90–0.98, P¼0.011), which may display significance in the future when additional studies are available for meta-analysis. In opposition, when NIV was related beside tracheal intubation for ventilator support weaning, NIV presented an important risk decrease in pneumonia frequency (RR 0.79; 95% CI 0.71–0.88, P,0.0001), by a meta-analysis of five relevant RCTs. In an original survey of 6869 pneumonia cases from 400 German ICUs, the mean pneumonia incidences were 1.58 and 5.44 cases per 1000 ventilator days for NIV and IMV, respectively, and 0.58 cases associated with no ventilation, which suggests that NIV increases pneumonia risk [10]. However, there existed no discrepancies in the balance of secondary sepsis and death among NIV and standard therapy. In opposition, previous investigations announced a lower incidence of pneumonia with NIV than with no ventilation. Several deficiencies in all these studies. First, NIV-associated pneumonia is unusual and possibly under-reported [10]. Although the issue of nosocomial pneumonia of NIV remains unsettled, NIV needs caution concerning aspiration risk. Pneumonia is a potential event during NIV and occurs developed to inhalation of external materials (i.e., condensed liquid in the ventilator circuit) or aspiration of gastric contents and secretions. Although unreported in RCTs, aspiration pneumonia has occurred in as many as 5% of NIV patients [11]. The risk of aspiration pneumonia is decreased by excluding patients with compromised upper airway capacity or with difficulty in removing secretions, by permitting at-risk patients nothing by the mouth until they are supported, and by placing the patient in the sitting or semi-sitting position during NIV. Caution should be taken in patients with unreasonable gastric distension, ileus, nausea or vomiting, or in those who are considered to be at high risk for gastric aspiration, for example in case of gastroesophageal reflux disease [11]. A nasogastric tube can be used, but it can conflict with mask fitting, improve air leaking, and add to discomfort.

Barotrauma

Barotrauma is a well-recognized complication of positive pressure ventilation. The risk of barotrauma is shallow during NIV and much lower than during invasive ventilation. Barotrauma has been reported in the presence of COPD, acute lung injury secondary to pneumonia, interstitial lung diseases, cystic fibrosis, and neuromuscular disorders [12]. Barotrauma risk can be decreased by adopting the following approaches: using pressure-controlled ventilation, especially in patients with low pulmonary compliance; keeping the peak inspiratory pressure as low as possible (i.e., 30 cm H_2O); optimizing the inspiratory and expiratory times to allow sufficient expiratory time to avoid auto-PEEP and breath stacking; applying a PEEP not exceeding auto-PEEP; and avoiding patient-ventilator desynchronization. When attempting to balance adequate ventilation with peak inspiratory pressure, some patients may manifest mild hypercapnia, which is acceptable as long as the patient remains asymptomatic [12].

Cardiovascular Comorbidities

Borel et al., noted that cardiovascular comorbidities are the principal determinants of death in subjects with obesity-associated hypoventilation managed by NIV. Cardiovascular comorbidities remain the primary determinant of death in these patients who are treated by NIV for sleep breathing abnormalities. Thus, NIV should be combined with other modalities of treatment such as rehabilitation programs including physical exercise, weight loss, lifestyle mode and relevant medication to additional decrease cardiovascular risk factors in subjects with obesity-associated hypoventilation [13]. The success of NIV in the treatment of acute cardiogenic pulmonary edema ACPE is related to a lower SAPS II (Simplified Acute Physiology Score II), admission at the emergency department, elevated PCO_2 at admission, improvement of the PO_2/FiO_2 index and the respiratory rate within the first hour. SAPS II and 3 should be customized with additional patient-risk factors to improve mortality prediction in patients undergoing NIV in intermediate care [14]. The recent guidelines from ERC/ATS recommend NIV, either bilevel NIV or CPAP, for subject affect to ARF due to ACPE (Acute cardiogenic pulmonary oedema) and raccomanded it in the pre-hospital setting [15].

Severe Decubitus and Skin Breakdown

Strategies to decrease the incidence of nasal skin lesions during NIV should be carefully considered from the beginning of therapy especially in patients with neuromuscular pathology who do not want invasive ventilation. The possibility to change the interfaces during the different daily activities is important to avoid skin breakdown in patients who need continuous NIV and refused invasive mechanical ventilation [16]. Skin infections that interfere with the continuation of NIV can occur in patients with chronic and immunocompromised diseases (Figure 1). A greater variety of different interface types, styles and materials have been developed by device manufacturers in recent years. This allows a suitable interface to be found for nearly every patient in most situations, but having to deal with many different interfaces and be able to select the most appropriate one can be challenging for clinical staff. The ability to try different mask types and sizes quickly may enhance tolerance as patients who do not adapt well to one type of mask may comply with another.

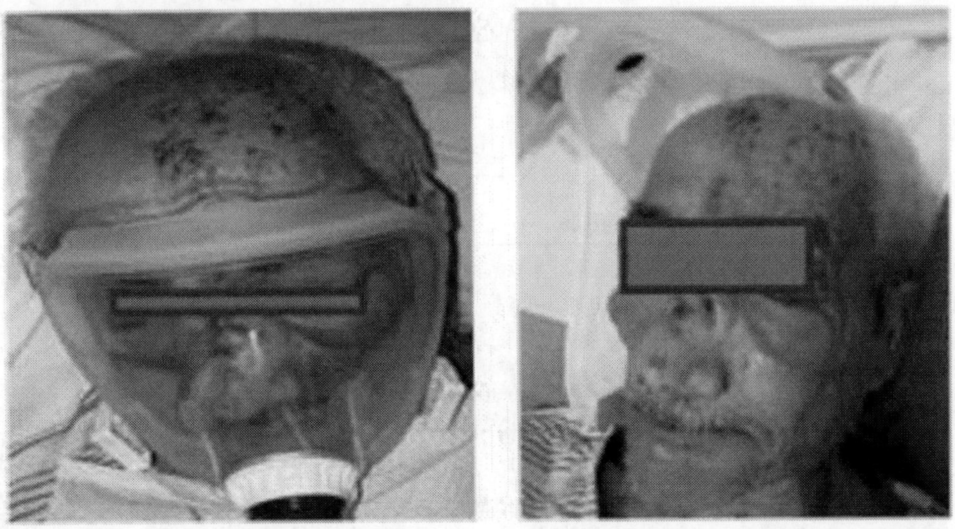

Figure 1.

Ventilator Failure

Cases of death following device failure are described. It is essential to realize that technical failures of the machines in these cases can be catastrophic. A headline from *The Times* newspaper of 14 August 2000—"*Power cut kills man on a home ventilator*"—is likely to strike a chill in the heart of anyone involved in providing home respiratory care. Simonds A. replay to this paper with a compelling summary. It is impracticable to guarantee total safety even in the hospital setting, Ventilators can break down, but engineering failure is uncommon and predictable. Included lies the difficulty—a significant part of any home care plan should be education of patients, families, and carers to help them use the equipment confidently and safely and to have a sensible plan of action once a problem arises [17].

Table 1. List of the most common machine technical failure alarms

Problem	**Consequence**	**problem management**
Powerfailure	Ventilator failure	Power allarm. Internal or external bactery
Ventilator malfunction	Ventilator failure	Regular manteinence. Bach up ventilator
Accidental disconnesion	Ventilator failure	Low pressure o volume alarms
Obstruction	Suboptimal ventilation	High pressure alarm set. Supports to prevent dragging. Secure connections
Mask fit	Pressure sore, leaks	Attenction to mask and alternate it. Low volume allarm
Tracheostomy problem obstruction	Failue of ventilation	Suction, change trachea, ambu ventilation
Falls out	Failure of ventilation	Improve fixation, ambu ventilation, small size tracheostomy tube
Medical problems	Acute deterioration and setting non appropiate	Rapid access to advice and evaluation of setting

Drugs

The benzodiazepines (BZD) are among the drugs most used by the population. Its contraindications include severe respiratory failure and sleep apnoea. BZD are the drugs most used by the community. Its contraindications incorporate severe respiratory failure and sleep apnoea. The primary purpose of Piñero-Zapata et al., was to verify whether there is a association within chronic benzodiazepine use and hospital mortality and up to 30 days later hospitalization. The study was managed on a retrospective cohort of 243 patients admitted to the emergency room at the General Hospital of the «Reina Sofia» University of Murcia during the year 2011. It was selected to have been treated with NIV during their hospitalization. The method used was a clinical history review looking for the code corresponding to the NIV process. The overall mortality was 20.6%. In patients with chronic consumption of BZD, it was 22.45% and 19.4% in patients who did not use these drugs. However, they failed to establish a important relationship between chronic benzodiazepine use and overall mortality [18].

Team Experience

NIV should be applied by a prepared and experienced team, with careful patient selection according to available guidelines and good clinical judgement, constantly taking into description the risk factors for NIV failure. Previously started, patients should be closely monitored in an ICU or step-down unit until appropriately stabilized, paying care not only to vital signs and gas exchange, but also to tolerance, comfort, air leaks, and patient-ventilator synergy [19]. When the team uses a ventilator, it is essential to know the device before working it. It is suggested to prefer a device that the team understands. The peculiar choice of device, adequate management of ventilatory support, a skilled team, and accurate clinical and instrumental monitoring are crucial to reducing the risk of complexities and mortality during NIV [19].

Proper Patient Selection NIV

Selection of proper patients is essential for the optimization of NIV success rates and reduce mortality. Usually, NIV must be commenced before laboratory data are available because subjects may decline during the stay and improve the risk of NIV failure. As represented in Figure 2, patients with respiratory distress and proper diagnosis should be judged for NIV [20]. The clinician must make two fundamental considerations: 1. whether the patient requires ventilatory assistance based on symptoms and signs of raised work of breathing or arterial blood gas disorders, and 2. whether such patients are candidates for NIV or should be immediately intubated. These enterprises are fundamental to the appropriate utilisation and importance of NIV and are based on the diagnosis, bedside notes, the clinician's judgment, and consideration of different guidelines. The timing of NIV beginning is essential too. NIV should be commenced early, as soon as indications appear, because delay may authorise further decline and enhance the probability of failure [21].

Predictors of NIV success or failure may additionally be valuable in electing patients (Table 3). The best predictor of success is a beneficial response to NIV in the first 2 h. In a prospective cohort study of nearly 800 COPD patients managed with NIV, Confalonieri et al., [22] recognised four factors—APACHE II score, pH, respiratory rate, and Glasgow coma score—that, when mixed in a chart, explained well predictive state at baseline. These factors had even more beneficial predictive condition after 2 h of NIV use; if all four factors were agreeable, the possibility of success was 97%; whereas if all were unfavourable, failure was a implicit confidence (99%).

Table 2. Selection guidelines for NIV in the acute setting

Appropriate diagnosis with potential reversibility
Establish need for ventilatory assistance
Moderate-to-severe respiratory distress and
Tachypnea (respiratory rate > 24/min for COPD, > 30/min for CHF); accessory muscle use or abdominal paradox
Blood gas derangement (pH < 7.35, Paco2 > 45 mm Hg, or Pao2/Fio2 < 200)
Exclude patients with contraindications to NIV
Respiratory or cardiac arrest
Medical instability (hypotensive shock, myocardial infarction requiring intervention, uncontrolled ischemia or arrhythmias)
Unable to protect airway
Unable to fit mask
Untreated pneumothorax
Recent upper airway or esophageal surgery
Excessive secretions*
Uncooperative or agitated*

* Relative contraindications.

Table 3. Factors associated with NIV success in the acute setting

Synchronous breathing with ventilator
Dentate
Less air leaking
Fewer secretions
Good tolerance
Respiratory rate _ 30/min*
Lower APACHE II score (_29)*
pH _ 7.30*
Glasgow coma score 15*
Pao2/Fio2 _ 146 after first hour if hypoxemic respiratory failure
COPD, CPE
No pneumonia, ARDS
Best predictor of success is a good response to NPPV within 1 to 2 h:
Reduction in respiratory rate
Improvement in pH
Improvement in oxygenation

How Can We Predict NIV Failure and High Mortality?

In summary, in hypoxaemic ARF, NIV failure is predicted by advanced age, high acuity illness on admission (i.e., Simplified Acute Physiology Score II, SAPS-II), acute respiratory distress syndrome, community-acquired pneumonia with or without sepsis, and multi-organ system failure. In hypercapnic ARF patients, failure is predicted by unimproved or worsened pH or respiratory rate, high-acuity illness at admission, and lack of cooperation. [23, 24, 25] Some laboratory indices are more sensitive than clinical findings. Specifically, an unimproved or worsened PaO_2 /FIO_2 ratio during a 1 h NIV accurately predicts NIV failure. Compared with the PaO_2 /FIO_2 ratio, however, the oxygenation index provides a superior estimate of lung function involvement and is a better predictor of NIV failure. Patient selection and monitoring are crucial to reduce NIV failure. NIV should not be used in patients suffering from claustrophobia, in respiratory arrest, with a low level of consciousness or who are unable to tolerate the NIV device because of agitation or uncooperativeness. NIV is contraindicated in patients who are unable to protect their airway due to a swallowing impairment or excessive secretions not sufficiently managed by clearance techniques, and after recent upper airway surgery. Such patients need prompt IMV that, when postponed, is associated with increased morbidity and mortality. All patients started on NIV should be monitored closely for signs of NIV failure until stabilized.

CONCLUSION

Several variables independently associated with NIV failure, such as higher SOFA score, SAPS II or 3, Lower APACHE II score, worsening of radiologic infiltrate and low oxygenation after 1h of NIV, were highly predictive of mortality. Careful selection is of major importance in patients with chronic obstructive pulmonary disease. In addition, special attention should be paid to patients with NIV-dependent neuromuscular disease or in the acute phase.

Higher organ system failure during NIV treatment, including metabolic acidosis, and variables related with worse initial response to the empiric treatment and NIV support were independently associated with NIV failure on multivariate analysis. These results indicate that the optimal management of these patients seems not restricted to appropriate support with NIV but should also include general support measures and effective empiric treatment. In the overall population, older age, NIV failure and higher organ system failure were independently associated with hospital mortality. Thus, further improvement of survival could be potentially achieved by combining adequate support against organ system dysfunction and optimal NIV management of patients. However, it is very important to evaluate each individual patient with the support of a multidisciplinary team and it must be borne in mind that despite the identified mortality predictors, each patient may have a complex and a completely unexpected response.

REFERENCES

[1] Oppersma E, Doorduin J, van der Heijden E H, van der Hoeven J G, Heunks L M. Noninvasive ventilation and the upper airway: should we pay more attention? *Crit. Care*. 2013;17(6):245. Published 2013 Dec 5. doi:10.1186/cc13141.

[2] Keenan S P, Mehta S: Noninvasive ventilation for patients presenting with acute respiratory failure: the randomized controlled trials. *Respir. Care* 2009, 54:116–126.

[3] Roy B, Samson N, Moreau-Bussière F, Ouimet A, Dorion D, Mayer S, Praud J-P: Mechanisms of active laryngeal closure during noninvasive intermittent positive pressure ventilation in nonsedated lambs. *J. Appl. Physiol.* 2008, 105:1406–1412.

[4] Thille A W, Rodriguez P, Cabello B, Lellouche F, Brochard L: Patient–ventilator asynchrony during assisted mechanical ventilation. *Intensive Care Med.* 2006, 32:1515–1522.

[5] Vignaux L, Vargas F, Roeseler J, Tassaux D, Thille A, Kossowsky M, Brochard L, Jolliet P: Patient–ventilator asynchrony during non-invasive ventilation for acute respiratory failure: a multicenter study. *Intensive Care Med.* 2009, 35:840–846.

[6] Mittal R K*: Motor Function of the Pharynx, Esophagus, and its Sphincters*. Morgan & Claypool Life Sciences: San Rafael, CA; 2011.

[7] Carlucci A, Richard J C, Wysocki M, Lepage E, Brochard L: Noninvasive versus conventional mechanical ventilation. An epidemiologic survey. *Am. J. Respir. Crit. Care Med.* 2001, 163: 874-880.

[8] Conti G, Antonelli M, Navalesi P, Rocco M, Bufi M, Spadetta G, Meduri G U: Noninvasive vs. conventional mechanical ventilation in patients with chronic obstructive pulmonary disease after failure of medical treatment in the ward: a randomized trial. *Intensive Care Med.* 2002, 28: 1701-1707.

[9] Ferrer M, Esquinas A, Leon M, Gonzalez G, Alarcon A, Torres A (2003) Noninvasive ventilation in severe hypoxemic respiratory failure: a randomized clinical trial. *Am. J. Respir. Crit. Care Med.* 168:1438-1444.

[10] Kohlenberg A, Schwab F, Behnke M, Geffers C, Gastmeier P. Pneumonia associated with invasive and noninvasive ventilation: an analysis of the German nosocomial infection surveillance system database. *Intensive Care Med.* 2010; 36: 971–8.

[11] Gay P C. Complications of noninvasive ventilation in acute care. *Respir. Care* 2009; 54: 246–57.

[12] Carron M, Gagliardi G, Michielan F, Freo U, Ori C. Occurrence of pneumothorax during noninvasive positive pressure ventilation through a helmet. *J. Clin. Anesth.* 2007; 19: 632–5.

[13] Borel J C, Burel B, Tamisier R, Dias-Domingos S, Baguet J P, Levy P, Pepin J L. Comorbidities and mortality in hypercapnic obese under domiciliary noninvasive ventilation. *PLoS One.* 2013;8(1):e52006.

[14] Martinez-Urbistondo D, Alegre F, Carmona-Torre F, Huerta A, Fernandez-Ros N, Landecho M F, García- Mouriz A, Núñez-Córdoba J M, García N, Quiroga J, Lucena J F. Mortality Prediction in Patients Undergoing Non-Invasive Ventilation in Intermediate Care. *PLoS One*. 2015 Oct 5;10(10):e0139702.

[15] Rochwerg B, Brochard L, Elliott M W, Hess D, Hill N S, Nava S, Navalesi P, Antonelli M, Brozek J, Conti G, Ferrer M, Guntupalli K, Jaber S, Keenan S, Mancebo J, Mehta S, Raoof S.. Official ERS/ATS clinical practice guidelines: noninvasive ventilation for acute respiratory failure. *Eur. Respir. J.* 2017;50:1602426.

[16] Fiorentino G, Annunziata A, Gaeta A M, Lanza M, Esquinas A. Continuous noninvasive ventilation for respiratory failure in patients with amyotrophic lateral sclerosis: current perspectives. *Degenerative Neurological and Neuromuscular Disease.* 2018;8:55-61.

[17] Simonds A K. Risk management of the home ventilator dependent patient. *Thorax.* 2006; 61(5):369-371.

[18] Piñero-Zapata M, Cinesi-Gómez C, Luna-Maldonado A. Mortality in patients with acute respiratory failure on chronic treatment with benzodiazepines. *Enferm, Clin.* 2013 May-Jun;23(3):89-95.

[19] M. Carron, U. Freo, A. S. BaHammam, D. Dellweg, F. Guarracino, R. Cosentini, P. Feltracco, A. Vianello, C. Ori, A. Esquinas, Complications of non-invasive ventilation techniques: a comprehensive qualitative review of randomized trials, *BJA: British Journal of Anaesthesia*, Volume 110, Issue 6, June 2013, Pages 896–914.

[20] Erik Garpestad, John Brennan, Nicholas S. Hill. *Noninvasive Ventilation for Critical Care. Chest Journal.* August 2007Volume 132, Issue 2, Pages 711–720.

[21] Nava S, Navalesi P, Conti G. Time of non-invasive ventilation. *Intensive Care Med.* 2006; 32:361–370.

[22] Confalonieri M, Garuti G, Cattaruzza M S, et al. A chart of failure risk for noninvasive ventilation in patients with COPD exacerbation. *Eur. Respir. J.* 2005; 25:348–355.

[23] Nava S, Hill N. Non-invasive ventilation in acute respiratory failure. *Lancet* 2009; 374: 250–9.

[24] Ferrari G, Olliveri F, De Filippi G, et al. Noninvasive positive airway pressure and risk of myocardial infarction in acute cardiogenic pulmonary edema: continuous positive airway pressure vs. noninvasive positive pressure ventilation. *Chest* 2007; 132: 1804–9.

[25] Carron M, Freo U, Zorzi M, Ori C. Predictors of failure of noninvasive ventilation in patients with severe community-acquired pneumonia. *J. Crit. Care* 2010; 25: 540.

In: Non-Invasive Mechanical Ventilation Complications ISBN: 978-1-53619-515-6
Editor: Antonio M. Esquinas

Chapter 37

Complications during Non-Invasive Mechanical Ventilation. Short and Long Term Outcomes

L. Olivencia Peña*, MD, PhD, M. Sevilla, MD and A. Fernández, MD, PhD
Intensive Care Unit, Granada, Spain

Abstract

Failure of Non Invasive Ventilation (NIV) can potentially be associated with prolonged invasive mechanical ventilation (MV) and increased mortality. Correct selection of patients for NIV treatment is essential, since the application of NIV should not delay endotracheal intubation but avoid it. The aim of this review is to analyze the determinants of outcomes in pathologies in which NIV has proven to be the treatment of choice.

Keywords: Noninvasive ventilation, outcomes, respiratory failure, critically ill

Introduction

NIV is considered a first-line treatment alongside conventional treatment in hypercapnic ARF in chronic obstructive pulmonary disease (COPD), and in ARF of acute cardiogenic pulmonary edema (CPAP), in the absence of contraindications. Importantly, failure of NIV can potentially be associated with prolonged invasive mechanical

* Corresponding Author's E-mail: l.olivencia@hotmail.com.

ventilation (MV) and increased mortality. The correct selection of patients for the use of NIV is essential, since the application of NIV should not delay endotracheal intubation but avoid it.

Outcomes of Non-Invasive Ventilation in Patients with Chronic Obstructive Pulmonary Disease (COPD)

The evidence of the benefits of NIV in hypercapnic ARF in patients with COPD has been widely demonstrated. In a registry carried out in American hospitals during the 1998 - 2008 period on the use of MV in patients with exacerbation of COPD, a progressive increase over the years of NIV use of 462% (from 1 to 4.5% of all admissions), along with a 42% decrease in the use of invasive MV (from 6 to 3.5% of all admissions) [1]. At European level, in 2008, a study was carried out on the use of NIV, with the treatment of hypercapnic ARI being the main indication of NIV (48%) [2]. Since then numerous studies have emerged confirming the benefits of non-invasive positive pressure ventilation (NIPPV) in COPD patients and hypercapnic ARF in terms of decreased need for intubation, hospital mortality, and hospital stay [3]. Different meta-analyzes have analyzed these results, observing a significant decrease in the need for intubation of 18 - 28% and in hospital mortality of 10 - 13% [4], together with a significant reduction in hospital stay of 2 - 5 days [4, 5]. Most patients included in the aforementioned studies had respiratory acidosis. The parameters associated with the success and failure of the technique are: adequate level of consciousness at the start of NIV and the improvement in pH, PaCO2 and level of consciousness after 1h are related to a good response to NIV in hypercapnic ARF in COPD patients [6]. In patients in whom NIV fails, the time range of NIV before intubation is very wide and that the increase in the duration of NIV before intubation is associated with a decrease in hospital survival. Hence the importance of the time window to assess the success or failure of the technique so that delays in intubation are avoided, which could be associated with a worse prognosis. The early start of NIV is essential in the success of the technique. The exhaustion of the patient, associated with a marked respiratory acidosis and eventual encephalopathy, should be avoided, since in these conditions there is a high risk of failure. The presence of pneumonia or acute respiratory distress syndrome are factors associated with failure of the technique.

Outcomes of Non-Invasive Ventilation in Patients with Acute Cardiogenic Pulmonary Edema (ACPE)

A clinical improvement (reduction of respiratory rate and dyspnea sensation) and gasometric improvement (increase in PaO2, reduction in PaCO2 and acidosis) have been observed faster with the application of NIV than with conventional oxygen therapy [7], the differences being observable from 30min after applying the technique.

Both NIPPV and CPAP show fast response times (from 30min) [8], with clinical resolution generally being earlier with the application of NIPPV, even reaching differences of almost one hour between the two techniques [9].

Similarly, physiologically based studies have shown that, although the use of CPAP is associated with a reduction in respiratory work in patients with acute cardiogenic lung edema, this effect is greater with the use of NIPPV. In the study by Nouira et al. [9], a subanalysis of patients with hypercapnia was performed. In these patients, the CPAP is compared with the NIPPV and no differences in the evolution of the patients are observed between the 2 techniques.

The hospital stay is not modified by the use of NIV in the ACPE with respect to conventional treatment, being this from 8 - 14d [7, 10].

Most of the randomized studies show a clear tendency to decrease the need for intubation with NIV treatment [10]. The different meta-analyzes [11-15] show a significant reduction in the percentage of intubations with the application of NIV compared to conventional oxygen therapy, both when considering CPAP and NIPPV. Both, both NIPPV and CPAP compared to conventional oxygen therapy have been shown to be effective in reducing the rate of intubation. The superiority of one technique over the other has not been demonstrated.

There is controversy over the impact of NIV on mortality hospitalization of patients with ACPE.

Most of the randomized studies, despite observing a tendency to lower mortality in the groups treated with NIV, have not demonstrated significant reductions thereof [7, 10], probably due to the low significance of the studies.

The different meta-analyzes [11-15] that compare the effect of NIV on hospital mortality with conventional oxygen therapy (despite the fact that they are based on studies with a small number of patients and with variability in design), coincide in detecting a significant decrease in hospital mortality with the use of NIV.

When the 2 ventilatory modalities are analyzed separately, the application of CPAP maintains a significant reduction in mortality compared to conventional treatment, with an absolute reduction of 13%, while the application of NIPPV is only associated with a tendency to such decrease, with an absolute reduction of 7% [14]. However, when comparing both techniques there are no significant differences.

Key Messages

1. Noninvasive ventilation (NIV) with conventional therapy improves the outcome of patients with acute respiratory failure due to hypercapnic decompensation of

chronic obstructive pulmonary disease (COPD) or acute cardiogenic pulmonary edema (ACPE).

2. In COPD, NIV improves gas exchange and symptoms, reducing the need for endotracheal intubation, hospital mortality and hospital stay compared with conventional oxygen therapy.
3. In ACPE, NIV accelerates the remission of symptoms and the normalization of blood gas parameters, reduces the need for endotracheal intubation, and is associated with a trend towards lesser mortality.
4. The early start of NIV is essential in the success of the technique.
5. The correct selection of patients for the use of NIV is essential, since the application of NIV should not delay endotracheal intubation but avoid it.

REFERENCES

[1] Chandra, D., Stamm, J. A., Taylor, B., Ramos, R. M., Satterwhite, L., Krishnan, J. A. et al. Outcomes of noninvasive ventilation for acute exacerbations of chronic obstructive pulmonary disease in the United States, 1998 - 2008. *Am. J. Respir. Crit. Care Med.*, 2012; 185: 152 - 9.

[2] Crimi, C., Noto, A., Princi, P., Esquinas, A., Nava, S. A European survey of noninvasive ventilation practices. *Eur. Respir. J.,* 2010; 36: 362 - 9.

[3] Plant, P. K., Owen, J. L., Elliott, M. W. Early use of non-invasive ventilation for acute exacerbations of chronic obstructive pulmonary disease on general respiratory wards: a multicentre randomised controlled trial. *Lancet,* 2000; 355: 1931 - 5.

[4] Peter, J. V., Moran, J. L., Phillips-Hughes, J., Warn, D. Noninvasive ventilation in acute respiratory failure a meta-analysis update. *Crit. Care Med.,* 2002; 30: 555 - 62.

[5] Quon, B. S., Gan, W. Q., Sin, D. D. Contemporary management of acute exacerbations of COPD: A systematic review and metaanalysis. *Chest,* 2008; 133: 756 - 66.

[6] Antón, A., Güell, R., Gómez, J., Serrano, J., Castellano, A., Carrasco, J. L. et al. Predicting the result of noninvasive ventilation in severe acute exacerbations of patients with chronic airflow limitation. *Chest,* 2000; 117: 828 - 33.

[7] Gray, A., Goodacre, S., Newby, D. E., Masson, M., Sampson, F., Nicholl, J. Noninvasive ventilation in acute cardiogenic pulmonary edema. *N Engl. J. Med.,* 2008; 359: 142 - 51.

[8] Ferrari, G., Olliveri, F., de Filippi, G., Milan, A., Aprà, F., Boccuzzi, A. et al. Noninvasive positive airway pressure and risk of myocardial infarction in acute cardiogenic pulmonary edema: continuous positive airway pressure vs. noninvasive positive pressure ventilation. *Chest,* 2007; 132: 1804 - 9.

[9] Nouira, S., Boukef, R., Bouida, W., Kerkeni, W., Beltaief, K., Boubaker, H. et al. Non-invasive pressure support ventilation and CPAP in cardiogenic pulmonary edema: A multicenter randomized study in the emergency department. *Intensive Care Med.*, 2011; 37: 249 - 56.

[10] Park, M., Sangean, M. C., Volpe Mde, S., Feltrim, M. I., Nozawa, E., Leite, P. F. et al. Randomized, prospective trial of oxygen, continuous positive airway pressure, and bilevel positive airway pressure by face mask in acute cardiogenic pulmonary edema. *Crit. Care Med.,* 2004; 32: 2407 - 15.

[11] Weng, C. L., Zhao, Y. T., Liu, Q. H., Fu, C. J., Sun, F., Ma, Y. L. et al. Meta-analysis: Noninvasive ventilation in acute cardiogenic pulmonary edema. *Ann. Intern. Med.*, 2010; 152: 590 - 600.

[12] Masip, J., Roque, M., Sánchez, B., Fernández, R., Subirana, M., Expósito, J. A. Noninvasive ventilation in acute cardiogenic pulmonary edema: Systematic review and meta-analysis. *JAMA*, 2005; 294:3124 - 30.

[13] Peter, J. V., Moran, J. L., Phillips-Hughes, J., Graham, P., Bersten, A. D. Effect of non-invasive positive pressure ventilation (NIPPV) on mortality in patients with acute cardiogenic pulmonary edema: A meta-analysis. *Lancet,* 2006; 367:1155 - 63.

[14] Winck, J. C., Azevedo, L. F., Costa-Pereira, A., Antonelli, M., Wyatt, J. C. Efficacy and safety of non-invasive ventilation in the treatment of acute cardiogenic pulmonary edema systematic review and meta-analysis. *Crit. Care,* 2006; 10: R69.

[15] Vital, F. M., Saconato, H., Ladeira, M. T., Sen, A., Hawkes, C. A., Soares, B. et al. Non-invasive positive pressure ventilation (CPAP or bilevel NPPV) for cardiogenic pulmonary edema. *Cochrane Database Syst. Rev.,* 2008. CD005351. doi:10.1002/14651858. CD005351.pub2.

In: Non-Invasive Mechanical Ventilation Complications ISBN: 978-1-53619-515-6
Editor: Antonio M. Esquinas

Chapter 38

Complications During Non-Invasive Mechanical Ventilation: Quality of Life

David Eugenio Jerves Donoso*
Pneumology Department, Hospital Santa Bárbara, Soria, Spain

Abstract

Non-invasive ventilation (NIV) appeared in 1927 as a result of the invention of the iron lung by Drinker and Shaw. Patients needing this type of treatment have shown to benefit from fewer hospital admissions, shorter stays, and fewer sleep breathing disorders; nevertheless, for some diseases like amyotrophic lateral sclerosis (ALS) or Duchenne muscular dystrophy, there are discrepancies concerning the utility of NIV with regards to the patient's quality of life. Noteworthy, since 1995, the WHO highlights the importance of quality of life as a significant factor for one's existence.

Accordingly, it is necessary to create specific tools to measure the quality of life of patients requiring chronic NIV.

Keywords: non-invasive ventilation (NIV), health-related quality of life (HRQoL), obstructive sleep apnea (OSA), amyotrophic lateral sclerosis (ALS)

Introduction

One of the relevant questions that arise regarding the utility of NIV is if its prolonged use can affect the patient's quality of life. For this reason, several tools (both generic and specific to respiratory diseases and ALS) have been used to assess quality of life.

* Corresponding Author's E-mail: davidjerves@hotmail.es.

However, more studies demonstrating their utility are still lacking, as most of them show important discrepancies.

Association Between Non-Invasive Ventilation and Quality of Life

According to the WHO (1995), quality of life is defined as "an individual's perception of their position in life in the context of the culture and value systems in which they live, and in relation to their goals, expectations, standards, and concerns" [1]. In 1996, Testa M. highlighted the need for evaluating health outcomes, which the author called "health-related quality of life" (HRQoL).

As determined by Plummer (1989), the goals of NIV are: extending life, enhancing the quality of life, providing an environment that will enhance the individual's potential, reducing morbidity, and improving physical and physiologic functions [2].

Patients with chronic respiratory insufficiency on NIV show a decrease in number of respiratory exacerbations and in hospital admissions per years, as well as an improvement of sleep breathing disorders; all of which have a positive effect on their quality of life [3].

Quality of life has generally been assessed through several questionnaires, both generic and specific to respiratory diseases and ALS. The most used ones are:

- Pictured Childs Quality of Life Self Questionnaire (Autoquestionnaire Qualité de Vie Enfant-Imagé, AUQUEI)
- Severe Respiratory Insufficiency Questionnaire (SRI)
- Impact on Family Scale (IFS)
- Family APGAR
- Goldberg Health Questionnaire [4]
- McGill Quality of Life Questionnaire (MQOL)
- Amyotrophic Lateral Sclerosis Functional Rating Scale (ALSFRS)
- Amyotrophic Lateral Sclerosis Assessment Questionnaire (ALSAQ-40) [5]
- St. George's Respiratory Questionnaire (SGRQ) [6]
- Chronic Respiratory Disease Questionnaire (CRDQ) [7]
- Short Form Health Survey (SF36)
- Sleep Apnea Quality of Life Index (SAQLI)
- Chronic Respiratory Disease Questionnaire (CRDQ)
- Amyotrophic Lateral Sclerosis Specific Quality of Life Instrument-Revised (ALSSQoL-R) [8]

Zamietra and collaborators performed a study using ALSSQoL-R before and after NIV on ALS patients, finding no significant differences regarding health-related quality of life [9].

The most frequent complications of NIV are: nasal blockage, poor tolerance of treatment pressure, and mask leak [10]. Moreover, the long-term use of oro-nasal Continuous Positive Airway Pressure (CPAP) is a potential cause of pneumoparotitis [11]; still, there is no evidence that these tools impair quality of life. Nonetheless, in 9 studies on muscular dystrophy (574 participants) by 59 doctors in UK, 13% of them believed that NIV impairs patients' quality of life [12].

In patients with stroke presenting obstructive sleep apnea (OSA), it has been observed that CPAP discontinuation was due to difficulties with CPAP use, facial weakness, motor impairment, and discomfort with use of full-face mask [13]. On the other hand, Batool-Anwar and collaborators did not observe any improvement in quality of life of patiens with mild OSA on CPAP [14]. Moreover, it has been shown that the use of antidepressants and CPAP-induced sleep disorders are predictors of poor adherence [15].

It Is Important to Consider That Any Procedure That a Patient Undergoes May Cause Complications, Which Can Be Mild, Moderate, or Severe

The main complications during NIV treatment are:

- Mask maladjustment and leak
- Facial erythema
- Claustrophobia
- Rash and other skin lesions
- Pressure ulcers
- Nasal congestion and obstruction
- Dryness of the nasal and oral mucosa
- Eye irritation
- Nose and ear pain
- Abdominal distension
- Dyssynchrony
- Aspiration
- Hypotension
- Pneumothorax

Under all circumstances, our main goal must be to improve the quality of life of patients on NIV through the minimization or avoidance of treatment-associated complications. To this effect, the following should be considered:

1. Establishing achievable goals
2. Choosing the most adequate technique for each single patient
3. Patients and their families must understand why the treatment is necessary, accept it, and collaborate at each stage of the proposed treatment
4. The medical and nursing staff, as well as the material and equipment supplier, must correctly follow-up each patient and solve any doubt that they or their families may have.
5. Using the appropriate parameters for each case.
6. Trying to establish use resting periods, provided the patient's pathology enables it.

It would be recommendable to develop questionnaires and/or specific scales to assess the quality of life and complications associated with NIV.

Furthermore, it would be beneficial to perform prospective, double-blind, clinical trials on a representative sample and with adequate internal and external validity, so that we can truly get insight into the long-term use of NIV and become aware of any possible associated decrease in the patients' wellbeing.

References

[1] The World Health Organization Quality of Life assessment (WHOQOL): position paper from the World Health Organization. *Soc. Sci. Med.* 1995;41(10):1403-9.

[2] Plummer A L, O'Donohue W J, Jr., Petty T L. Consensus conference on problems in home mechanical ventilation. *Am. Rev. Respir. Dis.* 1989;140(2):555-60.

[3] Guisela M. *Fisiología e indicaciones de la asistencia ventilatoria no invasiva.* Sociedad Chilena de Neumología Pediátrica. 2008. [*Physiology and indications for non-invasive ventilatory assistance.* Chilean Society of Pediatric Pneumology]

[4] Pamela S. *Calidad de vida relacionada en salud: Concepto y evaluación en pacientes con ventilación mecánica no invasiva*. Sociedad Chilena de Neumología Pediátrica. 2008. [*Health-related quality of life: Concept and evaluation in patients with non-invasive mechanical ventilation.*]

[5] Sanchez-Lopez C R, Perestelo-Perez L, Ramos-Perez C, Lopez-Bastida J, Serrano-Aguilar P. [Health-related quality of life in patients with amyotrophic lateral sclerosis]. *Neurologia*. 2014;29(1):27-35.

[6] Capparelli I, Fernandez M, Saadia Otero M, Steimberg J, Brassesco M, Campobasso A, et al. Translation to Spanish and Validation of the Specific Saint George's Questionnaire for Idiopathic Pulmonary Fibrosis. *Arch. Bronconeumol.* 2018;54(2):68-73.

[7] Ali S, Kabir Z. Domiciliary non-invasive ventilation and the quality of life outcome of patients suffering from chronic respiratory failure. *Ir. Med. J.* 2007;100(1):336-8.

[8] E. O A. *Efectividad de la ventilación no invasiva para el tratamiento de la insuficiencia respiratoria en pacientes con Esclerosis Lateral Amiotrófica*. 2016. [*Effectiveness of non-invasive ventilation for the treatment of respiratory failure in patients with Amyotrophic Lateral Sclerosis*]

[9] Zamietra K, Lehman E B, Felgoise S H, Walsh S M, Stephens H E, Simmons Z. Non-invasive ventilation and gastrostomy may not impact overall quality of life in patients with ALS. *Amyotroph. Lateral Scler*. 2012;13(1):55-8.

[10] Kennedy B, Lasserson T J, Wozniak D R, Smith I. Pressure modification or humidification for improving usage of continuous positive airway pressure machines in adults with obstructive sleep apnoea. *Cochrane Database Syst. Rev.* 2019;12:CD003531.

[11] Goates A J, Lee D J, Maley J E, Lee P C, Hoffman H T. Pneumoparotitis as a complication of long-term oronasal positive airway pressure for sleep apnea. *Head Neck.* 2018;40(1):E5-E8.

[12] Kinali M, Manzur A Y, Mercuri E, Gibson B E, Hartley L, Simonds A K, et al. UK physicians' attitudes and practices in long-term non-invasive ventilation of Duchenne Muscular Dystrophy. *Pediatr. Rehabil.* 2006;9(4):351-64.

[13] Palombini L, Guilleminault C. Stroke and treatment with nasal CPAP. *Eur. J. Neurol.* 2006;13(2):198-200.

[14] Batool-Anwar S, Goodwin J L, Kushida C A, Walsh J A, Simon R D, Nichols D A, et al. Impact of continuous positive airway pressure (CPAP) on quality of life in patients with obstructive sleep apnea (OSA). *J. Sleep Res*. 2016;25(6):731-8.

[15] Hussain S F, Irfan M, Waheed Z, Alam N, Mansoor S, Islam M. Compliance with continuous positive airway pressure (CPAP) therapy for obstructive sleep apnea among privately paying patients- a cross sectional study. *BMC Pulm Med.* 2014;14:188.

In: Non-Invasive Mechanical Ventilation Complications
Editor: Antonio M. Esquinas
ISBN: 978-1-53619-515-6

Chapter 39

Cost Associated with Non-Invasive Ventilation Complications

Elena Maria Jimenez Gonzalez[1,*], Cristina Palma Rodríguez[2] and Marta Ruiz Perez de la Blanca[2]

[1]Department of Emergency, Hospital de Alta Resolución de Alcalá la Real, Jaén, Spain

[2]Department of Emergency, Hospital Comarcal de Baza, Granada, Spain

Abstract

The use of non-invasive mechanical ventilation has become widespread for acute and chronic respiratory failure.

With its use, it is often possible to reduce the number of patients who require invasive mechanical ventilation, with the advantages that this entails, especially associated with avoiding some of the complications of the procedure.

This represents significant economic savings, because although non-invasive ventilation is not without risks, these are in any case less in number and in severity than those associated with invasive mechanical ventilation.

In this chapter we will review different studies carried out throughout history in which an attempt has been made to evaluate the benefits of non-invasive mechanical ventilation, as well as an economic analysis of its cost-effectiveness.

Keywords: non-invasive ventilation, economic resources, complications, healthcare costs, length of stay

[*] Corresponding Author's E-mail: elenamariajg@gmail.com.

Introduction

Endotracheal intubation and mechanical ventilation (MV) are techniques that have saved a large number of lives. However, it is known that the use of artificial routes is not without complications. Therefore, non-invasive ventilation (NIV) has been proposed in recent decades as an alternative approach in order to avoid/decrease a large number of these.

Its use is increasingly widespread and is used in multiple services: from emergencies to a large number of hospitalization plants such as pneumology, internal medicine or intensive care unit.

It has been successfully tested on various diseases. Although its best known use is in respiratory insufficiencies secondary to exacerbated COPD, it has also been used with guarantees in other pathologies such as cardiogenic edema, asthma attacks or neuromuscular diseases.

The incidence of complications with NIV is low, and it is usually acceptable taking into account its benefits as well as the economic savings that would be involved in avoiding invasive mechanical ventilation.

Complications of Non-Invasive Mechanical Ventilation

As we said, although the incidence of complications in non-invasive mechanical ventilation is low, it is not exempt from them. If it is true, that these are usually light and easily solvable as we will see below.

The most common are associated with the use of masks. They would be, for example, the appearance of tissue lesions due to pressure at the facial level, abdominal distension, aerophagia, nausea and vomiting due to the entry of air into the digestive system, dryness of the nasal and oral mucosa, accumulation of secretions secondary to the tightness of the mask facial with high flows (which can lead to risk of atelectasis, pneumonia or airway obstructions), intolerance to the mask (restlessness, anxiety) [1].

We will now carry out a breakdown according to the reason for the complication [2].

Associated with the Mask

Subjective discomfort can be high (up to 50%), but it is usually easily solved by changing or adjusting the mask. It is common to find skin disorders (between 5% and 30% to 50% have been described) [3], such as hypersensitivity rashes or localized infections. They usually respond well to topical steroid or antibiotic treatments.

More serious would be the appearance of ulcers in the nasal bridge, since although they usually improve with local cures, cases have been described in which skin grafts have been required for their treatment.

Another associated problem may be restlessness, anxiety, or claustrophobia associated with the use of non-invasive mechanical ventilation. For this, there are helmets or full face masks that usually reduce this sensation.

Aerophagia and sialorrhea can also be associated. They are symptoms that usually respond adequately to simethicone or anti-sialorrheic.

Arm edema and deep vein thrombosis have also been described as complications. This is due to the fact that in some cases the helmet is secured by two clamps to the armpits. The compression you exert can lead to venous and lymphatic disease with detected edema. This in affected patients could involve deep vein thrombosis of the axillary veins. Although, it is an easily avoidable complication using other types of masks or using devices in which the bands are attached to the bed [3].

Complications Related to Pressure and Flow

Some are included such as ear discomfort, sinus pain, or gastric insufflation. The noise can increase the patient's anguish, cause sleep disorders or cause alterations in the ear such as tinnitus. All of them are avoidable with a decrease in pressure, which must be adjusted according to the tolerance and comfort of the patient.

More serious complications associated with pressure would be pneumothorax and pneumocephalus, although these have been mentioned anecdotally.

Regarding side effects of the flow, we find nasal dryness, congestion or obstruction (nasal or sinus irritation). They usually respond to topical treatments such as decongestants, corticosteroids, and thermal humidification [2].

Eye irritation can be avoided by properly monitoring air leaks.

Aspiration and Mucus Plugging

Aspiration is one of the most important complications as it is potentially serious. The risk of aspiration pneumonia has been estimated in 5% of patients with NIV. Although it is true, this risk decreases considerably when patients with upper respiratory tract involvement or difficulty eliminating secretions are excluded [3]. For this reason, making a correct selection of patients is essential (avoiding patients with a low level of consciousness or with little collaboration in the technique). Some authors consider the previous placement of a nasogastric drainage to avoid this complication, although it is true that in the majority of studies analyzed to see the incidence of associated pneumonia, this is not done and even so the number of them continues to be minimal.

Mucus plugging can also be associated as a complication, although it does not usually occur when humidifications, hydrations and respiratory physiotherapy are performed regularly.

Inadequate Gas Exchange

It largely depends on the patient-ventilator synchrony. During NIV, activation and the respiratory assist cycle should be synchronized with the patient's respiratory efforts. However, in studies performed, patient-ventilator asynchrony has been observed in 15-54% of patients with acute respiratory failure [4].

Proper monitoring, as well as neurally adjusted ventilatory support, have been shown to improve this asynchrony by reducing activation and cycling delays.

Hemodynamic Compromise

Infrequent but serious complication. The pressure applied to the airway increases intrathoracic and right ventricular pressure. This can lead to decreased preload and ventricular filling. This continuous pressure in the airways decreases cardiac output and stroke volume in a pressure-dependent manner, and increases systematic vascular residences without changing heart rate and blood pressure [3].

Analysis of the Evidence on the Costs Associated with the Complications of Non-Invasive Mechanical Ventilation

We will now review the evidence associated with the complications of non-invasive mechanical ventilation.

In 2006, Iñigo and Esquinas conducted a retrospective analysis of patients treated with NIV. Of the 10 patients studied, none suffered complications associated with this process, nor did they require orotracheal intubation or transfer to an intensive care unit. They concluded in their study that NIV is a safe technique in selected patients with respiratory failure and that it is an effective method to avoid intubation and ICU stays with few adverse effects. These depend largely on the characteristics of the patient, the type of ventilator or the monitoring carried out [5].

In many cases, the use of non-invasive mechanical ventilation avoids the need for MV. Thanks to this, we achieve cost savings by avoiding potential complications of this technique such as ventilator - associated pneumonia (VAP). This complication results in longer stays in intensive care units, is associated with increased use of antibiotics, and results in increased mortality.

VAP is mainly due to germs such as Pseudomonas aeruginosa and methicillin-resistant Staphylococcus aureus (MRSA) and is the most frequent cause of mortality among nosocomial infections in patients admitted to intensive care units.

It is caused by the lower airway being a sterile area in healthy people. Tracheal intubation and MV break this down, causing secretions from the oral cavity to build up in the airway.

Studies have been conducted to see if NIV is associated with a lower rate of nosocomial pneumonia. A cohort of 320 patients who were in ICU for more than 2 days and required mechanical ventilation for one day or more was chosen [6].

They were divided into 4 groups according to the form of mechanical ventilation received: 38 required NIV and then endotracheal intubation, 23 received endotracheal intubation and then NIV. 1900 only endotracheal intubation and 60 only NIV.

Incidence rates of ventilator-associated pneumonia were 18% in the first group (NIV plus endotracheal intubation), 22% in the second group (endotracheal intubation and then NIV), 8% in endotracheal intubation and 0% in NIV.

The authors conclude that while these differences are significant, they could be attributed to the severity of the patients receiving each of the options as well as the risk to which they are exposed.

Therefore, in another similar study, an attempt was made to adjust patients according to the severity of the disease that made them need intubation [7]. We included 761 patients who required mechanical ventilation for more than 48 hours. Of these, 129 were ventilated with NIV, 607 by endotracheal intubation and 25 started NIV but later required intubation. In this study we concluded that the use of NIV not only reduced the risk of pneumonia associated with mechanical ventilation compared with endotracheal ventilation, but also reduced the risk of nosocomial infections as a whole, and this occurred regardless of the severity of the patient's illness.

Subsequently, in 2001, a prospective survey was conducted to assess the incidence of the use and effectiveness of non-invasive ventilation in clinical practice [8]. To this end, 689 patients requiring ventilatory support were included (581 by endotracheal intubation vs 108 with non-invasive ventilation). The reasons for requiring it were: 30% coma, 7% cardiogenic pulmonary edema, 48% hypoxemia, 15% hypercapnic acute respiratory failure. Patients in coma were subsequently excluded because NIV could not be used in them. This technique was used in 14% of patients with hypoxemia, 27% of those with pulmonary edema and 50% of those with hypercapnic acute respiratory failure. The incidence of nosocomial pneumonia (10% vs 19%, $p = 0.03$) and mortality (22% vs 41 p > 001) was lower in patients with NIV than those with endotracheal intubation.

Since it has been estimated that each VAP produced costs more than USD 40 000 in the USA [9], the use of NIV as a means of avoiding MV and its complications was already being considered in the late 1980s.

Initially, however, NIV was seen as a complex procedure that required more time from the professionals involved, as well as increased costs.

As a result of this approach, several studies emerged that sought to demonstrate the opposite, i.e., that NIV would effectively result in long-term cost savings (at the expense of reducing MV complications) and that it did not result in increased workload for professionals.

In 1997, Nava et al. [10] conducted a prospective trial in COPD patients to evaluate the human and economic resources needed to ventilate patients with NIV compared to those needed in another group requiring MV.

They concluded that although initially more time might be required from the professionals in the NIV group, this difference ceased to be significant after 48 hours. After that time, NIV was neither more expensive, nor slower, nor more time-consuming or personal than MV. Moreover, after the first few days, NIV consumed much less time than MV for doctors and nurses, so the idea that increased professional time was a problem during NIV seemed to be discarded.

Shortly thereafter, in the year 2000, Plant et al. [11], carried out a prospective, multicenter, randomized and controlled study in order to determine if the early introduction of NIV in a general respiratory patient room was effective in reducing the need for intubation and mortality associated with acute exacerbations of COPD.

For this, two groups were recruited, one which received standard therapy alone (oxygen therapy, nebulizers ...), and another in which NIV was also added.

It was found that although in both groups there was a reduction in pH and pCO2, this improvement was faster in the first hour in the NIV group. Similarly, in this group, the fall in respiratory rate at 4 hours was greater, as was the duration of dyspnea.

Regarding the consequences of these events, it was appreciated that the use of NIV significantly reduced the need for intubation (27.1% required in the standard group versus 15.3% in the NIV group). Similarly, in-hospital mortality was reduced (20.3% in the standard group versus 10.2% in the NIV group).

Therefore, it was concluded from this study that the early use of NIV in COPD patients with mild and moderate acidosis, led to a faster improvement of the physiological variables as well as fewer subsequent complications.

Three years later, the same authors carry out a new study with which they intended to model the costs that this intervention entailed in a real-life setting [12].

To do this, they carry out an incremental cost-effectiveness analysis, carried out together with a randomized controlled trial of 14 centers in which standard medical treatment was compared with the same plus NIV in patients admitted to the hospital with an exacerbation of COPD, respiratory acidosis and respiratory rate greater than 23 breaths per minute.

In this study, NIV was associated with a £ 49,362 reduction in costs as well as a 50% reduction in mortality. Mainly the cost savings were at the expense of reducing stays in intensive care units.

The mean costs were £ 2800 (95% confidence interval £ 1896 to £ 4388) for the group receiving standard treatment and £ 2155 (£ 1742 to £ 2966) for the non-invasive ventilation group. Therefore, an average saving of £ 645 is shown per patient receiving non-invasive ventilation (£ 2310 to £ 386).

For this reason, it was concluded that NIV is a more effective and less expensive strategy in this group of patients, reducing the risk of death and the number of admissions in the UCIS. Subsequently, the same group of authors carried out a new study in which they try to show whether the use of home NIV in groups of patients with stable COPD leads to a reduction in hospital admissions and general medical care, and therefore a saving in appearance economic [13].

To do this, they compared the effectiveness and costs of home NIV with conventional treatment in a group of patients with recurrent admissions for acidotic exacerbations of COPD. The average annual cost per patient before starting NIV at home was £ 13,163 (95% CI £ 8,695 to £ 17,631). However, one year after initiation, the cost was £ 4909 (95% CI: £ 2888 to £ 6930), which represents a saving of £ 8254 (95% CI: £ 4013 to £ 12 495 ($p = 0.002$). This saving is achieved thanks to a reduction in the rates of hospital admission and length of stay.

Years later, Clini et al. [14] carried out a trial comparing the cost of health care in COPD patients in whom NIV is used vs. patients in which only long-term oxygen therapy is used. Cost was calculated in 77 of the 90 patients included in the trial (NIV + Long-term oxygen therapy, $n = 35$; Long-term oxygen therapy, $n = 42$).

As results, it was appreciated that the average cost of medications and oxygen therapy was similar for both groups. However, considering the cost of hospitalization, this was lower in the group in which NIV was added, compared to the one that was not (8.25+/-10.29 vs. 12.50+/-20.28 EUR/patient/day, $p < 0.05$), which means a 34% saving in hospitalization costs. This difference is mainly due to the fact that the patients in whom NIV was used required a shorter stay in the ICU.

Therefore, they concluded that the addition of NIV does not increase costs in relation to the usual regimen with oxygen therapy, but even decreases them in COPD patients.

Although it is true, that the patients to whom NIV is applied should be carefully selected, since not in any patient with said pathology would it be a cost-effective alternative. It is thought that this therapeutic modality may also have a positive impact on the survival of these patients. However, this fact should be considered in long-term studies.

NIV is also a useful strategy for hospitals with fewer resources, since MV is an expensive technique with estimates of $ 29,000-110,000/QALY. This represents unreasonable and unacceptable expenses for low-income countries. Added to this is the shortage of beds in intensive care units, and of resources in general. In 2015, Shraddha et al. [15] published a study with the aim of comparing the cost-effectiveness ratio of the use of NIV vs. standard treatment in patients with respiratory failure due to COPD in India. In this study, they found that the mortality rate was 0.101 in the NIV group vs. 0.278 for the standard treatment group. Cost $ 78/QALY ($ 525.02/6.82) for standard treatment vs. $ 75/QALY (636.33/8.49). Although the NIV group was somewhat more expensive, it was more effective (increasing QALY by 1.67). They mention that the low cost/QALY estimate suggests that NIV could be considered as an additional opportunity in low-income countries where MV is not as widely available.

Therefore, it is evident from the review of these articles the great utility of NIV in patients with exacerbations of COPD. However, not only has the cost-effectiveness of this technique been studied in said pathology.

In 2003, Mars et al. measured it in Obstructive Sleep Apnea Hypopnea [16], concluding that the treatment with NIV (in this case nasal CPAP) of obstructive sleep apnea syndrome has a cost-effectiveness ratio in the same line than other therapeutic measures financed, such as antihypertensive drugs. The benefit is found in the improvement in the quality of life of these patients.

In 2005, Gruis and Cols measured the application of this system to patients with amyotrophic lateral sclerosis (ALS) [17]. In their study, they appreciate that in general, patients who received NIV experienced 0.59 QALY (quality-adjusted life years) at a cost of $ 1,773, compared to the patient who did not receive such treatment and who experienced a 0.54 QALY at a cost of $ 0, this assumed an incremental cost-effectiveness ratio of $ 33,801. In the absence of other studies, they conclude that their model suggests that NIV initiated at the time of diagnosis would be profitable if it demonstrated to improve HRQoL (health related quality of by 7-14%.

Regarding costs related to adaptation to NIV, in 2014, Pallero and Cols [18], evaluated the economic differences in patients adapted to the technique at hospital vs. outpatient level. For this, 53 patients with chronic respiratory failure secondary to restrictive chest disease, obesity-hypoventilation syndrome or neuromuscular disease were included. These patients were randomized to ambulatory adaptation (AA, n = 23) or hospital adaptation (HA, n = 25). The main outcome variable was the decrease in PaCO2 six months after the start of NIV, which resulted in 4.9 (2.3; 7.4) mmHg in AA (95% CI) and 3.3 (1.4; 5.1) mmHg in HA. The direct cost was calculated at 1,500 euros in AA patients vs. 2,692 in HA patients.

From this they conclude that adaptation to NIV in the outpatient setting is not inferior to that of the hospital in terms of therapeutic equivalence in these patients, while it can represent significant economic savings for the health system.

The cost-effectiveness of NIV for weaning has also been recently evaluated in patients admitted to the intensive care unit, concluding that the probability that weaning with NIV is profitable in relation to that produced without NIV ranges from 57-59% in the general population and between 82-87% for COPD patients, so it could also be considered a cost-effective application for this technique [19], although it is true that long-term studies are required to accurately assess the effectiveness of this technique.

CONCLUSION

In conclusion, there is current evidence to support the use of non-invasive ventilation in a large selected group of patients. Although it is a technique that is not without complications, these are mostly mild and affordable if the benefits they provide are taken into account.

As we have seen, we have numerous studies that demonstrate that this technique can reduce the need for endotracheal intubation, as well as its duration, and even reduce mortality in patients with acute respiratory failure due to exacerbations of COPD.

Likewise, its usefulness has been seen in other pathologies such as asthma, pneumonia, cardiogenic pulmonary edema, OSAS, ALS, weaning or acute respiratory failure after extubation.

Its use avoids MV on numerous occasions. With this, the complications that frequently occur with this invasive technique (such as ventilation-associated pneumonia) are significantly reduced, and doing so achieves significant cost savings. This saving, as we have seen throughout the chapter, occurs mainly associated with the reduced need for hospital stays (especially in intensive care units). Similarly, it has been associated with a decrease in morbidity and mortality in patients with acute and chronic respiratory failure, so it should be a technique that should be integrated into routine clinical practice.

REFERENCES

[1] Moya, Claudia Liliana Cruz. Complicaciones de la ventilación mecánica no invasiva en adultos en la unidad de cuidados intermedios. *Teoría y Praxis Investigativa* [Complications of non-invasive mechanical ventilation in adults in the intermediate care unit. *Investigative Theory and Praxis*], 2008, vol. 3, no 1, p. 13-20.

[2] Gay, Peter C. Complications of noninvasive ventilation in acute care. *Respiratory Care*, 2009, vol. 54, no 2, p. 246-258.

[3] Carron, M., et al. Complications of non-invasive ventilation techniques: a comprehensive qualitative review of randomized trials. *British Journal of Anaesthesia*, 2013, vol. 110, no 6, p. 896-914.

[4] Vignaux, Laurence, et al. Patient-ventilator asynchrony during non-invasive ventilation for acute respiratory failure: a multicenter study. *Intensive care medicine*, 2009, vol. 35, no 5, p. 840.

[5] Iñigo A, Esquinas A. Práctica clínica y metodología. *Revista Iberoamericana de Ventilación no Invasiva* [Clinical practice and methodology. *Ibero-American Journal of Non-Invasive Ventilation*]. 2007;5(9):7-10.

[6] Guerin, C., et al. Facial mask noninvasive mechanical ventilation reduces the incidence of nosocomial pneumonia. *Intensive Care Medicine*, 1997, vol. 23, no 10, p. 1024-1032.

[7] Nourdine, K., et al. Does noninvasive ventilation reduce the ICU nosocomial infection risk? A prospective clinical survey. *Intensive Care Medicine*, 1999, vol. 25, no 6, p. 567-573.

[8] Carlucci, Annalisa, et al. Noninvasive versus conventional mechanical ventilation: an epidemiologic survey. *American Journal of Respiratory and Critical Care Medicine*, 2001, vol. 163, no 4, p. 874-880.

[9] Rello, Jordi, et al. Epidemiology and outcomes of ventilator-associated pneumonia in a large US database. *Chest*, 2002, vol. 122, no 6, p. 2115-2121.

[10] Nava, Stefano, et al. Human and financial costs of noninvasive mechanical ventilation in patients affected by COPD and acute respiratory failure. *Chest*, 1997, vol. 111, no 6, p. 1631-1638.

[11] Plant, P. K., Owen, J. L., Elliott, M. W. Early use of non-invasive ventilation for acute exacerbations of chronic obstructive pulmonary disease on general respiratory wards: a multicentre randomised controlled trial. *The Lancet*, 2000, vol. 355, no 9219, p. 1931-1935.

[12] Plant, P. K., et al. Cost effectiveness of ward based non-invasive ventilation for acute exacerbations of chronic obstructive pulmonary disease: economic analysis of randomised controlled trial. *Bmj*, 2003, vol. 326, no 7396, p. 956.

[13] Tuggey, J. M., Plant, P. K., Elliott, M. W. Domiciliary non-invasive ventilation for recurrent acidotic exacerbations of COPD: an economic analysis. *Thorax*, 2003, vol. 58, no 10, p. 867-871.

[14] Clini, Enrico M., et al. Home non-invasive mechanical ventilation and long-term oxygen therapy in stable hypercapnic chronic obstructive pulmonary disease patients: comparison of costs. *Respiration*, 2009, vol. 77, no 1, p. 44-50.

[15] Patel, Shraddha P., Pena, Margarita E., Babcock, Charlene Irvin. Cost-effectiveness of noninvasive ventilation for chronic obstructive pulmonary disease-related respiratory failure in Indian hospitals without ICU facilities. *Lung India: official organ of Indian Chest Society*, 2015, vol. 32, no 6, p. 549.

[16] Mar, Javier, et al. The cost-effectiveness of nCPAP treatment in patients with moderate-to-severe obstructive sleep apnoea. *European Respiratory Journal*, 2003, vol. 21, no 3, p. 515-522.

[17] Gruis, Kirsten L., Chernew, Michael E., Brown, Devin L. The cost-effectiveness of early noninvasive ventilation for ALS patients. *BMC Health Services Research*, 2005, vol. 5, no 1, p. 58.

[18] Pallero, Mercedes, et al. Ambulatory adaptation to noninvasive ventilation in restrictive pulmonary disease: a randomized trial with cost assessment. *Respiratory Medicine*, 2014, vol. 108, no 7, p. 1014-1022.

[19] Petrou, S., et al. Is protocolised weaning that includes early extubation onto non-invasive ventilation more cost effective than protocolised weaning without non-invasive ventilation? Findings from the Breathe study. *PharmacoEconomics-Open*, 2020.

In: Non-Invasive Mechanical Ventilation Complications ISBN: 978-1-53619-515-6
Editor: Antonio M. Esquinas

Chapter 40

NON-INVASIVE MECHANICAL VENTILATION AND COMPLICATIONS: EDUCATION PROGRAMS PERSPECTIVES

Alejandro Úbeda MD, PhD, María Salgado MD and Antonio M. Esquinas MD
Intensive Care Unit. Hospital Punta de Europa, Algeciras, Spain
Intensive Care Unit. Hospital Morales Meseguer, Murcia, Spain

ABSTRACT

The education and training of medical personnel on NIMV is crucial to ensure success, reduce complications and improve outcomes for patients with respiratory failure.

Patients with respiratory failure who require NIMV are by definition critically ill patients; they need to be managed by experienced personnel with skills in respiratory therapy capable to deal with ventilator settings, patient response, respiratory equipment, and monitoring preventable NIMV failure. Understanding respiratory physiology, knowledge of how a ventilator works and interacts with abnormal patient physiology is vital.

Effective and safe use of NIMV depends on careful selections of the patient, but also trained personnel. Education programs ensure basic training in NIMV management, and these skill translate into improve patients care and better outcomes.

Although many educational centers give training on NIMV, mainly in the ICU and respiratory field, specialized courses are not as common as they should be. To acquire in-depth knowledge that would let physicians to understand and manage NIMV, specialized courses and training are needed.

Even though training programs should be adapted to previous knowledge, it is vital to put up skills in progressive manner to ensure understanding of NIMV related topics. All personnel involved in day-to-day care of patients requiring NIMV may get a minimum skill in the management of these patients; these include not only physicians but also nurses, respiratory therapist, and physiotherapists.

Keywords: noninvasive ventilation, education programs, complications

Introduction

The education and training of medical personnel on NIMV is crucial to ensure success, reduce complications and improve outcomes for patients with respiratory failure [1-3].

Patients with respiratory failure who require NIMV are in definition critically ill patients; they need to be managed by experienced personnel with skill in respiratory therapy capable to deal with ventilator settings, patient response, respiratory equipment, and monitoring preventable NIMV failure [4]. Understand respiratory physiology, knowledge of how a ventilator works and interacts with abnormal patient physiology is vital.

A multidisciplinary team formed by specialized nurses, respiratory therapists and physiotherapists working closely it would be ideal, since the quality of the interactions between them has an impact in the successful of non-invasive mechanical therapy.

Educations Programs: Influences on Outcomes with NIMV

To avoid the most common complications and ensure success of NIMV is crucial to select carefully the patients and those will be managed by experienced personnel. Literature suggests usage rates of NIMV around 70% in respiratory failure due to COPD and 20% in case of chronic heart failure (CHF). Some studies have found lower rates of use, only 10-15% of patients with COPD or CHF. This discrepancy may results in lack of clinicians knowledge and training [5].

Effective and safe use of NIMV depends on careful selections of the patient, but also trained personnel. Education programs ensure basic training in NIMV management, and these skill translate into improve patients care and better outcomes.

Selection of Patients

Using NIMV as ventilator support has a risk of failure, which means intubation and invasive mechanical ventilation. It's well known that delays in starting IMV has been associated with increased rates of morbidity and mortality. NIMV efficacy depends not only on severity and types of respiratory selections and the skills of physicians, but also on careful selection of the patient. These selection must be based on failure predictors to reduce risk of any complications and fail of NIMV [6].

These factors that predict failure at the time of initiating NIMV are:

- The level of pH few hours after initiating NIMV support.
- pCO_2 level: decrease in arterial pCO_2 reflects that the NIMV therapy is effective in improving alveolar ventilation.
- Work of breathing: respiratory rate, the use of respiratory accessory muscles, chest and abdomen movements.
- Vital signs: heart rate, blood pressure, mental estatus (consciousness).

Even if these predictive factors help physicians to select patients with better outcomes, an unsuccessful initial NIMV does not necessarily means a definitive failure of non-invasive support. A well trained personnel is capable to identify suboptimal therapies and detect air leaks, patients-ventilator asynchronies, and ventilator setting in terms of respiratory rates, inspiratory time or pressures that can cause failures of NIMV if are not solved.

Training Programs in Non-Invasive Ventilation

Training is the key to the successful implementation of any clinical skill. Although many educational centers give training on NIMV, mainly in the ICU and respiratory field, specialized courses are not as common as they should be. To acquire in-depth knowledge that would let physicians to understand and manage NIMV, specialized courses and training are needed.

In Europe training programs in NIMV are starting to be usual. The European Respiratory Society (ERS) conducts a project named HERMES (Harmonized Education in Respiratory Medicine for European Specialists) that try to conduct an initiative in respiratory medicine education [7]. This training must include knowledge-based learning supported by practical application, such as ventilator setting, role of interfaces, air leaks, asynchronies…

The British Thoracic Society (BTS) guidelines on NIMV management conclude that targeted educations must be based not only in learning but also in practical training, to ensure physician confidence/competence are acquired [8]. That also means a change in the traditional assessment tool of written examinations to evaluate knowledge.

Miller's model of clinical competence (*Figure 1*) heads for multiple assessment tools to complement training programs in NIMV education. This model suggests two ways to acquire professional competence. First, clinicians need to get the basis of the clinical skill: knowledge-based assessment, which can be acquired by lectures, clinical problems solving, etc. Second, physicians have to achieve a skill-based assessment by direct observation of procedures or technique skill in clinical settings, simulated based education programs among others [9].

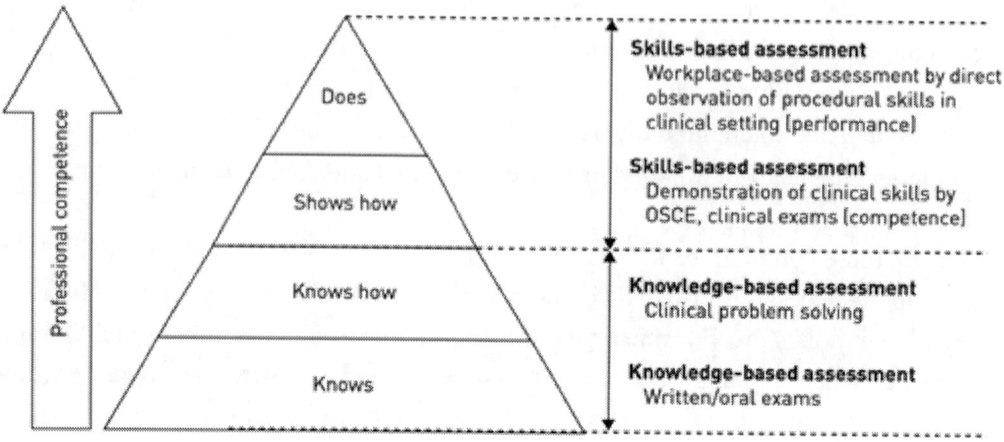

Figure 1. Miller's model of clinical competence.

Simulation Based Education for Non-Invasive Education

Simulation-based medical education is educational activity that use simulated components to replicate clinical practice, allowing subjects to respond to clinical problem under natural circumstances [10]. Although knowledge-based programs are relative easy to acquire via lectures and reviews, practical skills are more complicated to achieve. Simulated-based education is a useful tool in NIMV training programs and its implementation is widely spreading [11].

Contents on Training Programs in Non-Invasive Mechanical Ventilation

Even though training programs should be adapted to previous knowledge, it is vital to put up skills in progressive manner to ensure understanding of NIMV related topics. All personnel involved in day-to-day care of patients requiring NIMV may get a minimum skill in the management of these patients; these include not only physicians but also nurses, respiratory therapist, and physiotherapists.

Although these fact may slightly vary the contents of the training programs, there are basic skills that should be included (Table 1).

Physicians have to be capable to properly select patients who are likely to respond to NIMV successfully, as also promptly identify those ones who are likely to fail. They may acquired a confident management on NIMV being capable to identify patient-ventilator asynchronies and select the best fitted interface not only to ensure optimal patient comfort and prevent skin lesions, but also to reduce air leaks. Nurses may be competent to monitor NIMV, but also have the ability to identify and avoid any problems related to the patients or the monitor [12].

Table 1. Minimum content of NIMV training programs

Principles of respiratory failures	-Physiology and pathophysiology - Symptoms and signs of respiratory failure - Common respiratory diseases requiring NIMV - Hypoxic versus hypercapnic respiratory failure
Principles, function, and technology of NIMV	- Appropriate settings and staff - Types of ventilators - Selection of interfaces - Ventilator circuits
NIMV management	- Goals and strategies of NIMV - Prescription, set-up, and monitoring in NIMV - Definition and selection of the ventilator mode - Initial operation of the equipment - Analysis of flow and pressure curve - Recognition of patient-ventilator synchronization / desynchronization - Noninvasive and invasive cardiorespiratory monitoring in different set-ups
Problems related to NIMV	- Troubleshooting - Complications/treatment failure of NIMV - Problem-solving - Patient-ventilator synchronization with the NIMV - Management of secretions - Recognition of secretions
Other topics	- Air stacking, assisted cough, cough assist devices, bronchoscopy - Open issues and update on NIMV research development - Nasogastric tube insertion for NIMV treatment - Enteral feeding during NIMV - Optimal gas humidification during NIMV - Aerosol delivering during NIMV -Patient sedation during NIMV - Patient's needs and comfort measures - Management of oxygen therapy during NIMV - Management of oxygen therapy during pauses between NIMV cycles - Bronchoscopy during NIMV - NIMV in pulmonary rehabilitation programs, aerobic exercise training

KEY MESSAGES

1. Patient with respiratory failure who require NIMV is in definition a critically ill patient; those who need to be managed by experienced personnel with skill in respiratory therapy.
2. Education and training in NIMV have the potential to increase knowledge and skills of the staffs and improve success rates and outcome.
3. Physicians have to be capable to properly select patients who are likely to respond to NIMV successfully, as also promptly identify those ones who are likely to fail.
4. Personnel involved in care of patients requiring NIMV may get a minimum skill in the management of these patients; these include not only physicians but also nurses, respiratory therapist, and physiotherapists.
5. Educational programs are needed to ensure that physicians have enough competences and confidences in the management of NIMV. The lack of it is a barrier for optimal applications.

REFERENCES

[1] Bello G, De Pascale G, Antonelli M. Noninvasive Ventilation. *Clin. Chest Med.* 2016;37: 711-21.

[2] Karim H M R, Burns K E A, Ciobanu L D, El-Khatib M, Nicolini A, Vargas N, et al. Noninvasive ventilation: education and training. A narrative analysis and an international consensus document. *Adv. Respir. Med.* 2019; 87: 36–45.

[3] Esquinas R, Martín U J, Cordova F C, Criner G J, González Dí. Organización hospitalaria y formación clínica en ventilación mecánica no invasiva. In: *Esquinas R. ed. Tratado de ventilación mecánica no invasiva.* Práctica clínica y metodología. Aula Medica, Madrid 2006: 1129–1134. [Hospital organization and clinical training in non-invasive mechanical ventilation. In: Corners R. ed. *Non-invasive mechanical ventilation treatise.*]

[4] Elliot M W. Non-invasive ventilation: Essential requirements and clinical skills for successful practice. *Respirology* 2019;24:1156-64.

[5] Demoule A, Girou E, Richard J C, Taillé S, Brochard L. Increased use of noninvasive ventilation in French intensive care units. *Intensive Care Med.* 2006; 32: 1747–55.

[6] Carron M, Freo U, BaHammam A S, Dellweg D, Guarracino F, Cosentini R, et al. Complications of non-invasive ventilation techniques: a comprehensive qualitative review of randomized trial. *Br. J. Anaesth.* 2013; 110: 896-14.

[7] Artigas A, Noël J L, Brochard L, Busari J O, Dellweg D, Ferrer M, et al. Defining a training framework for clinicians in respiratory critical care. *Eur. Respir. J.* 2014; 44: 572-7.

[8] Davidson A C, Banham S, Elliott M, Kennedy D, Gelder C, Glossop A, et al. BTS/ICS guideline for the ventilatory management of acute hypercapnic respiratory failure in adults. *Thorax* 2016; 71 Suppl 2: ii1-35.

[9] Ziv A, Ben-David S, Ziv M. Simulation based medical education: an opportunity to learn from errors. *Med. Teach.* 2005; 27: 193–9.

[10] Mitchell S, Bloch K E, Butiene I, Cooper BG, Steenbruggen I, Hare A, et al. "Education is the passport to the future:" enabling today's medical teachers to prepare tomorrow's respiratory health practitioners. *Eur. Respir. J.* 2014; 44: 578–84.

[11] Hare A, Simonds A. Simulation-based education for non-invasive ventilation. *Breathe* 2013;9:367-70.

[12] Hill NS. Where should noninvasive ventilation be delivered? *Respir. Care* 2009; 54:62-70.

In: Non-Invasive Mechanical Ventilation Complications
Editor: Antonio M. Esquinas
ISBN: 978-1-53619-515-6

Chapter 41

GLOBAL HEALTH CARE IN NON-INVASIVE MECHANICAL VENTILATION COMPLICATIONS. ROLE OF INTEGRATED SOCIAL CARE, PSYCHOLOGICAL HOLISTIC MANAGEMENT AND PHYSIOLOGICAL ADAPTATIONS

***Cristina Palma Rodríguez*[1,*], *Marta Ruiz Pérez de la Blanca*[1] *and Elena María Jiménez González*[2]**

[1]Critical Care and Emergency Service Baza Hospital, Granada, Spain
[2]High Resolution Hospital Alcalá la Real, Jaén, Spain

ABSTRACT

For patients in need of ventilatory assistance, non-invasive mechanical ventilation has proven an increase in survival rate in patients with acute respiratory insufficiency or chronic obstructive pulmonary disease, as well as lees need for invasive ventilation. Nevertheless, as with any other technique, there are several contraindications and complications which we will explain in this chapter, as being aware of them and with the correct formation of the staff in charge we can make these complications to be recognized and we can take actions to palliate them.

Keywords: non-invasive mechanical ventilation complications, social care, adults, psychology

* Corresponding Author's E-mail: crispr_1988@hotmail.com.

INTRODUCTION

There are around 10-15% of these complications that derive in failure, and they are usually related to mask and or respirator adaptation problems, which can generate respiratory asynchronies that lead to inefficiency of the treatment. We can divide theses complications into four main groups:

1. Complications related to the mask or even the restraint mechanism.
2. Complications related to the pressure and flow, as well as air humidification.
3. Severe complications.
4. NIMV disconnect, psychological aspects.

COMPLICATIONS RELATED TO THE MASK OR RESTRAINT MECHANISM

This one is one of the most common ones, even though they are not the most severe. These problems mostly depend on the kind of mask it is used. The contact point in between the skin and the mask can cause *facial erythema* (20-34%), *cutaneous acneiform rash* (5-10%), *ulceration* (5-10%) and even necrosis, especially in the nasal bridge. Another complication could be irritative conjunctivitis. Usually caused by air leak over the conjunctiva, and the lacrimal liquid ecstasy derived from the overpressure over the nostrils (making the emptying very difficult). All these situations cause discomfort to the patient, one of the main problems of NIMV. This kind of situations happens in almost 50% of the cases, and can even cause claustrophobia. Also, related to the mask, there can be expectoration, secretions retainment, oral ingestion difficulty and rebreathing of expired air.

In order to avoid these complications, we should use the correct interface for each case, with masks having the correct size, we should not over tight the interface, so we do not cause any leak; for the ulcers, we can use hydrocolloid dressings at the contact zones, oil-based moisturizing creams in pressure points when the patient is having a resting moment without the interface (much needed to prevent this kind of complications). For the acneiform rash, we can even use topical solutions with steroids or antibiotics as doxycycline. For conjunctivitis, artificial tears and even specific treatments with collyrium if required. It is also very efficient to alternate in between facial and nasobuccal interfaces.

As we mentioned, rebreathing is one of the other main problems, it can induce hypercapnia, caused by an excessive dead space in the interface, we can solve this problem by choosing masks with the less possible dead space (whether facial or nasobuccal) and not closing the exhalation vents. When using ventilators without an expiratory valve, putting an anti-rebreathing valve is quite recommended.

Another less common kind of complications, but no less important, are those related to the harnesses, as there might be an accidental disengagement (leading to hypoxemia by alveolar derecruitment). There can also be an overpressure problem, causing thrombosis in the axillary vein (in cases using a Helmet kind interface, where the harness is placed under the axillae), in order to prevent this we should apply symmetrical pressure, so there are no leaks, but also taking into consideration the comfort of the patient.

Complications Related to the Pressure and Flow and Air Humidification

The pressure-related complications include *discomfort, ear and paranasal sinuses pain* (10-30%) by consequence of gastric pressure and insufflation (5-10%) which manifests as *abdominal distension, flatulence* or *nausea*, and related to the flow we can see an increase in *secretions, nasal congestion and obstruction* (20-50%) as well as *dry mouth and nose (10-20%).*

Usually, all these complications get better when decreasing the pressure, as most of them appear with inspiratory pressure over 20 cmH_20, but an optimal pressure for this matter has not been established.

To make the ear and paranasal sinuses pain and the dryness at these zones, we have to hydrate with physiological serum and aspirate the secretions when necessary. We also have to maintain the correct state of hydration and stimulate for the Valsalva manoeuvre to be realized, that keeps the eustachian tubes and other sinuses emptying holes permeable. When in pain, we can administrate analgesia. Also, it is recommended to start the ventilatory supply with relatively low pressures (8-12 cmH_2O), so we can increase this pressure progressively, according to patient tolerance.

For abdominal distension, usually, we can administrate simethicone (when it is painful) and reduce pressure, although it is typically a well-tolerated side effect that requires no adjustments. If needed, we can use a nasogastric tube to check permeability, warning the patient that this can cause vomiting; if the patient comes to suffer from nausea, we can administrate metoclopramide.

When humidification is insufficient, we can find the other adverse effects described (nasal and pharyngeal dryness), caused by an excessively dry air that alters the mucous and there is a bigger chance of mucus obstruction that originates difficult ventilation and can even obstruct the air vents. The mucous membrane alterations can get aggravated by the oxidative effect of a high O_2 concentration in the supplied air, by the pressure effect. Humidification is recommended every time the technique is going to be applied for at least 24 hours, and we will control the humidification levels until we reach de desired conditions. We will also control the mouth and nose hygiene exhaustively as much as possible.

Severe Complications

Severe complications are less common, and they occur approximately 5% of the cases. Amongst them, we can find bronchoaspiration, which appears in patients that present oral ingestion or through a nasogastric tube, and they are using a facial mask. The situation could get worse if the patient has received sedatives or has a neuromuscular disease. Also, vomit or secretions can stay in the mask, and if not noticed, it can lead to aspiration. In order to prevent this, we should start applying the technique one or two hours after ingesting. When not possible, one option is to do continuous enteral feeding through a transpyloric probe to minimize the vomits. We would try to keep a semi-sitting position, and we will warn the patient/familiars about the possibilities of vomiting and how to proceed to retire the mask if possible.

Another one of the complications is *pneumothorax*, even though it is not very frequent (and the risk increases with the ventilatory pressure), this is the reason why we should try and keep the less effective pressure possible, especially in patients with pulmonary bullae. If this happens, the thorax tube should be placed and cease the non-invasive mechanical ventilation or decrease the pressure.

Lastly, the *hemodynamic alterations* are some other of the possible complications, as there can be hypotension caused by the increase of intrathoracic pressure and a lower preload with a decreasing of the cardiac output. Some arrhythmias might appear caused by hypoxemia. Mostly, the NIMV is well tolerated, as it is usually used with low pressure; nevertheless, in patients with a compromised cardiac function, these complications might appear. In order to prevent these problems, it is essential to keep a routinary and continuous control both at the beginning of the therapy.

NIMV Disconnect, Psychological Aspects

This is an independent point due to its importance, as it might lead us to a failure of the technique (which occurs in 7-42% of the cases). Frequently, there is some intolerance by the patient because of mask rejection as the leading cause (up to 50% of the cases), *tolerance* is the technique failure's main prognostic factor. It is also crucial to correct possible asynchronies in between the ventilator and the patient, to avoid the asynchronies to appear it is imperative a good use of inspiratory and expiratory ventilator's triggers.

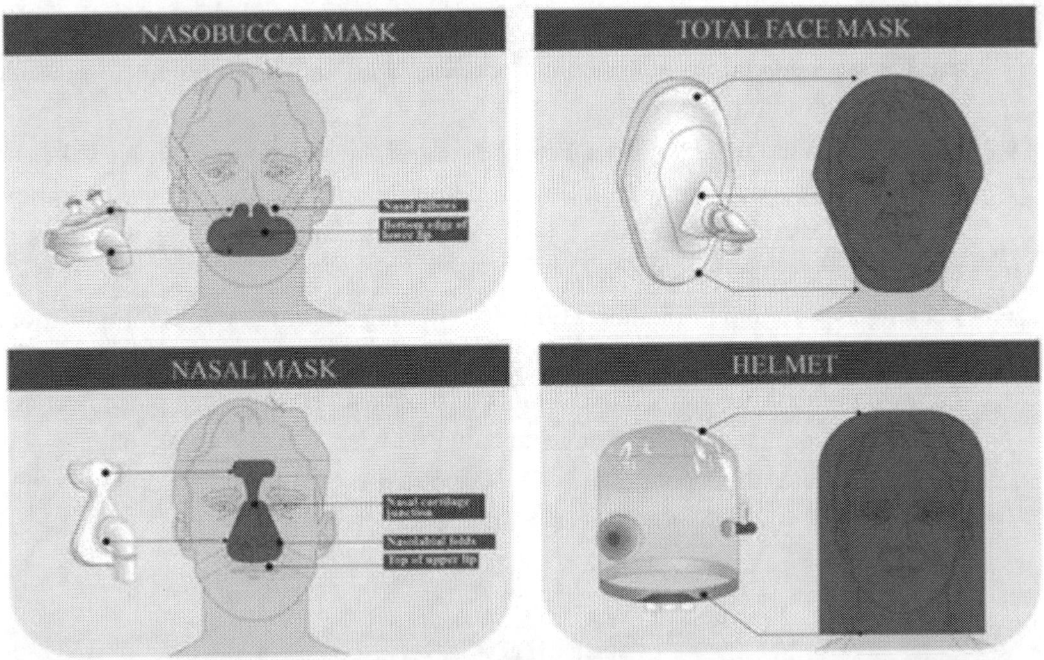

Figure 1.

Too many leaks could also cause the technique to fail, to reach a system without any leaks is almost impossible, but we do have to reduce the number of leaks to an acceptable level. Regarding this, it is essential to pick a good mask that reunites all the characteristics needed: good adaptability, little dead space, low weight, easy to put, and a good fit (Figure 1).

It is vital to reach the technique's success that the patient collaborates because, in most of the cases, the process generates anxiety, claustrophobia, and discomfort; this is why we should treat the patient kindly, being supportive and using correct verbal and non-verbal communication from the beginning. Offering useful information about the machines the patient is going to be connected to, techniques we are going to proceed with, and remembering the impossibility of talking during the assisted ventilation, but also providing them with resources and ways to communicate whether it is visually or by writing. We can allow the entrance of familiars always that is possible and intermittently.

KEY MESSAGES

- The NIMV has been proven to be an efficient treatment for patients in respiratory insufficiency, but, even being a non-invasive technique, it may lead to certain complications that we must know in order to prevent.

- Evaluating the use of the technique, as well as the correct interface (the type of mask, right colocation, minimizing leaks), as well as being vigilant to possible asynchronies with the ventilator.
- Explaining to the patient, previous to the start of the technique, if he is awake and aware, the procedure we will follow and how important it is their collaboration. We have to use techniques that avoid the patient's anxiety and helping them to adapt to the equipment.
- Keeping a close monitorization of the vitals, being alert of possible complications (bronchoaspiration, asynchronies, abdominal distension, pain...).
- To prevent the injuries in contact points of the mask, right padded placement and protection (forehead, nasal bridge and chin), keep a daily check on the skin health, and use of decongestants and emollients. We should evaluate resting periods every 4-6 horas for correct hydration and feeding of the patient.

References

[1] Mehta S, Hill N. State of art: noninvasive ventilation. *Am. J. Resp. Crit. Care Med.* 2001; 163: 540-77.

[2] Heili Frades S, Peces Barba G. Problemas en ventilación mecánica no invaiva: ineficacia y complicaciones. En: *Ventilación no invasiva* [Non-invasive mechanical ventilation problems: ineffectiveness and complications. In: *Non-invasive ventilation*] pp 45-61. Madrid: Neuromadrid, 2007; p 45-61.

[3] Morchón Simón D, González Rozas M. Complicaciones de la ventilación mecánica no invasiva. En: *Fundamentos de metodología y organización hospitalaria en ventilación mecánica no invasiva* pp 279-282. 3ª edición-Asociación y escuela internacional de ventilación mecánica no invasiva [Complications of non-invasive mechanical ventilation. In: *Fundamentals of methodology and hospital organization in non-invasive mechanical ventilation* pp 279-282. 3rd edition-Association and international school of non-invasive mechanical ventilation].

[4] Jalilie E, Afredo et al. X. Complicaciones y estándares de cuidado de la ventilación no invasiva [Non-invasive ventilation complications and standards of care]. *Rev. Chil. Enferm. Respire*. 2008; 24: 233-236.

[5] López Esteban E, Cachón Pérez JM. Complicaciones de la ventilación no invasiva. Prevención de complicaciones. En: *Cuidados de enfermería en ventilación mecánica no invasiva* pp 93-101. Asociación y Escuela Internacional de Ventilación Mecánica No Invasiva [Complications of non-invasive ventilation. Prevention of complications. In: *Nursing care in non-invasive mechanical ventilation* pp 93-101. Association and International School of Non-Invasive Mechanical Ventilation].

[6] Hill NS. Complications of noninvasive ventilation. *Respir. Care* 2000; 45: 480-1.

[7] Abad Corpa E, Hernández González M, Ortells Rodríguez MJ et all. Complicaciones de la ventilación mecánica no invasive [Complications of non-invasive mechanical ventilation]. *Enferm. Global* 2002; 1-12.

[8] Monge Cuevas A, Vinagre Romero JA. Complicaciones en pacientes con ventilación mecánica no invasiva [Complications in patients with non-invasive mechanical ventilation]. *Metas. Enferm. Sept.* 2015; 18(7); 13-18.

In: Non-Invasive Mechanical Ventilation Complications ISBN: 978-1-53619-515-6
Editor: Antonio M. Esquinas

Chapter 42

EVIDENCE-BASED RECOMMENDATIONS FOR DIAGNOSIS PREVENTION AND TREATMENT NON-INVASIVE VENTILATION COMPLICATIONS

Bruno Prata Martinez[1,2,3], Cassio Magalães Silva e Silva[1,3], and Mansueto Gomes Neto[1,3,*]

[1]Department of Physiotherapy, Federal University of Bahia, Salvador-Bahia, Brazil
[2]State University of Bahia, Salvador-Bahia, Brazil
[3]Physiotherapy Research Group at Federal University of Bahia, Salvador-Bahia, Brazil

ABSTRACT

Noninvasive ventilation is an important resource for preventing orotracheal. Noninvasive ventilation has the advantages of reducing patient discomfort, and procedural complications. However, noninvasive ventilation is associated with frequent uncomfortable or even life-threatening adverse effects (aerophagia, nasal skin injury, ventilator-induced lung injury; patient-ventilator asynchrony; nasal and eye irritation, bronchoaspiration risks, hypotension, and pneumothorax), and patients should be thoroughly screened beforehand to reduce potential severe complications. Even complications common to both noninvasive ventilation and invasive mechanical ventilation occur less frequently in patients undergoing noninvasive ventilation. Thus, noninvasive ventilation is associate with a reduced need for invasive mechanical ventilation and significant outcome and minor complications. Noninvasive ventilation should be applied by a trained and experienced team, taking constantly into account the potential complications.

Keywords: noninvasive ventilation, complications, critical care

* Correspondence Author's E-mail: Mansueto Neto netofisio@gmail.com.

INTRODUCTION

Noninvasive ventilation is an important resource for preventing orotracheal intubation [1, 2]; to assist in ventilatory weaning [3-4]; as well as to minimize dyspnea and enhance the rehabilitation of patients with chronic diseases [5]. Despite its advantages in several situations for the treatment of respiratory failure, when correctly indicated, there are complications and adverse effects during its use. Among some of these are aerophagia; nasal skin injury; claustrophobia; ventilator-induced lung injury; patient-ventilator asynchrony; nasal and eye irritation; bronchoaspiration risks; hypotension; pneumothorax and spread of aerosol infections [6-8].

In general, these complications are minor and can be reversed with early diagnosis and subsequent treatment. Some factors must be considered as type of fan; type of circuit used, patient characteristics and interface types.

The primary goal of non-invasive ventilation is to maintain adequate levels of arterial oxygen pressure (PaO_2) and carbon dioxide ($PaCO_2$); besides reducing the signs of increased respiratory work. Despite having similar effects to invasive mechanical ventilation, there are some differences listed below [8]:

1. Due to the inherent escape of NIV, these systems may not supply volumes and pressures in a similar way to invasive VM, even in fans with exhaust compensation systems;
2. As NIV is applied via the oronasal pharynx that connects with the esophagus and trachea, high esophageal pressures can lead to gastric distention;
3. The unprotected trachea is exposed to the risk of aspiration, in situations of stomach distention;
4. The lack of an artificial airway limits the effectiveness of airway aspiration; In single branch circuits,
5. there is a risk of rebreathing in CO 2; especially when using low pressures.

How to Diagnose and Treat Complications Associated WITH NIV

In situations where non-invasive ventilation is indicated, monitoring during the procedure is essential, as described by Ergan et al. [9] for the following aspects:

Table 1. Monitoring of NIV described by Ergan et al., [9]: Clinical

Clinical parameters	Comfort
	Interface tolerance
	Respiratory frequency
	Dyspnea and use of accessory muscles
	Level of consciousness
	Ability to protect airways superiors
	Gastric distension
	Disease severity score
	Delirium sedation score
Physiological parameters	Oxygen saturation
	Analysis of blood gases
	transcutaneous CO_2
	End-tidal CO_2
Ventilatory parameters	Respiratory frequency
	Total exhaled volume
	Escape
	PEEPi
	Patient-ventilator interaction
Cardiac parameters	Blood pressure
	ECG
	Echocardiography
Others	Radiological evaluation (chest radiography and computed tomography)
	Pulmonary and diaphragmatic ultrasound

In this monitoring, possible complications should be identified during the application of NIV so that actions can be taken to reverse or minimize them, and when possible to prevent their occurrence. The following will describe complications associated with NIV and forms of prevention and treatment.

Nasal Skin Injury

It occurs mainly when using the oronasal interface, which is the most used in respiratory insufficiencies, but can also occur while using the nasal interface. The nasal lesion occurs due to the pressure that the mask exerts at the base of the nose, to prevent air leakage during the technique and consequently asynchrony. These skin lesions can reach up to 50% of patients who undergo NIV [10] and the literature describes that it usually occurs in 4 to 6 hours of continuous use.

The occurrence of these injuries can influence failure during NIV and can be prevented as long as the team is trained and equipment is available at the hospital to perform the intervention [12].

Some intrinsic factors increase the risk of developing these injuries, such as [13]:

- Sensory impairment;
- Acute illness;
- Chronic illness;
- Hypoxia or very low blood pressure;
- Extremes of age;
- Low level of consciousness;
- Vascular disease;
- Malnutrition / dehydration;
- Chronic skin condition;

STRATEGY FOR PREVENTION AND TREATMENT

When adjusting the interface, it is necessary to use an appropriate size for the patient's face, as well as that the fixation of the clamps is at the minimum level of adjustment / pressure, which promotes an adequate sealing of the system, that is, no leakage [13]. This is because this escape is related to NIV failure due to an increase in the number of asynchrony and reduced tolerance due to inadequate supply of ventilatory demand. The ideal is the use of a flexible, soft and moldable interface to prevent injuries.

- In patients at high risk of developing skin lesions or in pain due to the existence of pressure ulcers, an alternative may be to switch to a totalface interface [14]. Another strategy to avoid these injuries is the use of other interfaces such as the helmet, in the places where the equipment is available [15]. Attention should be given to CO_2 rebreathing while applying the Helmet [16].
- In patients at high risk for ulcers or possibly needing more prolonged use of NIV, studies have shown that the use of protective pads at the base of the nose as hydrocolloids should be used to prevent the occurrence of injuries [17-18].
- In patients with signs of skin deterioration, the position of the interface should be changed every 10 minutes, with the assessment of the possible change in the interface. Regular skin assessment during NIV every 2 to 4 hours is essential to identify the risk of injury and the need for some preventive strategy in other patients [15].

Risk of Bronchoaspiration

Excessive secretion and the inability to expectorate it is another important failure factor for NIV [19]. A recent study demonstrated that the use of the cough machine increased the chance of success for NIV [20]. One of the justifications is that NIV is not intended to remove secretions. In this way, the cough machine promotes removal and later NIV is installed to reduce respiratory failure and / or to improve blood gases.

Aerophagia

Some patients during NIV use present abdominal distention secondary to aerophagia and this can lead to nausea and vomiting, in addition to increasing the risk of flare in NIV due to increased intra-abdominal pressure [19].

Strategy for Prevention and Treatment

Guide patients to breathe through their nose and when using the nasal interface, keep their mouth closed.

- In patients with high aerophagia, nasogastric tubes can be used to remove this excess air in the gastric cavity.
- In the presence of vomiting, the interface must be removed immediately, with bronchial hygiene therapy being performed. Reinstallation should be done carefully due to the risk of a new vomiting event.

Ventilator-Induced Lung Injury

Similar to the use of invasive mechanical ventilation, NIV can also trigger lung injury depending on the programmed parameters, the patient's level of effort and the existing lung disease. The mechanisms that lead to this injury are high transpulmonary pressures, excess pulmonary stretching through a tidal volume in addition to the physiological and cyclic alveolar opening and closing. As a consequence of this lesion, there is a systemic inflammatory response with increased capillary permeability and worsening oxygenation [21-22]. Another injury that can occur due to the use of NIV is that associated with excessive respiratory effort, also called self-inflicted lung injury (P-SILI), which generates high transpulmonary pressures due to negative pleural pressure, even with adequate ventilatory parameters. [23, 24].

Strategy for Prevention and Treatment

To avoid lung injury induced by mechanical ventilation, the target tidal volume (6 to 8 ml / kg) should be used, pulmonary distention pressures below 15 cm H 2 0 and transpulmonary pressures below 30 cm H 2 0. In patients with excessive respiratory effort and not improving after NIV, the need for sedation and orotracheal intubation should be discussed with a multidisciplinary team, so that it is not delayed and there is an increased risk of death for the patient.

Patient-Ventilator Asynchrony

It is a frequent complication that occurs in about 40% of patients who undergo NIV, being very related to the level of air leak and the support pressure levels used [25]. The main patient-ventilator asynchronies are ineffective triggering, self-triggering, double-triggering, late and early cycling. In this sense, treating these asynchronies is related to better patient comfort and a better chance of success in NIV [26]. For that, one must look at the ventilation parameters and the flow and pressure curves by time.

Strategy for Prevention and Treatment

Ineffective firing: it consists of the patient making a muscular effort and he is not able to trigger the sensitivity of the ventilator. It usually causes air trapping, reduced muscle strength and respiratory drive inhibited by high lung volumes. It is up to the professional to assess which cause is causing the ineffective shots so that the necessary ventilation parameters can be adjusted.

Double-shot: consists of reduced ventilator inspiratory time in relation to the patient's respiratory muscle effort. That is, in a inspiratory effort, two ventilatory cycles are triggered. The treatment is to promote ventilatory adjustments in order to increase the inspiratory time of the ventilator indirectly (by adjusting the support pressure and / or the cycling percentage). Preferably, it is decided to reduce the percentage of cycling, except that the tidal volume levels are below the target value.

Late cycling: in this asynchrony, the ventilator time is longer than the patient's inspiratory time. The treatment consists of making adjustments to the ventilator in order to reduce the ventilator time, by increasing the percentage of the cycle, that is, reducing the support pressure, if the volume is above the target.

Early cycling: in this asynchrony, the ventilator time is less than the patient's inspiratory time. The treatment is similar to that of the double shot.

Hypotension and Pneumothorax

Due to the increase in intra-thoracic pressure due to the positive pressure imposed by NIV on the respiratory system, there is an impact at the hemodynamic level with some drop in blood pressure, increased afterload and reduced preload [26]. This drop will be more related to the level of PEEP used, as well as the patient's cardiovascular function. Another complication that can occur with low frequency is pneumothorax [27], usually in patients who already have some history of previous pneumothorax.

Strategy for Prevention and Treatment

During the use of NIV, cardiovascular parameters should be monitored, as previously described. To assess the effects of this positive pressure, the main parameters at the bedside are blood pressure and heart rate.

Avoid positive airway pressure levels above the required value, especially in the PEEP variable.

If pneumothorax is suspected, it must be confirmed by imaging or ultrasound before the installation of NIV.

References

[1] Osadnik C R, Tee V S, Carson-Chahhoud K V, Picot J, Wedzicha J A, Smith B J. Non-invasive ventilation for the management of acute hypercapnic respiratory failure due to exacerbation of chronic obstructive pulmonary disease. *Cochrane Database Syst. Rev.* 2017 Jul 13;7:CD004104. doi: 10.1002/14651858.CD004104.pub4.

[2] Rochwerg B, Brochard L, Elliott M W, Hess D, Hill N S, Nava S, et al. Official ERS/ATS clinical practice guidelines: noninvasive ventilation for acuterespiratory failure. *Eur. Respir. J.* 2017 Aug 31;50(2). pii: 1602426. doi: 10.1183/13993003.02426-2016.

[3] Yeung J, Couper K, Ryan E G, Gates S, Hart N and Perkins GD. Non-invasive ventilation as a strategy for weaning from invasive mechanical ventilation: a systematic review and Bayesian meta-analysis. *Intensive Care Med.* 2018; 44:2192–2204.

[4] Ceriana P, Nava S, Vitacca M, Carlucci A, Paneroni M, Schreiber A, et al. Noninvasive ventilation during weaning from prolonged mechanical ventilation. *Pulmonology* 2019;25(6):328-333. doi: 10.1016/j.pulmoe.2019.07.006.

[5] Gomes Neto M, Duarte L F G, Rodrigues E S Jr, Bittencourt HS, Dos Santos N G, David B C, et al. Effects of noninvasive ventilation with bilevel positive airway pressure on exercise tolerance and dyspnea in heart failure patients. *Hellenic J. Cardiol.* 2018 Nov - Dec;59(6):317-320. doi: 10.1016/j.hjc.2017.11.005.

[6] van Rooyen F, Soltesz K. *Non-invasive ventilation-A century of experience.* Available from: https://www.draeger.com/Products/Content/niv-fibel-bk-9051941-en.pdf (Accessed on 10 September 2018).

[7] Rocha E; Carneiro E M. Benefits and complications of noninvasive mechanical ventilation for acute exacerbation of chronic obstructive pulmonary disease. *Rev. bras. ter. Intensive* 2008;20(2):184-189. https://doi.org/10.1590/S0103-507X2008000200012.

[8] MacIntyre N R. Physiologic Effects of Noninvasive Ventilation. *Respir. Care* 2019;64(6):617–628.

[9] Ergan B, Nasiłowski J, Winck J C. How should we monitor patients with acute respiratory failure treated with noninvasive ventilation? *Eur. Respir. Rev.* 2018; 27: 170101.

[10] Carron M, Freo U, BaHammam A S, Dellweg D, Guarracino F, Cosentini R, et al. Complications of non-invasive ventilation techniques: a comprehensive qualitative review of randomized trials. *Br. J. Anaesth.* 2013; 110: 896-914.

[11] Bambi S, Peris A, Esquinas AM. Pressure ulcers caused by masks during noninvasive ventilation. *Am. J. Crit. Care* 2016; 25: 6-16.

[12] Cabrini L, Esquinas A, Pasin L, Nardelli P, Frati E, Pintaudi M, et al. An international survey on non invasive ventilation used for acute respiratory failure in general non-monitored wards. *Respir. Care* 2015; 60: 586-592.

[13] Brill A K. How to avoid interface problems in acute noninvasive ventilation. *Breathe* 2014; 10: 230-242.

[14] Lemyze M, Mallat J, Nigeon O, Barrailler S, Pepy F, Gasan G, et al. Rescue therapy by switching to total face mask after failure of face mask-delivered noninvasive ventilation in do-not-intubate patients in acute respiratory failure. *Crit. Care Med.* 2013; 41: 481-488.

[15] Alqahtani J S, AlAhmari M D. Evidence based synthesis for prevention of noninvasive ventilation related facial pressure ulcers. *Saudi Med. J.* 2018; Vol. 39 (5): 443-452 doi: 10.15537/smj.2018.5.22058.

[16] Taccone P, Hess D, Caironi P, Bigatello L M. Continuous positive airway pressure delivered with a "helmet:" effects on carbon dioxide rebreathing. *Crit. Care Med.* 2004; 32: 2090-2096.

[17] Weng M H. The effect of protective treatment in reducing pressure ulcers for non-invasive ventilation patients. *Intensive Crit. Care Nurs.* 2008; 24: 295-299.

[18] Otero D P, Domínguez D V, Fernández L H, Magariño A S, González V J, Klepzing J G, et al. Preventing facial pressure ulcers in patients under non-invasive

mechanical ventilation: a randomised control trial. *J. Wound Care* 2017; 26: 128-136.

[19] Gay PC. Complications of noninvasive ventilation in acute care. *Respir. Care* 2009; 54: 246–257.

[20] Gonçalves M R, Honrado T, Winck J C, Paiva J A. Effects of mechanical insufflation-exsufflation in preventing respiratory failure after extubation: a randomized controlled trial. *Crit. Care.* 2012; 16(2): R48.

[21] Slutsky A S, Ranieri V M. Ventilator-induced lung injury. *N. Engl. J. Med.* 2013;369(22):2126-2136.

[22] Chiumello D, Carlesso E, Cadringher P, Caironi P, Valenza F, Polli F, et al. Lung stress and strain during mechanical ventilation for acute respiratory distress syndrome. *Am. J. Respir Crit. Care Med.* 2008;178(4):346-355.

[23] Grieco DM et al. Patient self-inflicted lung injury and positive end-expiratory pressure for safe spontaneous breathing. *Current Opinion in Critical Care.* 2019 DOI: 10.1097/MCC.0000000000000691.

[24] Brochard L. Ventilation-induced lung injury exists in spontaneously breathing patients with acute respiratory failure: yes. *Intensive Care Med.* 2017;43(2):250-252.

[25] Vignaux L, Vargas F, Roeseler J, et al. Patient-ventilator asynchrony during non-invasive ventilation for acute respiratory failure: a multicenter study. *Intensive Care Med.* 2009; 35: 840–846.

[26] Younes M, Brochard L, Grasso S, et al. A method for monitoring and improving patient: ventilator interaction. *Intensive Care Med.* 2007; 33: 1337–1346.

[27] Pinsky, MR, Guimond, JG. The effects of positive end-expiratory pressure on heart-lung interactions. *J. Crit. Care* 1991;6(1):1-15.

[28] Mehta S, Hill NS. Noninvasive ventilation. *Am. J. Respir. Crit. Care Med.* 2001; 163: 540–577.

About the Editor

Antonio M. Esquinas MD, PhD

Intensive Care Unit, Hospital Morales Meseguer, Murcia, Spain

Active member as director International Fellowship program of noninvasive mechanical ventilation, fellow of American Association Respiratory Care (AARC), Fellow American Collage Chest Physicians. (ACCP), Director international school noninvasive mechanical ventilation, director Non-Invasive Ventilation College of Experts. Principal research and academic publications are related acute respiratory failure, noninvasive and invasive mechanical ventilation (weaning mechanical ventilation, COPD exacerbation, hypoxemic respiratory failure and acute cardiac diseases. Published 667 articles and 40 edited books related with mechanical ventilation and noninvasive mechanical ventilation.

INDEX

A

B

C

D

E

F

L

M

N

O

P

T

U

V

W